PHENYLPROPANOLAMINE

Clinical Pharmacology and Therapeutics Series
Volume 5

OTHER VOLUMES IN THE SERIES

Maini and Berry: *Modulation of Autoimmunity and Disease,* 1981
Wartak: *Clinical Pharmacokinetics,* 1983
Huskisson: *Anti-Rheumatic Drugs,* 1984
Nwangwu: *Concepts and Strategies in New Drug Development,* 1984
Reidenberg and Erill: *Drug-Protein Binding,* 1985
Sarasua, Pederson, and Koehler: *Primer on Ligand Binding,* 1986

PHENYLPROPANOLAMINE

Risks, Benefits, and Controversies

Edited by
John P. Morgan, M.D.
Doreen V. Kagan
Jane S. Brody

Clinical Pharmacology and Therapeutics Series
Volume 5

PRAEGER

PRAEGER SPECIAL STUDIES • PRAEGER SCIENTIFIC

New York • Philadelphia • Eastbourne, UK
Toronto • Hong Kong • Tokyo • Sydney

Library of Congress Cataloging in Publication Data
Main entry under title:

Phenylpropanolamine : risks, benefits, and controversies.

(Clinical pharmacology and therapeutics series ; v. 5)
Includes bibliographies and index.
1. Phenylpropanolamine--Therapeutic use--Congresses. 2. Phenylpropanolamine--Toxicology--Congresses. 3. Central nervous system--Effect of drugs on--Congresses. 4. Cardiovascular system--Effect of drugs on--Congresses. I. Morgan, John P. II. Kagan, Doreen V. III. Series. [DNLM: 1. Phenylpropanolamine--adverse effects. 2. Phenylpropanolamine--therapeutic use. W1 CL764J v.5 / QV 129 P541]
RM666.P57P47 1985 615'.7 85-6590
ISBN 0-03-001437-9 (alk. paper)

Published in 1985 by Praeger Publishers
CBS Educational and Professional Publishing, a Division of CBS Inc.
521 Fifth Avenue, New York, NY 10175 USA

56789 052 987654321

Printed in the United States of America on acid-free paper

Orders from outside the United States should be sent to the appropriate address listed below. Orders from areas not listed below should be placed through CBS International Publishing, 383 Madison Ave., New York, NY 10175 USA.

Australia, New Zealand
Holt Saunders, Pty, Ltd., 9 Waltham St., Artarmon, N.S.W. 2064, Sydney, Australia

Canada
Holt, Rinehart & Winston of Canada, 55 Horner Ave., Toronto, Ontario, Canada M8Z 4X6

Europe, the Middle East, & Africa
Holt Saunders, Ltd., 1 St. Anne's Road, Eastbourne, East Sussex, England BN21 3UN

Japan
Holt Saunders, Ltd., Ichibancho Central Building, 22-1 Ichibancho, 3rd Floor, Chiyodaku, Tokyo, Japan

Hong Kong, Southeast Asia
Holt Saunders Asia, Ltd., 10 Fl, Intercontinental Plaza, 94 Granville Road, Tsim Sha Tsui East, Kowloon, Hong Kong

Manuscript submissions should be sent to the Editorial Director, Praeger Publishers, 521 Fifth Avenue, New York, NY 10175 USA

For our parents

FOREWORD

As chairman of a pharmacology department, I was asked by representatives of the Thompson Medical Company to organize a meeting on phenylpropanolamine. The company agreed that a proper conference would require participation by those who disapprove of the product as well as those who favor it, since both the safety and efficacy of the drug have engendered controversy. Dr. John Morgan, who has been interested in look-alike drugs, agreed to plan a symposium. He and his associate, Ms. Doreen Kagan, organized the meeting with careful thought and judgment. They invited not only those who support and those who object to the use of phenylpropanolamine but also those who are knowledgeable about adrenergic drugs but whose opinions about phenylpropanolamine were not known. Ample time was provided on the program for discussion. The Thompson Medical Company scrupulously honored the agreement that Dr. Morgan be solely responsible both for the program and for these published proceedings. The company also suggested and funded awards to graduate students for research proposals on adrenergic drugs. Faculty from medical schools, selected by Dr. Morgan, appraised the proposals and made the awards.

The conference was lively and, most of all, revealing. It is a worthy example of academic and corporate cooperation.

Jack Peter Green, M.D., Ph.D.

Professor and Chairman
Department of Pharmacology
Mount Sinai School of Medicine
of the City University of New York

ACKNOWLEDGMENTS

This book is largely based on presentations given at a conference entitled "Phenylpropanolamine: Examining Benefits and Risks" held in New York City on June 10 and 11, 1984. Chapters 1, 6, and 11 were developed after the conference and so were not presented there.

Many people encouraged and assisted us in organizing this symposium and in preparing the proceedings. We are grateful to Barbara Cooper, Charles Decicco, Pyser Edelsack, Ellen Felten, Jack Peter Green, M.D., Gail Jara, Robert Lantos, Robert Marlin, Leonard Meiselas, M.D., Patti Otani, Stephenie Ross, Maribel Salabarria, Linda Toppi, Francine Warner, the staff of the New York Academy of Medicine, and other supportive friends.

The conference sponsorship was shared by the City University of New York Medical School; the Department of Pharmacology of the Mount Sinai School of Medicine of the City University of New York; the California Society for the Treatment of Alcoholism and Other Drug Dependencies; and the Arnold and Marie Schwartz College of Pharmacy and Health Sciences of Long Island University.

Partial funding for the conference and for the publication of these proceedings was provided by Thompson Medical Company.

Note on Trademark Status

Information on the trademark status of many of the products mentioned in this book was gathered from the following sources: Self-medication: a guide to over-the-counter health care products. 1984. Oradell, NJ: Medical Economics; Physicians' desk reference for nonprescription drugs. 1980. Oradell, NJ: Medical Economics; Physicians' desk reference, 39th edition. 1985; 36th edition. 1982; 27th edition. 1973. Oradell, NJ: Medical Economics; Red-book: annual pharmacists' reference. 1983. Oradell, NJ: Medical Economics; telephone calls to manufacturers of specific products; and information supplied by contributing authors.

We regret that we were unable to obtain trademark information on the products listed below.

Altepose
Anahist
Antiadipositum
A.S.T.
B.C. Tablets
Comeback
Contac 500
Dimetapp Tablets L.A.
Easy-Mens
Elixamine
Eskornade
Formalin
Fugoa
Lunerin
Maranox
Minusin
Monhydrin
Mucron
Mydriatine
Neopiphen
Nilain
Pre-Mens
Recatol
Rinexin
Rinomar
Sinugard
Sinutabs S.A.
Slim-Rite
Soulls Slimming Tabs
Spindell
Statavar
Trimolets
Triogesic
Vita-Slim

CONTENTS

LIST OF TABLES

LIST OF FIGURES AND ILLUSTRATIONS

Figure | Page

BASIC AND CLINICAL APPLICATIONS

1

OVER-THE-COUNTER MEDICATION: AVAILABILITY AND ISSUES

John P. Morgan

INTRODUCTION

Fifteen years ago, 30 years after the introduction of phenylpropanolamine to clinical medicine in the United States, this was written:

> No serious toxicity has resulted from the use of phenylpropanolamine. Because of its safety, it is one of the few sympathomimetic drugs that can be incorporated in remedies sold without a prescription in the United States. (Aviado 1970, p. 241)

Recently in a letter to a journal of emergency medicine, these words, describing the same medicinal, appeared:

> The references cited in our paper included studies and reviews documenting 100 cases of untoward reactions. . . . we are familiar with an additional 50 cases. Our own cases include patients with altered mental states and hallucinations, ventricular tachycardia, one case of ruptured cerebral aneurysm [following ingestion of one capsule of Dietac™] and numerous hypertensive reactions. (Bernstein et al. 1983, p. 591)

How, after more than 30 years of use and the granting of a surprisingly comprehensive safety commendation in 1970, has phenylpropanolamine come to be currently regarded by many as a dangerous and widely misapplied chemical?

As will be documented in the conference proceedings that follow, phenylpropanolamine has been widely used since the 1930s in the United States. It has been available in both prescription and over-the-counter (OTC) cough, cold, and anti-allergy preparations. It entered the medicinal marketplace as a substitute for ephedrine because early studies suggested that it was less of a central nervous system (CNS) stimulant. Further, at clinical decongestant dosage it was thought to have minimal impact on the cardiovascular system. Despite its sympathomimetic character and its chemical resemblance to ephedrine, amphetamine, and other beta-isopropylphenylamines, it had important clinical distinctions. In one of the first pharmacological studies of phenylpropanolamine ever published, the authors compared the drug to its close chemical relative amphetamine: "The presence of the secondary alcoholic hydroxyl in phenylpropanolamine serves to decrease the toxicity to a degree that becomes significant therapeutically" (Hartung and Munch 1931). These remarks were based on findings that 300 times more phenylpropanolamine than amphetamine was required to cause death consistently in rabbits.

Prior to Aviado's 1970 review, the medical literature contained only a few papers on the human toxicity of phenylpropanolamine. These reported probable interaction with monoamine oxidase (MAO) inhibitors causing increased blood pressure (Duvernoy 1969; Humberstone 1969; Mason 1969; Tonks 1965), increased blood pressure associated with overdosage (Ostern and Dodson 1965; Salmon et al. 1965), and psychosis associated with phenylpropanolamine/antihistamine combinations (Kane and Green 1966). The reports not associated with MAO inhibitors were often confused because of the presence of other drugs and/or other diseases.

In the 1970s, the already important place of phenylpropanolamine in clinical medicine in the United States expanded further. For years, phenylpropanolamine had had some application as an anorexiant. Because it had been approved for nonprescription sales with this indication, its use grew rapidly. As many authors in these proceedings will note, the expansion of this market was unprecedented. Retail sales of phenylpropanolamine-containing diet aids exceeded $200 million in 1983.

THE APPEARANCE OF SIMULATED CONTROLLED SUBSTANCES ("LOOK-ALIKES")

After the curtailment of amphetamine by a series of government actions which diminished its diversion, the street stimulant market came to be dominated by "look-alikes." These are medicinal products made to resemble popular prescription formats, but containing only OTC drugs. Morgan, Puder, and Kagan (see chapter 9, this volume) have documented the appearance of phenylpropanolamine in these products in 1980-82 in combination with caffeine and ephedrine. This inclusion certainly increased human exposure to phenylpropanolamine, but of course such exposure was characterized by uncertain dosage, uncertain polypharmacy, and uncertain circumstances and thus was difficult to evaluate clinically.

The stage was therefore set for a mandatory reevaluation of phenylpropanolamine. For at least 30 years, ingestion of phenylpropanolamine had been extensive and evidence of its toxicity had been minimal. In the 1970s, this already extensive consumption increased further as OTC anorexiant sales and the stimulant look-alike market expanded. A series of case reports of adverse effects began to emerge in the mid-1970s and continued into the 1980s. These reports associated phenylpropanolamine with episodes of high blood pressure, cerebrovascular accidents, and CNS stimulation, including seizures, anxiety, and psychosis. At least 35 such accounts have been recorded.

Elsewhere, I have reviewed these articles in a context of the process by which associations are made between episodes of clinical adversity and possible drug toxicity (Morgan 1985). Briefly, the physician who generates a case report observes a non-unique clinical event. Hypertension, anxiety, and even psychosis may occur in the presence of not just one drug but many drugs; they occur in the presence of many diseases and they may even occur without any drug or any prior disease process being present at all. Therefore, the decision that events related in time (e.g., drug ingestion and anxiety) are causally related is not an easy one to make.

Stated another way, phenylpropanolamine ingestion and high blood pressure are extremely common events. When they appear together, how often is the linkage merely coincidental? The standard alerting mechanism--the case report--is of little help to us because it merely signals the association. If honestly presented, it usually also indicates why the relationship may not be valid (e.g., other drugs, other diseases, failure to verify the actual presence of the drug). Case studies and uncontrolled surveys (Norvenius, Widerlov, and Lonnerholm 1979; Dietz 1981) by their nature identify related phenomena. They cannot prove that such associations are other than coincidental. Case reports are like metaphors. They serve to sensitize us and make us vigilant regarding new associations, but they are not valuable in estimating the truth or the character of the relationships they signal.

ALTERNATIVE HYPOTHESES FOR THE RECENT, FREQUENT REPORTS OF PHENYLPROPANOLAMINE TOXICITY

Upon examining the failure of a group of clinical pharmacologists to agree with each other or the clinicians admitting patients as to the presence or absence of drug toxicity, Karch and Lasagna concluded that:

> Most reactions are difficult to categorize unequivocally as to cause due to the non-unique character of reactions, the presence of multiple drugs and the inability or failure to perform definitive cause-effect tests. . . . There are no standard guidelines for identifying ADR's [adverse drug reactions] and decisions on whether a specific reaction is drug related rest upon the clinical judgment of different physicians in different clinical environments, a situation guaranteed to produce divergence of opinion. (Medicine in the Public Interest 1974, p. 2. Reprinted with permission.)

The case reports, particularly those not associated with overdoses, may indicate the existence of a true relationship. One may accept that the early assessment of the safety of phenylpropanolamine was incorrect and that the wider exposure of the 1970s has given us a truer understanding of the drug's liabilities. Is there an alternative hypothesis? My previous remarks and the work of Lasagna and Karch would certainly suggest that bias in assigning blame to a drug might well exist. To cite an example, a parent assessing an adolescent child's poor school performance learns that the child is experimenting with marihuana. The parent is likely to attribute the poor performance to the psychotoxicity of marihuana. This assignment may be correct or incorrect. The automatic attribution of cause to marihuana is the result of bias and a context of preexisting distaste for this and other experimental, illegal drug use. Could the assignment of a series of non-unique clinical reactions to phenylpropanolamine likewise be biased? If the reports are biased, what factors could have caused clinicians to focus on the heretofore unnoticed drug product?

Three Reasons for Assignment Bias

1. The identification with amphetamine.

Phenylpropanolamine is identified with amphetamine and such identification provokes hostility. Amphetamine itself, once offered as a safe treatment for obesity, has become the prototype of a misused medicinal. Since phenylpropanolamine in some sense replaced amphetamine, reports claiming misuse are easily accepted because a context is prepared. The Thompson Medical Company's choice of the name "Dexatrim™" (perhaps to signal "Dexedrine®") may not have been a good marketing decision in the long run. Many reports have compared line structural drawings of amphetamine and phenylpropanolamine to emphasize their similarity. One paper was even published with ephedrine's structure incorrectly labeled as amphetamine (Bernstein et al. 1979). I do not identify this smugly but doubt that the comparison was closely examined because the associational point had been made.

2. The inclusion in simulated controlled substances.

Initially, the look-alike drugs were regarded with something close to amusement. In 1975-78, some workers in both law enforcement and drug abuse treatment expressed their pleasure that at least young people were not buying real amphetamine. However, as the merchandising of these fakes became more aggressive and their presence more manifest, a predictable aversion set in and the look-alikes were condemned at least as signposts on the road to real drug abuse and drug dealing. Ultimately, they were accepted as truly dangerous in addition to being merely offensive. The relatively recent inclusion of phenylpropanolamine in the look-alikes greatly contributed to the distaste for it. Surprisingly, an equal distaste did not develop for the other ingredients. Recent comment on the toxicity of caffeine and ephedrine has been minimal. Why the focus on phenylpropanolamine?

3. A bias toward anorexiants.

The aggressive and successful merchandising of OTC diet aids provoked bias, but the therapeutic claims were equally important in fomenting opposition. Since the abuse of amphetamine, most drugs used to suppress appetite have been suspect. Usually critics deny that anorexiants are effective. When proponents cite evidence of efficacy, critics state that the products have not been shown to be efficacious in the long run. If it is pointed out that anorexiants other than amphetamine and phenmetrazine have seldom been incriminated in abuse, critics claim that the cases will surely soon emerge and they recall the initial optimistic acceptance of amphetamine. After progressing many times through this conversation, one realizes that the critics and the culture have acquired a distinct, high-minded aversion to the use of drugs to diminish appetite. The common wisdom is that overweight Americans must reeducate themselves, and change their eating habits without reliance on medication. The harshest criticism of overmedication is directed against medication use that is thought self-indulgent. If there were more will power, we wouldn't need diet pills. If there were better attitudes, habits, or standards, we wouldn't need tranquilizers or sleeping pills. We ardently disapprove of the use of "little" psychoactive drugs and easily accept reports that they are dangerous, rather than deal with the difficult truth that their use is "merely" distasteful.

The phenylpropanolamine conference of 1984 and these proceedings have been constructed to illuminate these alternative interpretations: (1) that increased phenylpropanolamine exposure has uncovered serious risks or (2) that increased phenylpropanolamine awareness has provoked the application of bias. There are presentations from those who support one hypothesis or another regarding phenylpropanolamine toxicity. There are presentations of studies (animal, epidemiological, controlled trials) that should give a better developed context for the evaluation of case reports and earlier studies. I am not sure that a consensus will develop among those concerned, but I am sure that more appropriate information will be available for those who must make decisions (regulatory, marketing, clinical) about phenylpropanolamine.

A FEW WORDS ON NOMENCLATURE

The discussion of various phenylpropanolamine isomers and drug products in chapter 11 (see Morgan, this volume) may serve to clear up some confusion about what is truly a family of drugs. The text with few exceptions has been edited with an eye toward consistency and the following conventions.

The n-demethylated form of ephedrine was once identified as norephedrine and this name frequently occurs in the older medical literature. The trivial or generic name phenylpropanolamine was chosen because it signals the combining of a phenyl ring, an isopropyl alcohol, and an amine. Because such a product contains two chiral carbons, there are four possible isomers. There are two configurations each for norephedrine and norpseudoephedrine (see chapter 11, figure 11.2). These have in the past been referred to as "D" or "L" (for configuration) or as "d" or "l" (for optical activity). All of the phenylpropanolamine marketed in the United States has been a racemic mixture of d- and l-forms. To avoid confusion when this preparation is mentioned, it shall be labeled "(±)-phenylpropanolamine." This convention of "(+)" for "d" and of "(-)" for "l" shall be used for other isomers such as (+)-amphetamine, (-)-ephedrine, or (+)-cathine. Although both norpseudoephedrine and norephedrine could be called "phenylpropanolamine," such usage is avoided here. Unless specifically identified otherwise, phenylpropanolamine may be assumed to mean racemic (±)-norephedrine.

REFERENCES

Aviado, D. 1970. Phenylpropanolamine. In Sympathomimetic drugs, 240-43. Springfield, IL: Charles C. Thomas.

Bernstein, E. et al. 1983. Safety of phenylpropanolamine. Letter. Ann Emerg Med 12:591-92.

Dietz, A. J. 1981. Amphetamine-like reactions to phenylpropanolamine. JAMA 245:601-2.

Duvernoy, W. 1969. Positive phentolamine test in hypertension induced by a nasal decongestant. N Engl J Med 280:877.

Hartung, W. and J. C. Munch. 1931. Amino alcohols in the preparation and pharmacodynamic activity of four isomeric phenylpropanolamines. J Am Chem Soc 53:1875-79.

Humberstone, P. M. 1969. Hypertension from cold remedies. Letter. Br Med J 1:846.

Kane, F. J., Jr. and B. Q. Green. 1966. Psychotic episodes associated with the use of common proprietary decongestants. Am J Psychiatry 123:484-87.

Mason, A.M.S. and R. M. Buckle. 1969. "Cold" cures and monoamine oxidase inhibitors. Letter. Br Med J 1:845.

Medicine in the Public Interest. 1974. Adverse drug reactions in the United States: an analysis of the scope of the problem and recommendations for future approaches. Washington, D.C.: Medicine in the Public Interest.

Morgan, J. P. 1985. Phenylpropanolamine: an analysis of reported adverse reactions and overdosages. Fort Lee, NJ: Jack K. Burgess.

Norvenius, G., E. Widerlov, and G. Lonnerholm. 1979. Phenylpropanolamine and mental disturbances. Lancet 2:1367-68.

Ostern, S. and W. H. Dodson. 1965. Hypertension following Ornade ingestion. Letter. JAMA 194:472.

Salmon, P. R. 1965. Hypertensive crisis with Eskornade. Letter. Br Med J 1:193.

Tonks, C. M. and A. T. Lloyd. 1965. Hazards with monoamine oxidase inhibitors. Letter. Br Med J 1:589.

2

A HISTORY OF THERAPEUTIC USES OF PHENYLPROPANOLAMINE IN NORTH AMERICA

Harold I. Silverman

INTRODUCTION

First synthesized in 1910 (Kanfor, Haigh, and Dowse 1983), phenylpropanolamine (PPA), or (±)-norephedrine, has been pharmacologically and clinically evaluated repeatedly since its identification as a potentially useful sympathomimetic agent. The first half of this century saw only a handful of reports describing its properties and clinical applications. The drug received little attention outside the medical field prior to the late 1970s, when it began to gain popularity as a proven anorexiant agent.

This year marks the 75th anniversary of the recognition of phenylpropanolamine as a useful chemical entity. Unlike some other substances with similarly long histories of use, the medical history of phenylpropanolamine is not without controversy. This may be due to its clinical application in the treatment of obesity, drug therapy for which was and remains controversial. As an advocate of this drug, I believe that the weight of evidence attesting to its advantages and relative lack of adverse effects is sufficient to insure its continued use. Phenylpropanolamine, an official drug in the United States Pharmacopeia (USP XXI)--National Formulary (NF XVI) (1984a), is also recognized as a useful appetite suppressant in the current edition of the USP Dispensing Information (United States Pharmacopeial Convention 1984b) and has recently been reviewed by three separate Food and Drug Administration (FDA) expert advisory panels (Health and Human Services 1982a, 1982b; Health, Education and Welfare 1976).

In any current discussion of phenylpropanolamine, it must be emphasized that the literature abounds with misconceptions and with biased and anecdotal reports. There are a number of original studies which serve to attest to the drug's safety; some, unfortunately, are unavailable to the public (e.g., regulatory submissions known as New Drug Applications [NDAs], which are available for review only by FDA personnel). In addition, the literature rarely differentiates between the activities of the several norephedrine isomers. If a drug has four known isomeric forms, it is not unusual for the effects produced by one isomer to be wrongly attributed to another (Fairchild and Alles 1967).

HISTORY AND DEVELOPMENT

The initial pharmacological reports on the activity of phenylpropanolamine were provided by the renowned pharmacologist K. K. Chen, who is well-known for his introduction of ephedrine (also known as "Ma Huang") into Western medicine (Chen and Schmidt 1924; Chen, Wu, and Henricksen 1929; Chen and Schmidt 1930). Chen had investigated phenylpropanolamine in connection with a series of sympathomimetic amines chemically related to ephedrine. His early studies with phenylpropanolamine indicated that the drug would produce effects analogous to those of ephedrine. In subsequent clinical evaluations, it was reported that phenylpropanolamine was less likely to produce central nervous system (CNS) stimulation than was ephedrine or amphetamine, due to the substitution of a hydroxyl group on the beta-carbon (Goodman and Gilman 1960). Consequently, phenylpropanolamine's initial introduction into medicine was as a parenterally administered compound for the maintenance of blood pressure with significantly fewer side effects than ephedrine. However, as a pressor medication phenylpropanolamine was superseded by the more effective agents phenylephrine and epinephrine (Lilly and Company 1951) and is no longer used for this purpose. It should be noted that while a pressor effect of phenylpropanolamine has been demonstrated following intraperitoneal or intravenous administration, blood pressure has not been shown to be elevated by analogous doses given orally (Black 1937; Boyer 1938; Unger et al. 1967; Mitchell 1968; Silverman et al. 1980).

Marketed in 25 and 50 mg capsules and in 1% and 3% liquid solutions under the brand name Propadrine®, phenylpropanolamine was used as a nasal decongestant and for symptomatic treatment of allergic disorders due to hay fever, asthma, allergic rhinitis, urticaria, angioneurotic edema, and bronchospastic conditions accompanying allergic asthma. Additional uses included its application as an adjunct for the control of appetite in the dietary management of obesity. With regard to this latter application, phenylpropanolamine dosages suggested in New and Nonofficial Remedies (NNR), a former American Medical Association (AMA) publication (1954), ranged from 10 to 15 mg three times daily for young children to 50 mg two to three times daily for adults.

Use as an Anorexiant Agent

Phenylpropanolamine began to be used as an anorexiant following the appearance of an article by Hirsh (1939), in which he concluded that phenylpropanolamine was effective in controlling the appetite of patients on an antiobesity diet. Six additional studies conducted over the next ten years also concluded that phenylpropanolamine was safe and effective as an anorexiant (Kalb 1942; Cutting 1943; Colton 1943; Tainter 1944; Williams et al. 1948; Reilly 1950). Altepose, an antiobesity preparation containing 50 mg phenylpropanolamine in addition to 50 mg thyroid and 25 mg vinbarbital, was marketed for several years by Merck, Sharp, and Dohme as an adjunct to a restricted diet in the management of obese patients and was a popular prescription medication. The recommended dosage was one tablet one to three times daily before meals.

As an appetite suppressant and decongestant remedy, phenylpropanolamine was permitted to be sold without a prescription, as was ephedrine. The rationale for allowing over-the-counter (OTC) sale of these compounds relied partly on their usefulness as oral and topical nasal decongestants and oral bronchodilators in treating asthma and partly on the fact that directions for use were easily understood by consumers and could be followed without complications.

Given that a number of published reports attested to the effectiveness and relative safety of phenylpropanolamine and that phenylpropanolamine had been recognized as effective in the prestigious NNR publication of the AMA and could be sold on an OTC basis, several pharmaceutical firms initiated distribution of phenylpropanolamine as an anorexiant. Sales were vigorous and the use of the drug as an appetite suppressant continued to increase through the 1940s and 1950s. By the mid-1950s, millions of doses had been used in anorexiants, nasal decongestants, and bronchodilators.

EXAMINING ATTACKS ON PHENYLPROPANOLAMINE

It is significant that no adverse effects of phenylpropanolamine were reported during this early period, despite the fact that dosages were greater and advertising less controlled than they currently are. The 1957 edition of Sollmann's pharmacology text, A Manual of Pharmacology, stated that "no toxic effects [of phenylpropanolamine] have been reported clinically." Why, then, have several reports published in the last few years claimed adverse effects of phenylpropanolamine use? Are these purported side effects the result of even wider use of the drug or are they due to misuse, overuse, or use of norephedrine or ephedrine isomers other than phenylpropanolamine?

Subcommittee Hearings

In 1957, due to growing concern over extravagant claims designed to induce consumers to purchase weight-reducing drugs, the U.S. House of Representatives Legal and Monetary Affairs Subcommittee on Government Operations held four separate hearings focusing principally on advertising of appetite suppressants (U.S. Congress, House 1958). Various medical experts and representatives of the FDA, the Federal Trade Commission (FTC), the U.S. Post Office, and the National Better Business Bureau appeared as witnesses. Although medical experts contended that anorexiants should be used only under the supervision of a physician, FDA representatives "insisted that in doses permitted for OTC sale weight-reducing drugs were safe provided consumers adhere to package labelling directions" (U.S. Congress, House 1958). The then deputy director of the FDA advised the subcommittee that phenylpropanolamine in dosages of 25 mg was considered safe for nonprescription sale and that because of its long-term prior usage the FDA did not consider phenylpropanolamine to be a new drug. The sum and substance of the hearings with regard to phenylpropanolamine concerned not the safety or efficacy of the drug but rather the apparently excessive advertising claims made on its behalf. The subcommittee published its report, False and Misleading Advertising (Weight-Reducing Remedies), the following year.

The Controversial Fazekas Study

Soon thereafter the U. S. Post Office sponsored a clinical investigation, headed by Dr. J. F. Fazekas (Fazekas et al. 1959), to determine the effectiveness of phenylpropanolamine as a diet aid.* From the results of this study, conducted with 81 mentally deficient obese patients, the authors concluded that phenylpropanolamine did not possess any significant anorexiant potential. The Fazekas paper was used by various Federal agencies as evidence for the "ineffectiveness" of phenylpropanolamine as an appetite suppressant, and several phenylpropanolamine-containing products sold as anorexiants were seized.

From 1959, when the Fazekas article was published, until 1965, it appeared that phenylpropanolamine would be limited to use as a nasal decongestant, since its reputation as an anorexiant was now less than favorable. However, since the use of phenylpropanolamine as an appetite suppressant persisted, the FTC expanded the scope of its hearings to include questions of phenylpropanolamine's safety in addition to its efficacy. During an FTC-initiated hearing in the latter part of 1965 (Federal Trade Commission 1967), Dr. K. D. Campbell, a co-author of the Fazekas paper, made several statements which raised questions regarding the scientific merit of the Fazekas study. After extensive review, an FTC hearing examiner concluded that "if a normal person has a desire to lose weight then PPA taken in dosages of 25 mg three times a day . . . will be an effective appetite suppressant in the treatment of obesity" and further stated that "the errors, misstatements, inaccuracies and omissions in the Fazekas report take from the study a considerable degree of credibility which might otherwise be given to it" (Federal Trade Commission 1967). The Fazekas study was again repudiated in 1978 and 1979 during meetings of an FDA advisory review panel regarding weight control products (Health and Human Services 1979). Nevertheless, this same study—with admitted errors in its design, methodology, and conclusions—continues to be referred to in criticisms of phenylpropanolamine's anorexiant potential, notwithstanding recent clinical and pharmacological studies to the contrary.

---

*At that time I was a professor at Long Island University with a mild interest in antiobesity agents. I felt that the Fazekas paper was biased and composed a review article (Silverman 1963) that concluded that phenylpropanolamine was an effective anorexiant and was being wrongly criticized.

Confirmation of Safety and Efficacy by Three FDA Advisory Panels

A review of the safety, efficacy, and labeling of all OTC drugs by FDA advisory review panels was begun in 1972. Consequently, phenylpropanolamine was subjected to such review by three independent advisory panels over the next six years. Each panel concluded that phenylpropanolamine was safe for nonprescription or OTC use (Health and Human Services 1982a, 1982b; Health, Education and Welfare 1976).

Data on animal toxicological testing of phenylpropanolamine were submitted to the advisory review panel on OTC cold, cough, allergy, bronchodilator, and antiasthmatic drugs. Although a considerable amount of animal data was submitted (including tests of phenylpropanolamine in several species), phenylpropanolamine's long history of use in humans was judged by the panel to be sufficient confirmation of its safety. They concluded that:

> At therapeutic doses of phenylpropanolamine taken orally the incidence of side effects in adults and children is low. There have been isolated reports, however, of individuals experiencing idiosyncratic reactions of central nervous system stimulation and/or blood pressure rise following therapeutic doses. These effects would be expected in most individuals with acute overdoses of the drug. (Health, Education and Welfare 1976)

It should be noted that while advisory panel reports and company submissions to OTC panels provide much useful data, the FDA does not always evaluate them in other contexts where the data might prove to be important. For example, a study demonstrating the safety of phenylpropanolamine in combination with aspirin in moderate to high doses was submitted to the 1976 advisory panel (Pugliese 1976). Yet, in the preamble to the weight control products monograph published some six years later (Health and Human Services 1982a), the agency voiced concern over possible interaction of phenylpropanolamine with aspirin and other nonsteroidal anti-inflammatory agents because of a single case report suggesting an interaction of phenylpropanolamine with indomethacin and called for studies to resolve this issue—one that should never have been raised since a well-controlled safety study was already in their files.

Appetite suppressants were reviewed at no less than 33 separate meetings of the FDA's miscellaneous advisory panel over a period of more than three years. Studies were submitted showing phenylpropanolamine (and phenylpropanolamine combined with caffeine) to be an effective anorexiant. The statistical validity of these studies was confirmed by the panel's statistical consultant, Dr. R. D'Agostino, who also noted that the studies of phenylpropanolamine were significantly more reliable than many studies submitted to the panel in support of other drugs. The panel later voted to place phenylpropanolamine in Category I (for adequate safety and effectiveness) as an aid in weight reduction.

With the passage of time and acquisition of knowledge, confidence in the panel's evaluation of phenylpropanolamine as safe and effective has grown; witness the fact that American Home, Ciba-Geigy, and Menley & James (to name but a few), following the lead of the Thompson Medical Company, have seen fit to enter the weight control market with phenylpropanolamine products.

Misuse and False Advertising

Following the publication of monographs on the efficacy of phenylpropanolamine as a nasal decongestant and anorexiant, the use of the drug increased significantly. Commensurate with this increase in legitimate use, some entrepreneurs, extolling combinations of phenylpropanolamine, ephedrine or pseudoephedrine, and caffeine as legal stimulants, seized the opportunity to manufacture and distribute them. Unfortunately, the presence of these "triple combinations" and other similar products on the market precipitated an increase in anecdotal reports of adverse reactions, effects which were attributed to phenylpropanolamine alone rather than to the combinations of sympathomimetic agents. Doses were frequently excessive inasmuch as no dosage adjustments had been made to correct for the presence of more than one drug of the same pharmacological class.

While the FDA has never sanctioned a stimulant claim for phenylpropanolamine, some unethical manufacturers and wholesalers have persisted in labeling and advertising their phenylpropanolamine products as stimulants. This unfortunate and illegal practice reflects badly on the drug, despite the existence of numerous studies which show it not to be a stimulant. The only source for the claim that phenylpropanolamine induces stimulation is its structure and pharmacological classification, although in fact stimulation does not occur with conventional doses nor even with moderate overdoses. This has been confirmed at FDA advisory panel meetings (Health and Human Services 1978) and in animal studies (Griffiths, Brady, and Snell 1978; Maher

1984; Schuster and Johanson 1984), yet the myth of phenylpropanolamine as stimulant persists. It is always difficult to change a preconceived notion, even by submission of data.

Confusion with Other Isomers

Racemic phenylpropanolamine is frequently confused with a related stereoisomer, (+)-norpseudoephedrine, also known as cathine, which is a CNS stimulant. In semitropical regions it occurs naturally in the leaves of the shrub Catha edulis, or khat; people who live in some Indian, African, and Arabian Peninsular countries chew khat for its stimulant effect. Khat also contains another alkaloid, cathinone ((-)-alpha-aminopropiophenone), which is a relatively strong stimulant and, unlike caffeine, is chemically unstable (Klein 1979). Unfortunately the scientific and medical literature does not always distinguish between the several alkaloids in khat or emphasize the fact that its stimulant properties are not due to norephedrine (of which only trace amounts are found in khat) but rather to cathinone and cathine.

Cathine, as (+)-norpseudoephedrine, is used in European countries primarily as an anorexiant; appetite suppressants marketed in West Germany contain cathine, not phenylpropanolamine. Recatol, Fugoa, and Minusin, three of the more popular European OTC anorexiants, produce a definite stimulant effect in both animals and humans (Ibid.; Hamilton 1977).

Recent Data on Safety and Efficacy

During the past few years a number of studies have been conducted with phenylpropanolamine to examine its effects on the cardiovascular and neurological systems and to determine whether the increasingly frequent anecdotal reports of adverse reactions have any basis in fact. In the last ten or 12 years, more clinical and experimental studies have been done of phenylpropanolamine than of the great majority of currently available OTC medications.

I have now tabulated 34 phenylpropanolamine safety studies, which included as subjects over 300,000 people. Patients were studied for periods ranging from one day to six years. Oral daily phenylpropanolamine dosages varied from 25 to 200 mg given alone or in combination with other medications. Well over 50 investigators were involved in these studies, and all of them concluded that phenylpropanolamine showed no adverse effect on blood pressure or heart rate, and further that it was not a stimulant, that it lacked arousal potential, and that it was not euphorigenic. Psychometric studies at several institutions demonstrated an absence of dependence liability under test conditions employing profiles of mood states, addiction center inventories, and visual analog scales.

The original seven studies (Hirsh 1939; Kalb 1942; Cutting 1943; Colton 1943; Tainter 1944; Williams et al. 1948; Reilly 1950) and the NNR monograph (American Medical Association 1954) affirming phenylpropanolamine's anorexiant effectiveness have been complemented by at least 16 contemporary clinical investigations, five of which have been published (Hoebel et al. 1975a, 1975b; Griboff, Berman, and Silverman 1975; Altschuler et al. 1982; Noble 1982).

Among therapeutic agents intended to provide relief from nasal congestion due to the common cold, flu, hay fever, allergic sinusitis, and sinusitis, the drug Contac® is probably the best known worldwide. Contac® was originally approved by the FDA in 1961 under an NDA submitted by Menley & James Laboratories (New Drug Application 1961), and its active ingredients initially included 50 mg phenylpropanolamine, 4 mg chlorpheniramine maleate, and 0.2 mg belladonna alkaloids. Contac® and several other combination phenylpropanolamine dosage forms have been continuously marketed by Menley & James and its parent company, Smith, Kline & French. Reformulated and approved by the FDA in 1979 to contain 75 mg phenylpropanolamine and 8 mg chlorpheniramine maleate, this sustained-action nasal decongestant is typical of some 150 or more OTC products, billions of doses of which have been sold under numerous brand names for symptomatic relief of discomfort associated with the common cold and allergic disorders. With regard to prescription use, six phenylpropanolamine-containing products ranked in the "top 200" category of prescription drugs for 1980: Dimetapp®, Ornade®, Naldecon®, Tussornade®, Dimetane® expectorant, and Dimetane® expectorant DC (1980: Top 200 drugs 1981). These six products accounted for over 31 million prescriptions in 1980, which equal well over a billion individual doses when considering both original and refill prescriptions.

CONCLUSION

In conclusion, well-conducted clinical studies have repeatedly shown phenylpropanolamine to be safe and effective as a nasal decongestant and anorexiant. A billion or more doses of it have been used every year for the last 25 years, providing a safety record which, when judged on the basis of legitimately produced dosage forms, is remarkable for its relative absence of serious adverse effects. Such concerns as may exist regarding phenylpropanolamine's safety all too often have their origin in biased articles which place undue emphasis on unusual, idiosyncratic events or which wrongly claim it to be the cause of an adverse reaction to a multiple-ingredient formulation.

Concerns that hypertensive persons might not be able to use this drug safely have been assuaged by studies of it in hypertensive, obese, and asthmatic patients (Unger et al. 1967; Bradley 1982). That phenylpropanolamine lacks significant potential for abuse or habituation has been demonstrated in a series of animal and human studies both in the United States and abroad.

Phenylpropanolamine is a clinically dependable and safe anorexiant and nasal decongestant that, even when taken in significant overdose, produces no lasting sequelae and no tachyphylaxis and is devoid of abuse potential. Phenylpropanolamine may be aptly described as an anorexiant and decongestant well deserving of a second look.

REFERENCES

Altschuler, S. et al. 1982. Three controlled trials of weight loss with phenylpropanolamine. Int J Obes 6:549-56.

American Medical Association, Council on Pharmacy and Chemistry. 1954. New and nonofficial remedies, 234-40. Philadelphia: J. B. Lippincott.

Black, N. J. 1937. The control of allergic manifestations by phenyl-propanol-amine (Propadrin) hydrochloride. Journal--Lancet 57:101-2.

Boyer, W. E. 1938. The clinical use of phenyl-propanolamine hydrochloride (Propadrine) in the treatment of allergic conditions. J Allergy 9:509-13.

Bradley, M. H. 1982. Single-blind safety and efficacy evaluation of phenylpropanolamine hydrochloride plus caffeine, phenylpropanolamine alone, and placebo in exogenous obese patients with controlled hypertensive disease. Report on file. New York: Thompson Medical Company.

Chen, K. K. and C. F. Schmidt. 1930. Ephedrine and related substances. _Medicine_ 9:1-117.

———. 1924. The action of ephedrine, the active principle of the Chinese drug, "Ma Huang". _J Pharmacol Exp Ther_ 24:339-57.

Chen, K. K., C. K. Wu, and E. Henricksen. 1929. Relationship between the pharmacological action and the chemical constitution and configuration of the optical isomers of ephedrine and related compounds. _J Pharmacol Exp Ther_ 36:363-400.

Colton, N. H. 1943. The management of obesity with emphasis on appetite control. _Am J Med Sci_ 206:75.

Cutting, W. C. 1943. The treatment of obesity. _J Clin Endocrinol_ 3:85.

Fairchild, M. D. and G. A. Alles. 1967. The central locomotor stimulatory activity and acute toxicity of the ephedrine and norephedrine isomers in mice. _J Pharmacol Exp Ther_ 158:135-39.

Fazekas, J. F., et al. 1959. Comparative effectiveness of phenylpropanolamine and dextro amphetamine on weight reduction. _JAMA_ 170:1018-21.

Federal Trade Commission (FTC). 1967. Hearing examiner J. B. Poindexter. Docket no. 7176. March 16.

Goodman, L. S. and A. Gilman. 1955. _The pharmacological basis of therapeutics_, 2nd ed., 479, 533. New York: Macmillan.

Griboff, S. I., R. Berman, and H. I. Silverman. 1975. A double-blind clinical evaluation of a phenylpropanolamine-caffeine-vitamin combination and a placebo in the treatment of exogenous obesity. _Current Therapeutic Research_ 17:535-43.

Griffiths, R. R., J. V. Brady, and J. D. Snell. 1978. Relationship between anorectic and reinforcing properties of appetite suppressant drugs: implications for assessment of abuse liability. _Biol Psychiatry_ 13: 283-90.

Hamilton, C. 1977. Effects of phenylpropanolamine on food intake in rhesus monkeys. Report on file. New York: Thompson Medical Company.

Health and Human Services, Food and Drug Administration (FDA). 1982a. Establishment of a monograph for weight control drug products for over-the-counter human use. FDA docket no. 81N-0022. Federal Register 47:8466-84. February 26.

———. 1982b. Over-the-counter oral health care and discomfort drugs: establishment of a monograph. FDA docket no. 81N-0022. Federal Register 47:22711-22930. May 25.

———. 1979. Advisory Panel on Miscellaneous Internal Drugs. Summary minutes of the 27th meeting. January 19-20.

———. 1978. Advisory Panel on Miscellaneous Internal Drugs. Summary minutes of the 24th meeting. August 4-6.

Health, Education and Welfare, Food and Drug Administration (FDA). 1976. Establishment of a monograph for over-the-counter cold, cough, allergy, bronchodilator and antiasthmatic drug products. FDA docket no. 76N-0052. Federal Register 41:38401. September 9.

Hirsh, L. S. 1939. Controlling appetite in obesity. J of Medicine (Cincinnati) 20:84-86.

Hoebel, B. G. et al. 1975a. Appetite suppression by phenylpropanolamine in humans. Obesity and Bariatric Medicine 4:192-97.

Hoebel, B. G. et al. 1975b. Body weight decreased in humans by phenylpropanolamine taken before meals. Obesity and Bariatric Medicine 4:200-206.

Kalb, S. W. 1942. The effect of amphetamine (benzedrine) sulfate, propadrine and propadrine hydrochloride in combination with sodium delvinal on the appetite of obese patients. J Med Soc NJ 39:584-86.

Kanfor, L., J. M. Haigh, and R. Dowse. 1983. Phenylpropanolamine hydrochloride. In Analytical profiles of drug substances, edited by K. Florey, vol. 12. New York: Academic Press.

Klein, M. 1979. Review: analysis of khat constituents by the U.N. laboratory (Geneva, Switzerland). _Microgram,_ XII, No. 10:185-96. October.

Lilly (Eli) and Company. 1951. _De re medica,_ 3rd ed., 422-31. Indianapolis: Eli Lilly.

Maher, T. J. 1984. A comparison of the central nervous system stimulatory activity of various anorexiants. Report on file. New York: Thompson Medical Company.

Mitchell, C. A. 1968. Possible cardiovascular effect of phenylpropanolamine and belladonna alkaloids. _Current Therapeutic Research_ 10:47-53.

New Drug Application (NDA). 1961. Submitted for Contac by Menley & James Laboratories, no. 12-686. Original approval September 7.

1980: Top 200 Drugs. 1981. _Pharmacy Times_ April: 17-25.

Noble, R. E. 1982. Phenylpropanolamine and blood pressure. _Lancet_ 1:1419.

Pugliese, P. T. 1976. Sine-Aid II: human safety study. Draft of unpublished data. FDA docket no. 76N-0052. _Federal Register_ 41. September 9.

Reilly, W. A. 1950. The treatment of obesity in children. _American Practitioner_ 1:228.

Schuster, C. R. and C. E. Johanson. 1984. Anorectic drugs, efficacy, reinforcing and discriminating aspects; studies in rhesus monkeys and man. Paper presented at the annual meeting of the Federation of American Societies for Experimental Biology. April.

Silverman, H. I. 1963. Phenylpropanolamine--misused? or simply abused? _Am J Pharm_ 135:45-54.

Silverman, H. I. et al. 1980. Lack of side effects from orally administered phenylpropanolamine and phenylpropanolamine with caffeine: a controlled three-phase study. _Current Therapeutic Research_ 28:185-94.

Sollman, T. 1957. _A manual of pharmacology,_ 8th ed., 507. Philadelphia: W. B. Saunders.

Tainter, M. L. 1944. Actions of Benzedrine and Propadrine in the control of obesity. J Nutr 27:89-105.

Unger, D. L. et al. 1967. Effect of an antiasthmatic compound on blood pressure of hypertensive asthmatic patients. Ann Allergy 25:260-61.

United States Congress, House. 1958. False and misleading advertising: weight reducing remedies. 33rd report by the Committee on Government Operations, 85th Congress, no. 2553. August 12.

United States Pharmacopeial Convention (USP). 1984a. United States Pharmacopeia (USP XXI)—National Formulary (NF XVI). Rockville, MD: United States Pharmacopeial Convention.

———. 1984b. USP Dispensing Information, 4th ed. Rockville, MD: United States Pharmacopeial Convention.

Williams, R. H. et al. 1948. Obesity and its treatment with particular reference to the use of anorexigenic compounds. Ann Intern Med 29:510.

3

THE BASIC PHARMACOLOGY OF PHENYLPROPANOLAMINE IN RELATIONSHIP TO OTHER PHENYLALKYLAMINES

Murray Weiner

INTRODUCTION

The major reason for interest in the pharmacology and animal behavioral effects of phenylalkylamine derivatives such as phenylpropanolamine (PPA) is the potential correlation of this information with the important clinical characteristics of these drugs. These correlations might help us arrive at objective and rational conclusions about the relative utilities and risks of the drugs. This review will not attempt to examine all pharmacologic reports on phenylpropanolamine. Instead, the pharmacologic data to be reviewed have been selected for their possible relevance to clinical and social problems.

There is considerable variation between sympathomimetic agents in both the incidence and the severity of abuse and untoward reactions. This logically follows from the evidence that they do not produce parallel effects on various physiological systems and subsystems. Thus, although it is tempting to deal with these agents as a class rather than individually, that approach would be sure to sacrifice important truths. The situation may be summarized by the saying: the simple truth may be simple, but the whole truth is often very complex.

PHENYLPROPANOLAMINE STRUCTURES AND ISOMERS

The structures of some important analogs of phenylpropanolamine are presented in table 3.1 and figure 3.1. While the term phenylpropanolamine applies to all the structures in figure 3.1, the material marketed in the United States as phenylpropanolamine is in fact racemic (±)-norephedrine. In contrast, the phenylpropanolamine sold in Europe and

FIGURE 3.1

The norephedrines

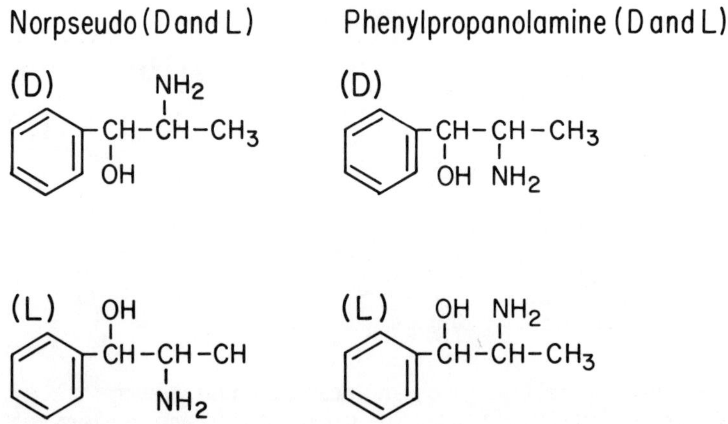

<u>Source</u>: Compiled by the author.

TABLE 3.1

Phenyl propyl amine sympathomimetic analogs

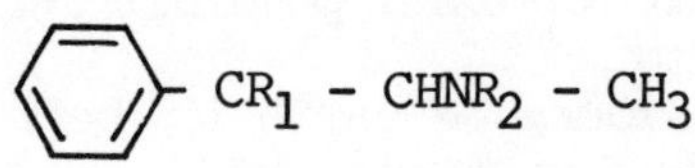

Generic name	R_1	R_2	Descriptive name
amphetamine	-H -H	-H -H	phenyl propane amine
ephedrine	-H -OH	-H $-CH_3$	phenyl propanol methyl amine
norephedrine	-H -OH	-H -H	phenyl propanol amine
diethylpropion	=O	$-C_2H_5$ $-C_2H_5$	phenyl ketopropyl diethylamine

<u>Source</u>: Compiled by the author.

Australia and referred to in foreign reports is often the (+)-norpseudoephedrine isomer, a pharmacologically distinct agent. Two adjacent carbons in ephedrine (a methylamine) and norephedrine (a primary amine) are chiral, yielding four stereoisomeric forms, schematically illustrated in figure 3.1; in contrast, amphetamine with only one chiral carbon has only two optical isomers. Although the marked variance in activity between (+)- and (-)-amphetamine is well-recognized, the differences in activity between the four isomers of ephedrine and norephedrine are often not considered. (For further discussion of this issue, see Morgan, chapter 11, this volume.)

PHENYLPROPANOLAMINE PHARMACOLOGY AND CLINICAL EFFECTS

Phenylpropanolamine is well-absorbed after oral administration. However, absorption can be altered by a variety of factors, particularly the presence of adsorbants such as activated charcoal (Tsuchiya and Levy 1972). In human beings, about 80% to 90% of the administered dose is excreted unchanged in the urine within 24 hours, with a urinary elimination half-life of about four hours. Plasma level studies show a similar half-life (Wilkinson and Beckett 1968; Mason and Amick 1981). There is some hepatic conversion to an active metabolite (4-hydroxy norephedrine) in rodents, which may complicate extrapolation of animal-derived pharmacokinetic information to clinical problems. Most regulatory questions about the action of different doses and formulations have been evaluated primarily on the basis of double-blind comparisons of activities rather than blood or urinary concentration patterns (Health and Human Services 1982).

The primary effects of sympathomimetics such as phenylpropanolamine are outlined in table 3.2. In clinical use of any of these drugs, the efficacy of the drug must be balanced against the possible risks and adverse effects associated with its use and the severity of the clinical problem being addressed.

Standard textbooks generally provide incomplete evaluations of many clinical and pharmacologic actions of sympathomimetic phenylalkylamines. A classic text on sympathomimetic drugs (Aviado 1970) does not mention anorexia as an effect of phenylpropanolamine. The 1980 edition of Goodman and Gilman presents a table summarizing the actions of this class of drugs, including phenylpropanolamine, but the column indicating central nervous system (CNS) and anorexiant activity has no entry for phenylpropanolamine, even though it has been used for many years as an over-the-counter (OTC) anorexiant and has been shown to cause reduced food intake and weight loss when administered in clinically tolerated doses (Health and Human Services 1982).

TABLE 3.2

Pharmacologic effects of sympathomimetics

Systems	Effects
Central nervous system	Stimulant (psychomotor, locomotor) Analgesic Drug-seeking ("addicting") Anorexiant
Cardiovascular system	Vasoconstriction Increased blood pressure, heart rate, cardiac output, etc.
Metabolic	Increased basal metabolic rate Accelerated blood sugar/carbohydrate metabolism Accelerated blood lipids/fat metabolism Accelerated gastrointestinal motility/secretions Decreased weight
Other	Mydriasis Decreased uterine contractility

Source: Compiled by the author.

Another pharmacology text (Levine 1973) discusses these agents as CNS stimulants under the heading "the amphetamines and cocaine" and states that the various members of this group "differ significantly in many of their phamacologic actions but are remarkably similar in their subjective effects, toxic symptoms and present day pattern of abuse." This qualitative similarity in both animal pharmacology and clinical experience is often assumed to indicate a common capacity for adverse effects and abuse. However, the evidence is clear that quantitative differences in potency are critical determinants of abuse potential and adverse CNS effects. There is an extensive literature of behavioral studies in animal and clinical models documenting these CNS dissimilarities (Tedeschi and Tedeschi 1968; Thompson and Johanson 1981).

Another major site of phenylpropanolamine activity is the cardiovascular system. The constriction of specific vascular beds, particularly in the nasopharynx, by topical or systemic applications of phenylpropanolamine is of proven clinical utility. Although other cardiovascular effects of phenylpropanolamine were once considered desirable in the treatment of hypotension and shock, they now represent primarily a source of concern as potential side effects.

Anorexiant Pharmacology

The discussion of the value of anorexiant drugs is based on the health risks associated with being overweight. There is little doubt that obesity adversely influences mortality and morbidity. Calculations based on insurance company data suggest that a given total amount of overweight in a population--whether it be modest overweight in many people or severe obesity in a few--is associated with a corresponding degree of increase in mortality (Weiner 1974). Diminished mortality statistics are observed with weight control, proportional to both the degree and duration of the weight loss achieved.

The complexities of and uncertainties about the mechanisms that control appetite and their relation to weight control are too great to cover completely in this limited review. Of key importance are the hypothalamic appetite centers and the factors that may affect them, including blood sugar levels, carbohydrate and fat metabolism, and gastrointestinal motility and secretions. Recently, appetite differences were observed between rats inbred for high versus low levels of red cell 2,3-diphosphoglycerate (DPG), the allosteric effector of oxygen-hemoglobin dissociation (Brewer 1984). The group inbred for high DPG was more active in bar pressing for food and had a significantly higher level of glycolytic intermediates. The greater bar pressing for food may have reflected a difference in learning capacity rather than appetite. In addition, the high-DPG (more active) animals also had lower cholesterol levels than their low-DPG counterparts whose oxygen-hemoglobin was more stable. Whether these correlations reflect an association between tissue oxygen availability and appetite is an unanswered question.

Patients who have experienced eating problems during severe active hepatitis sharply distinguish between the sensation of revulsion at the thought of food related to their inability to eat and normal satiation. Similarly, drugs like phenylpropanolamine that reduce the desire for food or lead to early satiation are clearly different from agents like 1,1-dichloro-2,2-bis(p-chlorophenyl)ethane (DDD) that, when used to treat metastatic adrenal tumors (Hutter and Kayhoe 1966), effectively eliminate the ability of some patients to accept food by mouth.

Animal Models and Route of Administration

In animal experiments, when weight change or food consumption is measured as an index of appetite, what is really being studied? In chronic drug safety studies of a wide variety of agents, reduced food intake is often the first evidence that toxic dose levels have been reached. Screening programs for new anorexiants to determine non-toxic and effective doses have been notoriously unsuccessful. Many effects, such as sedation, nausea, and dyskinesia, can cause reduced food intake in animals but have no relevance to appetite and satiation as clinical problems.

One method of evaluating the relevance of animal models designed to imitate presumed mechanisms of human obesity is to compare the range of effective doses of several known anorexiants in human beings and in animals. If a model appears valid, it is then often used to assess clinical anorexiant potential. For example, Sigell (1964) found a remarkable correlation between the human anorexiant potency of four agents and their efficacy in obese (gold thioglucose-induced) mice.

The pharmacological factors within an animal evaluative model include drug disposition (absorption, distribution, metabolism, excretion), the influence of a drug on a matrix of organ systems, the status of receptors (a complex, dynamically changing factor), and the nature and intensity of end organ responses. To expect similarity in these factors in species as dissimilar as man and mouse is asking too much. In view of the known differences in disposition of drugs in these species, a close quantitative correlation should be considered more a coincidence than a reflection of similarity.

In fact, merely changing the route of administration of a drug can alter both its metabolic patterns and its relative potency, even in the same species. With diethylpropion, for example, the metabolites generated after subcutaneous dosage are almost exclusively ketodesethyl derivatives, whereas considerable amounts of hydroxyl derivatives are generated after oral administration (table 3.3) (Wright et al. 1975). Phenylpropanolamine, which could constitute a hydroxylated des-diethyl derivative of diethylpropion, is not found in man following diethylpropion administration. The dosages studied (400 mg orally and 600 mg subcutaneously) were selected on the basis of their being equipotent; i.e., in studies of human volunteers under controlled conditions, oral diethylpropion was more potent (Jasinski, Nutt, and Griffith 1974). Jasinski, Nutt, and Griffith (Ibid.) also found the ratio of potency between amphetamine and diethylpropion to be clearly affected by the route of administration. This may be related to the previously discussed difference in metabolites produced after oral versus subcutaneous administration. The greater activity of oral diethylpropion in man suggests first-pass conversion to a more active metabolite, consistent with the "street" observation that intravenous diethylpropion is not popular (Cohen 1977).

TABLE 3.3

Plasma concentrations
after administration of diethylpropion

Substance		Plasma concentrations (ng/ml) hours after dose		
		0.5	2	6
Diethylpropion	PO	200	310	96
	SC	230	1,000	340
Alpha-keto metabolites	PO	300	520	504
	SC	1,270	800	610
Alpha-hydroxy metabolites	PO	0	570	950
	SC	0	220	530

Legend: PO: 400 mg orally; SC: 600 mg subcutaneously

Source: Wright, G. J. et al. 1975. DEP and its metabolites in the blood plasma of the human after subcutaneous and oral administration. Reprinted from Drug Metab Rev 4, page 267, by courtesy of Marcel Dekker, Inc.

Incomparability of Toxicities

An outstanding example of a significant pharmacologic effect seen with only some, and not other, sympathomimetic agents is the marked pulmonary hypertension produced in animals and man by aminorex, but not by most other anorexiants. This effect (figure 3.2) was carefully studied in animals (Brunner and Stepanek 1971; Stepanek and Zak 1975) only after clinical cases of cor pulmonale had been observed in aminorex-treated obese human subjects (Gurtner et al. 1968).

FIGURE 3.2

The effect of aminorex on pulmonary artery pressure

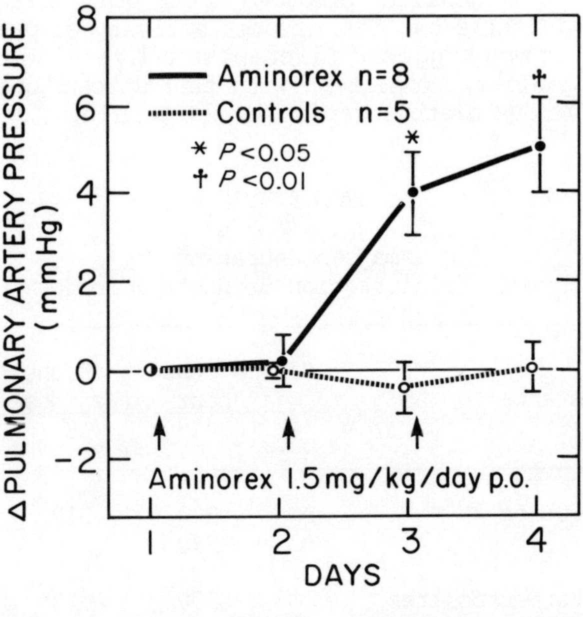

Source: Brunner, H. and J. Stepanek. 1971. Effects of aminorex on the pulmonary circulation of the dog. In The correlation of adverse effects in man with observations in animals: proceedings of the European Society for the Study of Drug Toxicity, vol. XII, edited by S. B. De C. Baker, 123-32. Amsterdam: Excerpta Medica. Reprinted with permission.

As for the more common cardiovascular effects of sympathomimetics, there is no doubt that phenylpropanolamine in sufficiently large doses is capable of both alpha- and beta-agonist action, with a potential of causing hypertension, tachycardia, and arrhythmias. Phenylpropanolamine is generally considered to be similar to ephedrine, although somewhat more active as a vasoconstrictor and less active as a CNS stimulant. It is also apparently less active than ephedrine in beta-mediated sympathetic responses.

The key question is with what degree and frequency undesired effects occur at clinically useful doses of phenylpropanolamine in man. Since information is available about undesired cardiovascular responses to decongestant and anorexiant doses of phenylpropanolamine (Health and Human Services 1982), animal studies of relative potencies are of little utility.

DRUG AND DISEASE INTERACTIONS

Another major question concerning any active and widely consumed agent, whether it be over-the-counter or prescription, is the effect of its use in the presence of disease or other drugs. Dose-response data generated under controlled conditions may not be wholly applicable. The complex chemistry of the body in health and disease, the variety of ingested foods, as well as other medications all contribute to the variation in response to any drug. Even when this scope of response is understood, the reactions of a particular subject rarely can be predicted or controlled. However, certain drug interactions can be detected and studied, and some of these can be avoided. Others are of little if any clinical significance and are best considered components of the differences between individuals.

Obviously, acceptable doses of other sympathomimetics added to phenylpropanolamine can become unacceptable by summation of effect (Rumack 1982). There is evidence that the administration of general anesthetics may sensitize the myocardium to the potential for phenylpropanolamine-induced cardiac arrhythmias. The hypotensive effect of guanethidine may be reduced by concurrent use of phenylpropanolamine. Phenothiazines may antagonize the anorexiant effect of phenylalkylamines, while monoamine oxidase (MAO) inhibitors may potentiate their sympathomimetic effects (U.S. Pharmacopeial Convention 1984). Practicing physicians can benefit from an awareness of these possibilities.

More subtle drug interactions may also occur, such as those alleged with indomethacin or other agents that influence the prostaglandin system. An altered response to norepinephrine-releasing action has been suggested. However, there is little evidence of serious consequences in the considerable clinical experience of the coadministration of aspirin with phenylpropanolamine, pseudoephedrine, or ephedrine.

With a new agent, animal studies are critically important in deciding what clinical approaches are appropriate. As data based on human use of the drug become available, the potential of animal pharmacologic studies to contribute to the solution of clinical questions correspondingly declines. Given the current status and history of phenylpropanolamine, it would be irrational to base decisions about current human toxicological issues on animal pharmacologic findings. The major contribution to be made by pharmacologists at this point is to illuminate the mechanisms underlying clinical findings. The interplay between pharmacologic, psychosomatic, and cultural components can be the critical determinant of an observed response to a drug. Both the pharmacologist and the practitioner need to bear this in mind when drawing clinical conclusions from pharmacologic observations.

REFERENCES

Aviado, D. M. 1970. Sympathomimetic drugs. Springfield, IL: Charles C. Thomas.

Brewer, G. W. 1984. Genetic approaches to producing different O_2 affinities in hemoglobin. Paper presented at symposium. O_2 transport by the red blood cell: 12th Katzir Katchalsky conference. Tours, France. April 12.

Brunner, H. and J. Stepanek. 1971. Changes in pulmonary artery pressure in dogs. Proceedings of the European Society for the Study of Drug Toxicity, Excerpta Medica International Congress Series, vol. XII, edited by S. B. De C. Baker, 123-32. Amsterdam: Excerpta Medica.

Cohen, S. 1977. DEP: an infrequently abused anorexic. Psychosomatics 18:28-33.

Goodman, L. S. and A. Gilman. 1980. The pharmacological basis of therapeutics, 6th ed. New York: MacMillan.

Gurtner, H. P. et al. 1968. Haufen sich die primar vascularen formen des chronischen cor pulmonale? Schweizerische Medizinische Wochenschrift 98:1579.

Health and Human Services, Food and Drug Administration (FDA). 1982. Establishment of a monograph for weight control drug products for over-the-counter human use. FDA docket no. 81N-0022. Federal Register 47:8466-84. February 26.

Hutter, A. M., Jr. and Kayhoe, D. E. 1966. Adrenocortical carcinoma: results of treatment with o,p'DOD in 138 patients. Am J Med 41:581-92.

Jasinski, D. R., J. G. Nutt, and J. D. Griffith. 1974. Effects of diethylpropion and d-amphetamine after subcutaneous and oral administration. Clin Pharmacol Ther 16:645-52.

Levine, R. 1973. Pharmacology. Boston: Little, Brown.

Mason, W. D. and E. N. Amick. 1981. High-Pressure Liquid Chromatographic analysis of phenylpropanolamine in human plasma following derivitization with o-phthalaldehyde. J Pharm Sci 70:707.

Rumack, B. H. 1982. PPA: a potentially hazardous drug. Ann Emerg Med 11:332.

Sigell, L. T. 1964. Experimentally induced obesity in mice as a model for the evaluation of anorexigenic agents. Ph.D. thesis, University of Oregon Medical School.

Stepanek, J. and T. Zak. 1975. Two year per oral study of aminorex in the dog. Z Kardiol 64:768-81.

Tedeschi, D. H. and R. E. Tedeschi. 1968. Importance of fundamental principles in drug evaluation. New York: Raven Press.

Thompson, T. and Johanson, C. E., eds. 1981. Behavioral pharmacology of human drug dependence. National Institute on Drug Abuse research monograph no. 37. Washington, D.C.: U.S. Government Printing Office.

Tsuchiya, T. and G. Levy. 1972. Relationship between effect of activated charcoal on drug absorption in man and its drug absorption characteristics in vitro. J Pharm Sci 61:586-89.

United States Pharmacopeial Convention. 1984. USP Dispensing Information, 4th ed., 183, 890. Rockville, MD: United States Pharmacopeial Convention.

Weiner, M. 1974. Open discussion. In _Obesity: causes, consequences, treatment_, edited by L. Lasagna, 98-100. New York: Medcom Press.

Wilkinson, G. R. and A. H. Beckett. 1968. Absorption, metabolism and excretion of the ephedrines in man. _J Pharmacol Exp Ther_ 162:139-47.

Wright, G. J. et al. 1975. DEP and its metabolites in the blood plasma of the human after subcutaneous and oral administration. _Drug Metab Rev_ 4:267.

4

PHENYLPROPANOLAMINE PREPARATIONS, MARKETING, AND ECONOMICS: U.S. AND ABROAD

Albert I. Wertheimer

INTRODUCTION

Phenylpropanolamine (PPA) is a medicinal chemical used in decongestants and anorexiants. This report will concentrate on the market for diet aids since the decongestant market is more complex, with numerous formulations of decongestants alone and in combination with antihistamines and analgesics available both over-the-counter (OTC) and by prescription. A brief examination of the medicinal market as a whole will help put the phenylpropanolamine market into perspective. According to Drug Topics (Glazer and Chi 1983), spending for prescription drugs in all categories of outlets was $16.2 billion in 1982 and was $3.3 billion for OTC drugs purchased in pharmacies. However, since OTC products are also sold in grocery, discount, department, and health and beauty aid stores, door-to-door, and by mail order, the total OTC market can be estimated at perhaps $7 billion or more.

THE PHENYLPROPANOLAMINE MARKET IN THE UNITED STATES

OTC Diet Aid Preparations

The OTC weight control market consists of a small number of products reported to work in different ways. Phenylpropanolamine, a sympathomimetic agent related to ephedrine and amphetamine, functions to reduce appetite. The market also includes bulk producers, such as methylcellulose, carboxymethylcellulose, psyllium hydrophilic mucilloid, agar, and karaya gum, that purportedly produce a sense of fullness, decreasing the desire to eat. Because of its numbing effect on taste, benzocaine has been combined with methylcellulose in some weight control products, usually chewable wafers. Other entries in this market are glucose and vitamin preparations designed to exert an inhibitory influence on the appetite center. Low-calorie, nutritionally balanced foods in cans or powders to be reconstituted with water are part of this market as well (American Pharmaceutical Association 1979).

The OTC diet aids business is big business. Simmons Market Research Bureau (1981) reported that 9.5 million adults used OTC weight loss products in 1981. Drug Topics (Glazer and Chi 1983) reported that in 1982 more than $381 million was spent for OTC diet aids in all outlets (table 4.1), about $175 million (46%) in drugstores.

TABLE 4.1

Spending for diet aids in all retail outlets in 1982

Weight reduction products	Total sales ($ million)
Reducing preparations	228.8
Metered calorie products	62.3
Synthetic sweeteners	61.3
Powder, liquid protein preparations	28.8

Source: Adapted from Glazer, M. and J. Chi. 1983. Drug Topics' 35th annual report on consumer spending. Drug Topics 127:2. Reprinted with permission of Drug Topics, Medical Economics Co. July 4, 1983.

There are nearly 30 entrants in the $229 million OTC market for reducing preparations. These firms spent almost $40 million in advertising in 1983 (Leading National Advertisers 1984). Persons familiar with this market estimate that approximately 30% of revenue from sales at the manufacturer's level is spent on advertising and promotion (Ross 1984).

The leader in this field is Thompson Medical Company, whose Dexatrim™ Reducing Capsule family has scored enormous success. The company estimates that its products account for approximately 69% of the retail sales of diet aid products in food and drug stores. Its advertising and consumer promotion expenses amounted to 29% of revenue from sales in 1983 (Thompson Medical Company 1984b). Jeffrey Martin's Ayds™ reducing candy, CIBA's Acutrim™ tablets, and Menley & James' Dietac™ capsules are the additional major products in the national market.

Until 1983, there had been a recent decline in sales of phenylpropanolamine appetite suppressant products. For example, Thompson Medical Company (1984a) reported annual retail sales as:

Year	Sales ($ Million)
1980	86.2
1981	75.1
1982	72.8
1983	94.7

Prescription Diet Aid Products

Prescription diet aids are also of economic importance. The leading products are Tenuate® by Merrill, Ionamin® by Penwalt, Fastin® by Beecham, Didrex® by Upjohn, and Tepanil® (Leading Antiobesity Preparations 1983). The Pharmaceutical Data Service (1984) has reported that, for the year ending December 1983, 6.2 million prescriptions were written for drugs in their category 18200, Anti-Obesity and Related Products. At an assumed retail price of $12 per prescription, this retail market can be estimated at about $74.4 million.

Regulation of the Market for Diet Aids

The prescription diet aids market had previously been dominated by a number of amphetamine products and derivatives. These drugs, including racemic amphetamine (Benzedrine®), dextroamphetamine (Dexedrine®), and methamphetamine (Desoxyn®, Obedrin®-LA), were the first to be widely prescribed for appetite suppression (Publishing Sciences Group 1977). However, what was considered wide-scale abuse and misuse of these products led the U.S. Food and Drug Administration (FDA) to establish manufacturing quotas for the production of amphetamine and to decrease the number of label indications. Some state laws have further restricted their use. One can only speculate as to how much of the previous, robust prescription anorexiant market has moved to the OTC sector. There is a great deal of speculation about the interchangeability of prescription and OTC anorexiant products, but few data exist.

Nor has the OTC market been free of recent federal involvement. In January 1972, the FDA announced the establishment of independent expert panels to review the ingredients used in nonprescription drug products and to recommend their classification according to safety and efficacy. Upon completion of a panel's review and recommendations regarding a particular substance, a report is published by the FDA in the Federal Register and public comments are invited. After this, the Commissioner of the FDA either accepts or rejects the recommendations in the report or takes a position based upon a modified form of the recommendations. The FDA then publishes its tentative final monograph. After a period during which public comments are again invited, the FDA publishes its final monograph setting forth the classification of the substance. Ingredients found to be safe and effective are placed in Category I and allowed to be used for their specified therapeutic purposes. Category II ingredients are those found to be either ineffective or unsafe and their use is prohibited. If available data are insufficient or in conflict, an ingredient is placed in Category III and allowed to be utilized in nonprescription drugs until publication of the final monograph. The Commissioner of the FDA has estimated that review of the panel's recommendations will continue for several more years.

In 1979, the Advisory Review Panel on Over-the-Counter Miscellaneous Internal Drug Products of the FDA concluded that phenylpropanolamine, benzocaine, and phenylpropanolamine in combination with caffeine should be placed in Category I as safe and effective ingredients in diet aids, within certain dosage limitations. The panel recommended that vitamins not be used in appetite suppressants. On February 26, 1982, the FDA published the report, together with an invitation for public comments.

Controversy Surrounding Phenylpropanolamine Diet Aid Products

Having been given this relatively clean bill of health or at least a green light from the FDA, the phenylpropanolamine industry might be expected to be joyous and optimistic, but that has not been the entire story for this controversial chemical. Certain individuals and groups have expressed disagreement with the FDA panel recommendation as published. For example, staff members from Ralph Nader's

Health Research Group (HRG) wrote in their 1983 book, Over the Counter Pills That Don't Work:

> Today, the most tempting items are those flat little boxes that dangle enticingly from drug store and supermarket shelves and promise "Fast Weight Loss" . . . . Despite the [FDA] panel's decision, it is our opinion that PPA poses a substantial hazard for its users, and has not succeeded in proving its effectiveness. (Kaufman et al., 1983, p. 81)

Because of this, HRG strongly recommends that weight loss aids that contain phenylpropanolamine not be used.

Another critic of phenylpropanolamine, Congresswoman Mary Rose Oakar (D-Ohio), introduced H.R. 4675 into the second session of the 98th Congress on January 26, 1984. This bill would require the FDA to remove from the OTC market all diet drugs containing phenylpropanolamine (U.S. Congress 1984).

Moreover, there has been much recent speculation that the FDA is considering Category III status for phenylpropanolamine. It is not known when the FDA's final monograph will be published or what form it will take, or how long it will be between publication, receipt and consideration of comments, and the FDA's final decision (Thompson Medical Company 1984b).

Phenylpropanolamine in Cough/Cold Preparations

Although many critics think that phenylpropanolamine in diet aid preparations has been implicated in some recent cases of morbidity, little is said about phenylpropanolamine in equal or even greater dosages used in cough and cold preparations. In 1982, 412,000 pounds of phenylpropanolamine were produced in the United States (Cozel et al. 1983). The vast majority of the product is employed as a decongestant in cough and cold remedies. Standard & Poors (1983) estimated that U.S. retail sales of cough and cold medications were $1.3 billion in 1982. Many of these products contain phenylpropanolamine (table 4.2). There have been relatively few recent criticisms or claims of toxicity attributed to the phenylpropanolamine contained in these products.

TABLE 4.2

Prescription and over-the-counter cough/cold products containing phenylpropanolamine available in 1984

Product	Form*	Unit dose* (mg)	Daily maximum adult dose† (mg)	Daily maximum child dose† (mg)
Prescription				
Anatuss syrup	L	12.5	—	—
Anatuss syrup with codeine	L	12.5	—	—
Anatuss tablets	T	25	—	—
Broncon® C.R. tablets	T	15	45	—
Codimal® expectorant	L	25	150	37.5-75
Conex	L	12.5	—	—
Conex with codeine	L	12.5	—	—
Dehist	C	75	—	—
Dimetapp® elixir	L	5	40	5-20
Dimetapp Extentabs®	T	15	45	—
Drize®	C	75	150	—
Dura-Tap/PD™ capsules	C	10	—	—
Dura-Vent™ capsules	C	75	—	—
Dura-Vent™/A capsules	C	75	—	—
E.N.T. syrup	L	5	—	—
E.N.T. tablets	T	50	—	—
E-Tapp elixir	L	5	—	—
Entex®	C	45	180	—
Entex® liquid	L	20	160	40-120
Entex® LA	T	75	150	—
Fiogesic® tablets	T	25	150	100
Histalet® Forte tablets	T	50	150	75
Hycomine® pediatric syrup	L	12.5	—	75
Hycomine® syrup	L	25	150	—

*The key for form of product is as follows:
- C: capsule (unit dose/capsule)
- L: liquid/syrup (unit dose/5 ml)
- T: tablet (unit dose/tablet)
- D: pediatric drops (unit dose/ml)

†A dash indicates either that dosage information was not provided in the source or that the product is not recommended for this age group.

TABLE 4.2 (continued)

Product	Form*	Unit dose* (mg)	Daily maximum adult dose† (mg)	Daily maximum child dose† (mg)
Kronohist Kronocaps	C	50	—	—
Naldecon® pediatric drops	D	5	—	5-20
Naldecon® pediatric syrup	L	5	—	10-40
Naldecon® syrup	L	20	80	40
Naldecon® tablet	T	40	120	60
Nolamine®	T	50	150	—
Norel Plus capsules	C	25	—	—
Ornade® Spansule® capsules	C	75	150	—
Phenate	T	40	—	—
Poly-Histine expectorant, plain	L	12.5	—	—
Poly-Histine expectorant with codeine	L	12.5	—	—
Poly-Histine-D capsules	C	50	—	—
Poly-Histine-D elixir	L	12.5	—	—
Propagest™	T	25	150	75
Propagest™ syrup	L	12.5	150	37.5-75
Protid	T	20	—	—
Rhindecon™	C	75	—	—
Rhindecon-G™	C	50	—	—
Rhinolar™	C	75	—	—
Rhinolar-Ex™	C	75	—	—
Rhinolar-Ex 12™	C	75	—	—
Ru-Tuss® with hydrocodone	L	3.33	40	13.3
Ru-Tuss® tablets	T	50	100	—
Ru-Tuss® II capsules	C	75	225	—
Rymed® capsules	C	45	—	—
Rymed® liquid	L	20	—	—
Rymed®-Jr. capsules	C	22.5	—	—
Rymed®-TR capsules	C	75	—	—
S-T Forte™ syrup and sugar-free syrup	L	5	20	10
Sinubid®	T	100	200	100
Sinulin®	T	37.5	150	—
Symptrol™	C	50	—	—
T-Dry capsules	C	50	100	—
T-Dry Jr. capsules	C	25	100	50
Tavist-D®	T	75	150	—

TABLE 4.2 (continued)

Product	Form*	Unit dose* (mg)	Daily maximum adult dose† (mg)	Daily maximum child dose† (mg)
Triaminic® expectorant with codeine	L	12.5	150	37.5-75
Triaminic® oral infant drops	D	20	—	§
Triaminic® timed-release tablets	T	50	150	—
Triaminic-DM® cough formula	L	12.5	150	37.5-75
Triaminic Juvelets®	T	25	150	75
Tuss-Ornade® liquid	L	12.5	150	37.5-75
Tuss-Ornade® Spansule® capsules	C	75	150	—
<u>Over-the-counter</u>				
A.R.M.® allergy relief medicine	T	37.5	150	—
Advanced Formula Dristan® capsules	C	12.5	150	75
Alka-Seltzer Plus®‡	T	24	192	96
Allerest® children's chewable tablets	T	9.4	—	75.2
Allerest® headache strength	T	18.7	149.6	74.8
Allerest® sinus pain formula	T	18.7	149.6	—
Allerest® tablets	T	18.7	149.6	74.8
Allerest® timed release	C	50	150	—
Bayer® children's cold tablets	T	3.125	—	12.5-50
Bayer® cough syrup for children	L	9	—	36-72
Cheracol Plus®	L	8.33	150	—
Children's CoTylenol®	L	6.25	—	31.25-62.5
Children's CoTylenol®	T	3.125	—	31.25-62.5

§4 drops/2 lb weight.
‡Phenylpropanolamine as bitartrate.

TABLE 4.2 (continued)

Product	Form*	Unit dose* (mg)	Daily maximum adult dose† (mg)	Daily maximum child dose† (mg)
Comtrex® multi-symptom cold reliever	C	12.5	150	75
Comtrex® multi-symptom cold reliever	L	4.2	150	75
Comtrex® multi-symptom cold reliever	T	12.5	150	75
Congesprin® liquid cold medicine	L	6.25	—	25-50
Contac® continuous action decongestant capsules	C	75	150	—
Contac Jr.®	L	9.375	—	56.25
Coricidin® cough syrup	L	12.5	150	37.5-75
Coricidin® extra strength sinus headache tablets	T	12.5	100	—
Coricidin 'D'® decongestant tablets	T	12.5	150	62.5
Coricidin® Demilets®	T	6.25	—	75
Coricidin® Medilets®	T	6.25	—	75
Coryban®-D capsules	C	25	—	—
Cremacoat™ 3	L	12.5	150	37.5-75
Cremacoat™ 4	L	12.5	150	75
Daycare® capsules	C	12.5	100	50
Daycare® liquid	L	4.17	100	50
Dorcol® pediatric cough syrup	L	6.25	—	37.5-75
Formula 44D®	L	12.5	150	37.5-75
4-Way® cold tablets	T	12.5	150	75
Halls® Mentho-Lyptus® decongestant cough formula	L	18.75	150	75
Head & Chest™	C	25	150	—
Head & Chest™	L	12.5	150	37.5-75
Head & Chest™	T	25	150	75
Headway® capsules	C	18.75	150	75
Headway® tablets	T	18.75	150	75
Naldecon-CX® suspension	L	18	144	36-72
Naldecon-DX®	L	9	—	36-72
Naldecon-EX®	D	9	—	9-36

TABLE 4.2 (continued)

Product	Form*	Unit dose* (mg)	Daily maximum adult dose† (mg)	Daily maximum child dose† (mg)
Ornacol®	C	25	100	—
Ornex®	C	18	144	72
Pertussin® Complex D® cough and cold formula	L	12.5	150	75
Pyrroxate® capsules	C	25	150	—
Robitussin-CF®	L	12.5	150	37.5–75
St. Joseph® cold tablets for children	T	3.125	100	18.75–75
Sinarest® extra strength tablets	T	18.7	149.6	—
Sinarest® tablets	T	18.7	149.6	74.8
Sine-Off®	T	18.75	150	75
Sine-Off® extra strength	C	18.75	150	—
Sine-Off® extra strength	T	18.75	150	—
Sine-Off® extra strength, no drowsiness formula	C	18.75	150	—
Triaminic® chewables	T	6.25	—	50
Triaminic® cold syrup	L	12.5	150	75
Triaminic® cold tablets	T	12.5	150	75
Triaminic® cough formula	L	12.5	150	37.5–75
Triaminic® expectorant	L	12.5	150	37.5–75
Triaminic-12® tablets	T	75	150	—
Triaminicin® tablets	T	25	100	—
Triaminicol® multi-symptom cold syrup	L	12.5	150	75
Triaminicol® multi-symptom cold tablets	T	12.5	150	75
Trind® liquid	L	12.5	100	6.25–50
Trind-DM® liquid	L	12.5	100	6.25–50
Tussagesic® suspension	L	12.5	150	37.5–75
Tussagesic® tablets	T	25	75	—
Ursinus® Inlay-Tabs®	T	25	100	—

Source: Compiled by the author. Data on prescription drugs derived from Physicians' desk reference. 1984. 38th ed. Oradell, NJ: Medical Economics. Data on OTC products derived from Self-medication: a guide to over-the-counter health care products. 1984. Oradell, NJ: Medical Economics.

SYNTHETIC DRUGS OUTSIDE THE UNITED STATES

Synthetic drugs are also being increasingly marketed throughout the world, including being exported to developing countries, whose national control measures are considered by many to be inadequate. As many as 20,000 pharmaceutical preparations are registered in some developing countries, with about 1,000 containing psychotropic ingredients. Many are sold over-the-counter, without a prescription.

World Health Organization Recommendations

The World Health Organization (WHO) evaluates the safety and efficacy of many psychotropic and narcotic drugs and also recommends controls when a threat to public health has been demonstrated (World Health Organization 1983). It derives its mandate from two conventions: (1) the 1961 Single Convention on Narcotic Drugs (with its 1972 modifying protocol), which covers hard drugs, such as cocaine, morphine, and opium; and (2) the 1971 Convention on Psychotropic Substances, which covers psychotropic drugs, both synthetic and those obtained from natural sources. WHO evaluations are considered particularly important for developing countries, since many of them import psychotropic drugs but lack the trained personnel with the expertise to make the determinations themselves (O'Connell 1981).

Six anorexiant drugs have been placed under international control following recommendations by the WHO: benzphetamine, mazindol, phendimetrazine, phentermine, amfepramone, and phenmetrazine. According to a WHO expert group, there is evidence that these six products are abused, are dependence-producing, and consequently "constitute a public health and social problem" (Ibid.). The effects of their use have been shown to be similar to substances already controlled, particularly (±)-amphetamine. The WHO recommendations were endorsed by the 30-member United Nations Commission on Narcotic Drugs at its 30th session in Vienna in February 1983.

The Commission on Narcotic Drugs also concluded that three other weight-reducing products--clortermine, chlorphentermine, and fenfluramine--should not be subject to international control, although their use will continue to be monitored. There is insufficient evidence that these drugs have "amphetamine-like abuse liability" or that significant public health and social problems arise from their use.

TABLE 4.3

International differences in phenylpropanolamine product availability

Country	Availability OTC	Availability Rx	Treatment Decongestant	Treatment Anorexiant	Dosage limits (mg)	Comments
North America						
Canada	N	Y	Y	N	N	Combination products.
United States	Y	Y	Y	Y	N	Alone/combination products. Anorexiants available only OTC.
Western Europe						
Austria	N	Y	Y	N	N	For rhinitis only.
Denmark	N	N	N	N	NA	
Finland	N	Y	Y	N	N	
France	Y	N	Y	N	N	Combination products.
Greece	Y	Y	Y	N	N	
Italy	Y	Y	Y	N	N	
Malta	N	Y	Y	N	N	
Netherlands	N	Y	Y	N	N	10 ml packages of nose drops only.
Norway	N	Y	Y	N	N	Alone/combination products.
Spain	Y	Y	Y	N	N	OTC diet products include protein, carbohydrates, vitamins, minerals, fiber
Sweden	N	Y	Y	N	N	
Switzerland	N	Y	Y	N	N	Combination only.
United Kingdom	Y	Y	Y	N	50/dose; 150/day	

Legend: Y: yes; N: no; NA: information not available.

TABLE 4.3 (continued)

Country	Availability OTC	Availability Rx	Treatment Decon-gestant	Treatment Anor-exiant	Dosage limits (mg)	Comments
West Germany*	Y	N	Y	Y	N	Advertising not directed to general public. Warnings appear on packages.
<u>Eastern Europe</u>						
Hungary	N	Y	Y	N	N	
U.S.S.R.	N	N	N	N	NA	
<u>Asia and Pacific</u>						
Australia	N	Y	Y	N	N	
Japan	Y	Y	Y	N	90/day	Combination products.
New Zealand	N	Y	Y	N	N	
Singapore	Y	Y	Y	N	N	
South Korea	Y	Y	Y	Y	N	No extraordinary labeling or cautions.
Taiwan	Y	Y	Y	Y	N	Alone in prescription products; combination in OTC products.
Thailand	Y	Y	Y	Y	N	Higher security category. Available only in pharmacies. Alone/combination products.
<u>Middle East and Africa</u>						
Djibouti	Y	Y	Y	N	NA	Combination products.
Israel	N	Y	Y	N	N	Combination products.
South Africa	N	Y	Y	N	N	
United Arab Emirates	Y	Y	Y	N	N	Cannot be advertised for diet purposes.

*Here the correspondent probably includes norpseudoephedrine under the category phenylpropanolamine.

<u>Source</u>: Compiled by the author.

Worldwide Availability of Phenylpropanolamine

I recently sent a brief questionnaire to colleagues in 30 countries asking if phenylpropanolamine was sold there and, if so, whether as an OTC or prescription product. Questions were also asked about advertising restrictions, the availability of other OTC sympathomimetic drugs, and the existence of any special cautions, restrictions, or size or strength limitations. Replies received from 27 nations and additional data on two other countries revealed a wide variation in international practices governing the accessibility of phenylpropanolamine (table 4.3).

Although it appears that phenylpropanolamine is contained in numerous cough and cold preparations in many countries, it is less widely available in anorexiant products since the diet aid market exists in only a limited number of nations. Overweight and obesity are conditions rarely encountered in much of Southeast Asia, Africa, and parts of Central and South America. Therefore, the lack of diet aid products in many countries may indicate an insufficient market as much as, if not more than, limitation by regulatory actions.

CONCLUSIONS

The increasing use of phenylpropanolamine throughout the world has generated a broad spectrum of opinion regarding its safety. Criticism has most frequently been directed against the use of phenylpropanolamine in diet aid products, even though it is also widely available in cough/cold preparations. How then can we reconcile the conflicting opinions of the supporters and critics of phenylpropanolamine? After reviewing the material discussed here and other reports and publications, I find credible, logical, and convincing arguments on both sides of the issue. Phenylpropanolamine is clearly effective as indicated and, taken as recommended, it does not appear to be more dangerous than many other drugs available over-the-counter. The major problem arises when a patient voluntarily exceeds the recommended dosage to gain a greater degree of appetite suppression or weight loss. If this destructive behavior can be prevented by improved package labeling and instructions, then no additional or special precautions will be required. However, if an extraordinary number of toxicities relating to the anorexiant use of phenylpropanolamine are seen, then it is suggested that phenylpropanolamine be the first candidate for a new category of drugs, called third-class drugs, already used in much of the world. This class of drugs would not require a doctor's prescription, but would only be available through a pharmacy in which a qualified pharmacist personally oversaw the transaction, was convinced on the basis of professional judgment that the patron had a legitimate need for the product, and was satisfied that the purchaser understood the use of the product.

REFERENCES

American Pharmaceutical Association. 1979. Handbook of nonprescription drugs, 6th ed., 222-24. Washington, D.C.: American Pharmaceutical Association.

Cozel, M. et al. 1983. United States International Trade Commission, organic chemicals: U.S. production and sales data, 1982. No. 1422:103. Washington, D.C.: United States International Trade Commission Publication.

Glazer, M. and J. Chi. 1983. Drug Topics' 35th annual report on consumer spending. Drug Topics 127:2.

Kaufman, J. et al. 1983. Over the counter pills that don't work, 81. Washington, D.C.: Public Citizen Health Research Group.

Leading Antiobesity Preparations. 1983. Drug Topics 127:9.

Leading National Advertisers. 1984. D217 Reducing aids, 204. New York: Leading National Advertisers.

O'Connell, K. 1981. UN controls on anorectic drugs. Australian Journal of Pharmacy 62:348.

Pharmaceutical Data Service. 1984. Therapeutic category product detail report. Phoenix: Pharmaceutical Data Service. January.

Physicians' desk reference. 1984. 38th ed. Oradell, NJ: Medical Economics.

Publishing Sciences Group. 1977. AMA drug evaluations, 3rd ed., 487. Littleton, MA: Publishing Sciences Group.

Ross, I. 1984. Telephone conversation with author. June 6.

Self-medication: a guide to over-the-counter health care products. 1984. Oradell, NJ: Medical Economics.

Simmons Market Research Bureau. 1981. Study of media and markets--health care products and remedies, 25. New York: Simmons Market Research.

Standard & Poors. 1983. Industry survey--health care, H21. New York: Standard & Poors.

Thompson Medical Company. 1982. Annual report. New York: Thompson Medical Company.

———. 1984a. Annual report. New York: Thompson Medical Company.

———. 1984b. Form 10-K, submitted to the United States Securities and Exchange Commission. February 21.

United States Congress, House. 1984. To require that diet drugs containing phenylpropanolamine be dispensed only upon prescription. HR 4675, Jan. 26. Hon. Mary Rose Oakar (D-Ohio).

World Health Organization. 1983. The use of essential drugs, 34. Technical report series no. 685. Geneva: World Health Organization.

5

PHENYLPROPANOLAMINE AS AN ANOREXIANT AGENT IN WEIGHT CONTROL: A REVIEW OF PUBLISHED AND UNPUBLISHED STUDIES

Michael Weintraub

INTRODUCTION

Scientists attempting to analyze the anorexiant efficacy of phenylpropanolamine (PPA) face many of the same difficulties as do those trying to assess its safety; that is, a variety of methodological problems make clinical studies of the effects of phenylpropanolamine hard to interpret. Nonetheless, in even the most seriously flawed of these clinical trials, we can find some material helpful for interpretation, evaluation, and action.

In this paper, I will first briefly outline a method that can be used to analyze clinical studies of the anorexiant efficacy of phenylpropanolamine. I will then summarize the procedures and results of a number of these trials, first some studies of the effects of phenylpropanolamine alone, then others investigating phenylpropanolamine combined with caffeine. These trials have been further divided between published reports subjected to peer review and unpublished studies which various companies marketing phenylpropanolamine have made available to me. Published and unpublished reports provide a complementary set of advantages and disadvantages. Published reports are, of course, readily available and have been reviewed by both experts and journal editors. Too often, however, the reviewers have not been critical enough. The advantage of unpublished reports is that they are generally more detailed and frequently contain raw data. Unfortunately, they are often inaccessible to interested physicians, scientists, consumers, and consumer advocates.

After examining these studies, I will then critically discuss their methodologies and findings and suggest improvements in study design and execution. Finally, I will review and comment on the effectiveness of phenylpropanolamine as an agent in the field of anorexiant therapy.

EVALUATING PHENYLPROPANOLAMINE CLINICAL TRIALS

A Method

The approach used in this article to evaluate the literature on the anorexiant efficacy of phenylpropanolamine is based on a system initially devised by Lionel and Herxheimer (1970) and then developed further at the University of Rochester by William Wardell and myself with help from John P. Morgan and Louis Lasagna. A number of versions of this evaluative system have been published (Weintraub 1982a, 1979; Wardell and Weintraub 1981) and the basic system is presented annually in a postgraduate course on clinical pharmacology and drug development at the University of Rochester. The evaluation uses a checklist (Weintraub 1979) with sections focusing on:

1. general aspects of the clinical trial—aim, phase, type, design, and both major and subsidiary objectives;
2. participant population--type, recruitment, inclusion/exclusion criteria, comparability of treatment groups, generalizability on the basis of the population, and consent;
3. treatments--those compared, the rationale for the dose, dose form, route of administration, dose interval, ancillary therapy, duration of therapy, setting, and source of medication;
4. experimental design details--controls, treatment assignment, run-in/wash-out periods, and timing of assessments;
5. compliance--participant and investigator;
6. data collection--observers' collection methods and measurements used to assess efficacy and adverse effects;
7. bias control--blinding;
8. data analysis--treatment group comparability, missing data, dropouts, dropins, compliance, and statistical tests; and
9. overall assessment--fatal errors, conclusions, and risk/benefit analysis.

This checklist provides the context in which the following studies will be discussed.

Phenylpropanolamine Consumers and Their Goals

To view phenylpropanolamine studies from a realistic perspective, we should know who the consumers of over-the-counter (OTC) weight reduction products are, what their goals are, and what the duration of self-treatment is likely to be. In not fully considering these factors, previous critics of the efficacy literature on phenylpropanolamine have often attributed unrealistic and inappropriate therapeutic goals to those using phenylpropanolamine.

Data on file at the Food and Drug Administration (FDA) indicate that typical purchasers of OTC phenylpropanolamine weight reduction aids are mildly overweight, the majority being 4.5 kg or less above ideal weight as defined by the 1983 Metropolitan Life Insurance Company Tables. They are likely to be in excellent health. Nearly all are women less than 45 years old. The most common duration of therapy is slightly less than two weeks with an average use of approximately three weeks. Numerous studies have shown that the purchaser's therapy goal is relatively minor weight loss, usually prompted by a pending social event or following a vacation or other period of increased food intake.

Most OTC medications are used to decrease symptoms. The symptom in the case of users of diet aids seems to be the discomfort resulting from self-imposed caloric restriction. People who take phenylpropanolamine use it to suppress appetite, enabling them to decrease food intake more easily.

These data, derived from consumer surveys, are probably not completely accurate. Nonetheless, in more precisely characterizing the likely consumer population, these surveys more closely reflect users' goals of self-therapy than do the weight loss standards attributed to them by outside critics. In doing so, these data provide a more valuable perspective from which to evaluate the efficacy of phenylpropanolamine.

STUDIES OF THE EFFECTS OF PHENYLPROPANOLAMINE ALONE

A Published Study of Phenylpropanolamine as an Appetite Suppressant (Crossover Design)

Hoebel et al. (1975a)

The basis for the use of phenylpropanolamine in treating obesity is that it reduces appetite. A study by Hoebel et al. (1975a) confirms this effect. In this double-blind, crossover study, several groups of subjects, including both obese and nonobese people, were given 25 mg of phenylpropanolamine or a matching placebo 30 minutes before a test meal. Participants had not eaten for two hours prior to taking the treatment medication. A concealed cylinder containing a liquid food was used to measure consumption as an indication of appetite. The subjects could take as much as they wished of the liquid through a straw. In the first experiment, participants drank 390.5 ml of liquid after phenylpropanolamine versus 535 ml after placebo. This difference was statistically significant. In a second study, changes were made in the method of administering the liquid diet, and participants ingested 669 ml on phenylpropanolamine and 707 ml on placebo. This difference was also statistically significant. The investigators did not discuss the reasons the amount ingested was much greater in the second study. Participants also noted a subjective decrease in appetite with phenylpropanolamine compared with placebo.

A Published Study of Phenylpropanolamine without Caffeine as a Weight Reduction Aid (Crossover Design)

The rest of the studies that will be discussed in this paper examine not only the appetite suppressant properties of phenylpropanolamine but also its effectiveness in weight reduction. The following five studies are investigations of the effects of phenylpropanolamine alone; listed by author, they are summarized in table 5.1.

Hoebel et al. (1975b)

A double-blind crossover study by Hoebel et al. (1975b) included 70 subjects, 20 men and 50 women, between 18 and 64 years of age. For their participation, volunteers received a small payment and a month's supply of medication. Twenty-five were 0.5 to 6.8 kg overweight, 35 were 6.9 to 11.5 kg overweight, and the remainder were either well within the desirable weight range or even underweight. Initial weights ranged between 51 and 119 kg.

The study consisted of two consecutive two-week treatment periods. During the first period, participants were randomly divided into two groups, one of which took 25 mg of phenylpropanolamine and the other a placebo 30 minutes before each meal; in the second period, the two groups switched treatments. No caloric restriction was prescribed or suggested. In the first two weeks of the study, participants in both groups lost weight (an average total of 0.91

TABLE 5.1

Clinical trials of phenylpropanolamine alone

Study (date)	Study design	Comparison agent	Daily mg dosage		Study length in weeks	Number of subjects (dropouts)		Weight loss (gain) in kg/week	
			single	total		PPA	placebo	PPA	placebo
Hoebel et al. (1975b)	Crossover	Placebo	25	75	2 2	70 total completed		0.46 0.32	0.28 (0.05)
Sebok (1977b)	Parallel	Placebo	50	100	6	36(6)	36(12)	0.47	0.27
Noble and Kalkhof (1981)	Parallel	Placebo	75	75	6	120(1)	123(8)	0.73	0.45
Noble and Respess (1981)	Crossover*	Placebo	50	50	6/-*	173(68)	88(36)	0.67	0.47
Settel (1965)	Crossover	Placebo	25	75	3/3	42(12) total		0.67	0.32

*First six weeks only of study analyzed (as parallel group study).
Source: Compiled by the author.

kg on phenylpropanolamine, 0.56 kg on placebo). In the second two-week period, participants who had initially been on phenylpropanolamine and then switched to placebo gained very slightly, while those on phenylpropanolamine formerly on placebo lost, on average, an additional 0.64 kg.* Participants on phenylpropanolamine reported less hunger and decreased food intake, particularly with the evening meal, than did those on placebo. Their afternoon and evening snacks also decreased. Apparently none of the participants left the study.

This study illustrates some of the problems in using crossover designs for weight control studies. For example, neither group returned to baseline status before beginning the second phase of the study, thus rendering the groups no longer comparable. Also causing difficulty in interpretation was the heterogeneity of subjects; some were actually underweight and inappropriate for inclusion in a weight loss study. Although a diet was neither suggested nor prescribed, it is obvious that decreased intake occurred in both treatment groups, particularly in the first two weeks. To diminish variation in caloric restriction, an individualized diet would have been valuable.

Overall, however, the results of this study indicate that phenylpropanolamine was more effective than placebo in helping participants lose weight.

Unpublished Studies of Phenylpropanolamine without Caffeine as a Diet Aid (Parallel Group Design)

Sebok (1977b)

Sebok (1977b) conducted a clinical evaluation of the anorexiant activity of Vita-Slim compared to placebo in the treatment of outpatients with exogenous obesity who were placed on restricted diets. Seventy-two subjects between 19 and 65 years of age and at least 7% over ideal weight took part in this six-week, parallel group, double-blind study with randomized treatment assignment. Participants received a 1,250 calorie-restricted diet and took 50 mg of phenylpropanolamine with kelp and vitamins or matching placebo at 10 a.m. and again at 4 p.m. Although participants on phenylpropanolamine lost an average of 2.8 kg compared to 1.6 kg

---

*Note that in table 2 of the published Hoebel et al. (1975b) paper there is an error in the percentage weight change calculations.

for those on placebo, this difference was not statistically significant, nor was a difference found in the subjective measures of appetite suppression. Eighteen participants (25%) left the study, six from the phenylpropanolamine treatment group and 12 from the placebo group. One participant on phenylpropanolamine cited a lack of efficacy and another noted an adverse effect as reasons for leaving the study.

Noble and Kalkhof (1981)

Following the same parallel group design, Noble and Kalkhof (1981) undertook a six-week, double-blind comparison of Dietac™ capsules containing 75 mg of phenylpropanolamine in a sustained-release form and a matching placebo. Complete details of the protocol, the ancillary therapy administered, and the patient population characteristics were not available for review. We can still evaluate the data, hoping that the large study groups of 120 on phenylpropanolamine and 123 on placebo (with minimal dropouts) will minimize the possible bias introduced.

At the end of the study, the participants receiving phenylpropanolamine had lost, on average, a total of 4.4 kg versus 2.7 kg by those receiving placebo, a statistically significant difference. Importantly, the order of magnitude of weight loss by the phenylpropanolamine group approximates that desired by a typical phenylpropanolamine user.

Unpublished Studies of Phenylpropanolamine without Caffeine (Crossover Design)

Noble and Respess (1981)

Noble and Respess (1981) performed a crossover study designed to last 12 weeks. This study compared Dietac™ (50 mg of phenylpropanolamine) and placebo in a double-blind design. The investigators prescribed a sustained-release phenylpropanolamine preparation or matching placebo to be taken once daily. Initially, 173 patients were enrolled on active medication and 88 on placebo; the intended crossover was to have consisted of three treatment groups. However, the study broke down after six weeks and the crossover was not carried out.

There were important differences not only in the number but also in the types of patients entered by the two investigators. Nonetheless, if we accept the premise that the patient populations were generally comparable, a broad assessment is possible. The 105 participants who received phenylpropanolamine (68 of the original 173 having dropped out) lost, on average, 4.0 kg in six weeks and the 52 on placebo (not including the 36 dropouts) lost 2.8 kg.

Settel (1965)

Settel (1965) studied 30 people in a double-blind, crossover study of phenylpropanolamine versus placebo in randomized treatments. According to the limited data available, participants lost 0.67 kg/week on phenylpropanolamine and 0.32 kg/week on placebo.

STUDIES OF THE EFFECTS OF PHENYLPROPANOLAMINE PLUS CAFFEINE

The remaining studies described in this article analyze the effects of phenylpropanolamine plus caffeine and can be located according to author in table 5.2.

Published Studies of Phenylpropanolamine plus Caffeine Versus Placebo (Parallel Group Design)

Griboff, Berman, and Silverman (1975)

In a four-week, parallel group study, Griboff, Berman, and Silverman (1975) compared a phenylpropanolamine/caffeine/vitamin combination to a placebo. The 77 participants in this study were between 11% and 57% over ideal body weight. Participants took a preparation containing phenylpropanolamine (25 mg) plus caffeine (100 mg) and multivitamins, or matching placebo, with an eight-ounce glass of water three times per day 30 minutes prior to each meal. The median total weight loss for the 24 females on placebo was 0.91 kg compared to 1.82 kg for the 25 females on phenylpropanolamine plus caffeine and vitamins; these weight loss results for females were significantly different at the $p < .05$ level by the one-sided Wilcoxon rank sum test (Wilcoxon and Wilcox 1964). The median total weight loss for the nine males on placebo was 2.05 kg and 3.64 kg for the eight males on phenylpropanolamine; this difference was not statistically significant. The investigators did not analyze data from dropouts, although they were included in a separate table.

It is difficult to assess the overall value of the phenylpropanolamine/caffeine/vitamin combination in this study since we are only given the median and range of the weight loss. Nevertheless, the trend for greater weight loss on active medication than on placebo by participants completing the study is impressive.

A secondary goal of the study was to assess the relationship between the test medication and subjects' perception of anorexiant effect. Nearly half the participants on the phenylpropanolamine preparation (47%) versus only 26% of those on placebo noted a decrease in appetite.

Altschuler et al. (1982): Sebok

In the first of three studies discussed by Altschuler et al. (1982), Sebok compared the anorexiant activity of 35 mg of phenylpropanolamine plus 140 mg of caffeine versus placebo given twice daily. Participants in this six-week, parallel group study ranged from 8.8% to 32% over ideal body weight.* Of the 72 people who entered the study, 56 completed it. Subjects took their test medication at 10 a.m. and 4 p.m.; no additional dietary advice was given. Mean total weight loss on phenylpropanolamine plus caffeine was 2.1 $\pm$ 0.32 kg (mean $\pm$ standard error of the mean) versus 0.94 $\pm$ 0.31 kg on placebo, a statistically significant difference. No participants who left the first of the three studies discussed in this paper complained of a lack of efficacy.

Weight loss on phenylpropanolamine plus caffeine in this study was less at six weeks than in the other two trials Altschuler et al. (1982) described, both of which will be discussed immediately below. This is surprising since the total daily dose of phenylpropanolamine in the trial was greater than that in the mazindol-controlled study and only 5 mg less than in the diethylpropion-controlled study. There are many possible reasons for the differences in weight loss, including (1) the lack of a specific caloric restriction diet in two of the studies (Sebok; Altschuler); (2) the presence of a placebo in the Sebok trial, which might bias against modest clinical effects; and (3) differences in the patient populations in each study. Of the three groups evaluated, for example, participants in the Sebok study had the least to lose to reach ideal body weight.

---

*There were errors in the published report, which indicated that the dose of phenylpropanolamine was 37.5 mg and that participants were at least 12% over ideal body weight.

TABLE 5.2

Clinical trials of phenylpropanolamine plus caffeine

Study (date)	Study design	Comparison agent (single/total mg dosage)	Daily PPA/caffeine mg dosage		Study length in weeks	Number of subjects (dropouts)		Weight loss (gain) in kg/week	
			single	total		PPA/ caffeine	comparison agent	PPA/ caffeine	comparison agent
Griboff, Berman, and Silverman (1975)	Parallel	Placebo	25/ 100*	75/ 300*	4	28(3)† 9(1)§	30(6)† 10(1)§	0.46† 0.91§	0.23† 0.51§
Altschuler et al. (1982)									
Sebok	Parallel	Placebo	35/ 140	70/ 280	6	36(8)	36(8)	0.35	0.16
Altschuler	Parallel	Mazindol (2/2)	50/ 200	50/ 200	6	34(7)	33(5)	0.61	0.68
Conte	Parallel	Diethylpropion (25/75)	25/ 100	75/ 300	8	31(6)	31(8)	0.39	0.45
Conte (1977)	Parallel	PPA alone (50/100)	50/ 200	50/ 200	8	32(7)	30(12)	0.77	0.62
Sebok (1977a)	Parallel	Placebo	35/ 140	70/ 280	6	35(9)	35(12)	0.48	0.32
Jolly (1972)	Parallel	Placebo	‡	‡	12	32(11)	31(18)	0.57	0.30

Conte (1978)	Parallel	Placebo	25/ ?	75/ ?	6	31(11)	31(8)	0.49	0.30
Altschuler (1980)	Parallel	Placebo	25/ ?	75/ ?	6	42(10)	23(5)	0.43	0.28
Noble (1977)	Parallel	Diethylpropion (75/75)	75/ 200	75/ 200	8	30(6)	30(9)	0.45**	0.51**
Noble and Pertschuck (1981)	Crossover††	Placebo	50/ 200	50/ 200	6/-††	175(74)	87(49)	0.43	0.27
Bohensky (1973)	Crossover	Dextro-amphetamine (15/15) Placebo	25/ 100	75/ 300	4/4	60 total completed		0.90	1.05§§ 0.28‡‡
Bradley (1982)	Crossover	PPA alone (75/75) Placebo	25/ 100	75/ 300	2/2	12(2)		0.64	0.86*** 0.29‡‡

*Compound included PPA/caffeine/vitamin.
†Data for women subjects only.
§Data for men subjects only.
‡Exact dosage not available.
**Medians.
††First six weeks only of study analyzed (as parallel group study).
§§Dextroamphetamine.
‡‡Placebo.
***PPA alone.
Source: Compiled by the author.

Published Studies of Phenylpropanolamine plus Caffeine Versus Prescription Anorexiants (Parallel Group Design)

Altschuler et al. (1982): Altschuler

In the comparative study by Altschuler of phenylpropanolamine plus caffeine versus mazindol (Sanorex®) discussed in the Altschuler et al. (1982) publication, 67 people entered the six-week, double-blind, parallel group clinical trial. Twelve (18%) dropped out, one from lack of efficacy in each group. The total daily dose was 50 mg of phenylpropanolamine plus 200 mg of caffeine or 2 mg of mazindol given once per day at 10 a.m. The treatment groups were roughly comparable, although participants' weights varied between 53.6 and 111.5 kg. These data come from the investigator's report to the sponsor. There are inconsistencies, however, between the published paper and the actual data reported to the sponsor relating to the percentage over ideal body weight.

Only the 55 participants who completed the study were evaluated. These participants lost, on average, a total of 3.68 $\pm$ 0.46 kg on phenylpropanolamine plus caffeine and 4.08 $\pm$ 0.35 kg on mazindol. There was no statistically significant difference in weight loss between treatments. However, by the Wilcoxon rank order test (one tail) (Wilcoxon and Wilcox 1964), weight loss from baseline to week six within both treatment groups was statistically significant. Both phenylpropanolamine plus caffeine and mazindol helped people lose weight. Two patients on phenylpropanolamine plus caffeine achieved a greater than 10% weight loss in the six weeks of the study; none did so on mazindol.

Altschuler also collected data on appetite suppression which were not published but were included in the investigator's report to the sponsor. As late as week six, nearly three-quarters of the participants receiving either medication reported moderate or complete suppression of appetite.

Altschuler et al. (1982): Conte

The third study discussed in the Altschuler et al. (1982) publication was a comparison by Conte of the anorexiant activity of Anorexin™ and diethylpropion in obese outpatients. In this eight-week, parallel group trial, 25 mg of phenylpropanolamine plus 100 mg of caffeine and vitamins were compared with 25 mg of diethylpropion (Tenuate®). Participants took the study medications three times per day with an eight-ounce glass of water, 30 minutes prior to breakfast, lunch, and dinner (for a total dose of 75 mg of phenylpropanolamine and 300 mg of caffeine or 75 mg of diethylpropion per day). Subjects were also provided with a 1,250 calorie diet. Initial weights ranged from 15% to 30% over ideal body weight.

Although 62 patients initially entered the study, only 48 were evaluated for anorexiant efficacy. The mean total weight loss on phenylpropanolamine plus caffeine was 3.10 $\pm$ 0.38 kg versus 3.61 $\pm$ 0.65 kg for the diethylpropion group, not a statistically significant difference. However, there was a significant difference from baseline to the eight-week point for both the phenylpropanolamine plus caffeine and the diethylpropion groups. Several participants lost 10% or more of their initial body weight. Of the subjects who were evaluated, only three on diethylpropion and one receiving phenylpropanolamine plus caffeine failed to lose weight.

In this eight-week study, 22.6% of the participants dropped out. (The total dropout rate was somewhat higher than in the phenylpropanolamine plus caffeine versus mazindol trial, in which 17.9% of the participants had left by the end of the study, which was shorter by two weeks.) Several of the participants had failed to lose weight at the time they withdrew from the phenylpropanolamine versus diethylpropion study; however, there was a net mean weight loss by dropouts from both treatment groups. These latter data were not included in the published results (Altschuler et al. 1982), but are found in the report of the investigator to the manufacturer.

An Unpublished Study of Phenylpropanolamine plus Caffeine Versus Phenylpropanolamine Alone (Parallel Group Design)

Conte (1977)

In an eight-week, parallel group study, Conte (1977) compared phenylpropanolamine alone (50 mg) versus phenylpropanolamine (50 mg) plus caffeine (200 mg), taken once daily. Participants were also placed on a 1,250 calorie diet. Sixty-two subjects entered the study, but only 43 completed the full eight weeks of treatment, for a dropout rate of 30.6%. Four patients noted lack of efficacy as the reason for leaving the study, while two others refused to follow the diet program.

The treatment groups differed in several important ways. There were five males in the phenylpropanolamine plus caffeine group versus one in the phenylpropanolamine alone group. The phenylpropanolamine plus caffeine subjects were an average of nearly seven years younger. Participants receiving phenylpropanolamine plus caffeine were, on average, more than 9 kg heavier and had a mean percentage over ideal body weight 5.3% greater than the phenylpropanolamine alone group. At week eight, participants on phenylpropanolamine alone had lost an average total of 4.95 kg and those on phenylpropanolamine plus caffeine 6.14 kg. Only 34.8% of the phenylpropanolamine alone group versus 60% of the phenylpropanolamine plus caffeine group noted complete to moderate appetite suppression. However, none of the differences in efficacy measures were statistically significant. Since being male and being significantly over ideal body weight are both predictors of initial successful outcome in weight control studies (Weintraub et al. 1981), the incomparability of the treatment groups may have seriously influenced the data, preventing demonstration of a difference, if one existed.

Unpublished Studies of Phenylpropanolamine plus Caffeine Versus Placebo (Parallel Group Design)

Sebok (1977a)

Sebok (1977a) carried out another study of phenylpropanolamine (35 mg) plus caffeine (140 mg) versus placebo, given twice daily. In this six-week, double-blind, parallel group study, participants were initially 10% to 40% over ideal body weight. All participants were advised to follow a 1,250 calorie diet. Forty-nine of the 70 subjects who entered the study completed the entire six weeks (a 30% dropout rate). Four people on phenylpropanolamine plus caffeine left the study because of adverse effects, while two on placebo did so. In addition, one placebo participant left due to lack of efficacy. The average total weight loss for the 26 remaining subjects on phenylpropanolamine plus caffeine was 2.9 kg versus 1.9 kg for the 23 on placebo. Dropouts on phenylpropanolamine plus caffeine also lost more weight than did dropouts on placebo. The difference in weight loss between the phenylpropanolamine plus caffeine and placebo groups was not statistically significant, and no significant decrease in appetite was demonstrated.

Jolly (1972)

In a 12-week, double-blind, parallel group study, Jolly (1972) studied phenylpropanolamine plus caffeine versus placebo. Sixty-three patients entered the study; 34 actually completed it. Eleven people dropped out from the phenylpropanolamine plus caffeine group and 18 from the placebo group. Dietary intervention was individualized so that participants were advised to eat 60% of the calories needed to maintain ideal body weight. The mean total weight loss on active medication was 6.8 kg versus 3.6 kg for the placebo participants. The FDA Advisory Committee reporting in the Federal Register on weight control drug products for OTC human use cited this study as one of the four judged "adequate to establish the effectiveness of the combination of phenylpropanolamine hydrochloride and caffeine for time periods ranging from 4-12 weeks" (U.S. Department of Health and Human Services 1982). Unfortunately, I was not able to obtain the full details of this study.

Conte (1978)

The methodology used by Conte (1978) to carry out another phenylpropanolamine plus caffeine study deserves comment. In this trial, participants were given phenylpropanolamine (25 mg) or matching placebo three times per day. The medication was dispensed in cubes to be added to coffee or tea. Thus, a combination of phenylpropanolamine or placebo and a varying dosage of caffeine was studied. In this study, too, there was a high dropout rate (19 of the initial 62 subjects, or 30.6%) over the six-week trial period. Many of the dropouts did not report back for the first clinic visit, perhaps indicating that they had been inappropriate choices for entry into the study. The median weight loss for each group was not statistically significant. Participants on phenylpropanolamine plus caffeine had a median total weight loss of 2.95 kg versus 1.80 kg in the placebo group. Dropouts from the phenylpropanolamine plus caffeine group lost approximately 1.4 kg and those on placebo approximately 0.7 kg before leaving the study.

The data indicated that weight loss in the placebo participants had stopped after four weeks, whereas the phenylpropanolamine participants continued to lose weight over the next two weeks. An initial response to placebo with early flattening of the weight loss curve is a common finding in weight control studies. High motivation and enthusiasm may help placebo participants lose weight over the first several weeks of the study. However, without the assistance of medication, people trying to lose weight usually cannot maintain this initial drive. Other factors may begin to retard weight loss as well. Commonly, differences between drug and placebo become apparent only after several weeks of a clinical trial.

Altschuler (1980)

Another unusual dosage form of phenylpropanolamine was studied by Altschuler (1980). Participants in his six-week clinical trial added four drops of phenylpropanolamine solution (25 mg per drop) or matching placebo to coffee or tea three times per day, 30 minutes prior to each meal. Participants were 18 to 70 years old and at least 3% over ideal weight. The study design restricted the randomization so that nearly twice as many subjects received phenylpropanolamine plus caffeine as received placebo. Thus, 42 participants received phenylpropanolamine plus caffeine (ten of whom, or 23.8%, dropped out) and 23 were on placebo (five of whom, or 21.7%, dropped out). The phenylpropanolamine plus caffeine group contained more males and weighed an average of 4.45 kg more than the placebo group. All participants were given a 1,250 calorie diet. The investigators analyzed data only from those who completed the study. On average, the phenylpropanolamine plus caffeine treatment group lost a total of 2.57 kg and the placebo group 1.68 kg ($p < .04$ by an unspecified statistical test).

The appetite suppressant effects of phenylpropanolamine plus caffeine were also measured in this study. At six weeks, 19% of those on phenylpropanolamine plus caffeine had moderate to complete appetite suppression versus none on placebo, results which support the anorexiant efficacy of phenylpropanolamine.

An Unpublished Study of Phenylpropanolamine plus Caffeine Versus Diethylpropion (Parallel Group Design)

Noble (1977)

In an unpublished study, Noble (1977) compared the anorexiant activity of phenylpropanolamine (75 mg) plus caffeine (200 mg) in a sustained-release preparation versus diethylpropion (75 mg). The medications were taken once each day at 10 a.m. with a full glass of water. All patients were given a 1,250 calorie diet plan to follow. This was an eight-week, parallel group, clinical trial that 60 patients entered. The protocol indicated they should be at least 15% over ideal body weight; however, the actual range was from 10% to 30%. The phenylpropanolamine plus caffeine participant group initially weighed 6.3 kg (8.2%) more than the diethylpropion treatment group. Forty-five participants completed the study and were analyzed. Fifteen (25%) dropped out, nine on diethylpropion and six on phenylpropanolamine plus caffeine. Dropouts included two participants in each treatment group who were not evaluated because they unilaterally decreased the medication dose during the course of the study. Only median total weight loss data for each group was made available. Over the eight weeks of the study, the median total weight loss in the phenylpropanolamine plus caffeine group was 3.6 kg and in the diethylpropion group 4.1 kg.

An Unpublished Study of Phenylpropanolamine plus Caffeine Versus Placebo (Crossover Design)

Noble and Pertschuck (1981)

In a double-blind, within-participant trial, Noble and Pertschuck (1981) compared sustained-release capsules containing 50 mg of phenylpropanolamine and 200 mg of caffeine to placebo, taken once daily. This study was designed as a three-group, crossover trial in which one-third of the patients were to receive placebo in the first six weeks and the phenylpropanolamine plus caffeine combination for the second six weeks. A second group was to receive the reverse and the third group was to take the phenylpropanolamine plus caffeine combination in both six-week periods. The investigators did not plan a wash-out period between treatments. The study broke down at the end of six weeks and only the first half of the crossover was analyzable. In addition, if patients missed more than two consecutive visits, they were excluded from the analysis.

Missing data presented an extremely important problem in this study. Only 101 of the original 175 patients on active medication and 38 of the 87 on placebo actually completed the six weeks without significant protocol violation. It is difficult to tell whether the groups were truly comparable at either the beginning or end of the study. For patients who continued through to the end of week six, there was a mean total weight loss of 2.6 kg on active medication versus 1.6 kg on placebo.

Unpublished Single-Blind Studies of Phenylpropanolamine plus Caffeine

Bohensky (1973)

Using as subjects 60 people from his private practice, Bohensky (1973) compared phenylpropanolamine plus caffeine,

(+)-amphetamine, and placebo in a four-week, single-blind, crossover clinical evaluation. Participants on phenylpropanolamine (25 mg) plus caffeine (100 mg) lost an average total of 3.6 kg, those on (+)-amphetamine lost 4.2 kg, and those on placebo lost 1.1 kg during the four weeks. These results support the weight reduction efficacy of phenylpropanolamine. However, the single-blind nature of this study diminishes its value.

Bradley (1982)

To test the safety and efficacy of phenylpropanolamine plus caffeine, phenylpropanolamine alone in a time-release formulation, and placebo, Bradley (1982) carried out a study in obese patients with controlled, stable hypertensive disease. The study was single-blind, the treatment sequence was the same for all patients, and the treatment schedules were different in each two-week sequence. These factors, working together, probably unblinded the study totally and may have provoked order effects as well. Two patients failed to complete the second and third portions of the study. Although both the basic premise and the study design are quite interesting, the data are difficult to analyze and the design is probably so flawed that the results are not interpretable.

CRITICISMS OF STUDY DESIGN AND METHODOLOGY

Although in the trials reviewed here phenylpropanolamine-treated participants experienced a consistently greater weight loss than did subjects treated with placebo, faulty design and execution of the clinical trials decreased the likelihood of demonstrating phenylpropanolamine's efficacy. Some of these problems are discussed below.

Inappropriate Weight Range

The participants in the studies ranged from those low in weight to those morbidly overweight. Given that people who purchase phenylpropanolamine are generally mildly overweight, the extremely heterogeneous study population in these reports does not reflect phenylpropanolamine consumers. People who are 50% to 70% overweight may require a different type of therapeutic intervention than mild caloric restriction and an OTC appetite suppressant.

Improper Choice of Diet

An improper dietary regimen--either the absence of dietary guidelines or an excessively rigid approach to caloric restriction--increased the difficulty in demonstrating a true effect of phenylpropanolamine in many of these trials. In most of the studies, a 1,250 calorie diet was prescribed. This was inappropriately low for many of the less overweight participants. For example, a calculation based on the data from one of the studies chosen at random demonstrates that intake on a 1,250 calorie diet would range from 16 to 26 calories/kg of ideal weight and from 11.5 to 21.3 calories/kg of actual weight. Depending on the participant's ideal weight, it is either extremely difficult to maintain an 11 or 12 calorie/kg diet or to lose weight on a 25 calorie/kg diet. Only in the Jolly study (1972) was an attempt made to adjust the diet to the participant's ideal body weight. Future studies of phenylpropanolamine should follow a similar procedure and individualize the caloric restriction plans as has been done in other weight control studies (Weintraub et al. 1984).

Inconsistent Handling of Dropout Data

Dropouts were also problematic in these studies. Not only was the dropout rate frequently high, but the data that were gathered from those leaving a study were often handled inappropriately. In some of the studies, a large percentage of the participants never returned for the first follow-up visit. This represents a defect in the participant selection process. A second reason for dropping out, particularly by those in a placebo group, was that the subjects became discouraged with their failure to lose weight. Participants may also have dropped out because of the often inappropriate nature of the diet regimen prescribed. In other cases, subjects may have left the study once they had achieved their own goal for weight loss.

Often data from the dropouts were collected but not included in the main analysis. There are a number of widely accepted statistical techniques for utilizing data from dropouts. The end point method, for example, analyzes the data to the point the patient withdraws. Individual graphs of weight loss versus time are plotted, the areas under the curves are calculated, and the means of each treatment group are compared. A second approach is to continue the dropout's final measured weight as the datum for each subsequent time point. A third approach penalizes the treatment group by using the dropout's baseline weight for the final assessment. Although this approach is rarely used, it may be the most realistic since most participants regain lost weight after withdrawing from a study.

Treating dropouts as if they had never entered the study (as was done in most of the studies described here) is illogical and can confound the results, obscuring a true difference. Participants doing well on placebo tend to stay in and those doing poorly to withdraw from the study. Thus, not using data from dropouts tends to enhance the placebo effect since it selects for placebo successes, and significant differences between active therapy and placebo may disappear. Conversely, not analyzing patients who left the phenylpropanolamine group will likely reduce evidence of the treatment effect since some of those dropouts will have achieved their weight loss goal. If one of the conventions were used to analyze phenylpropanolamine data with dropouts included, a true medication effect might be more clearly demonstrated.

Inappropriate Crossover Designs

The crossover designs in several of the studies discussed here are, in my opinion, inappropriate for weight loss trials. A basic premise of crossover studies is that the participants return to their baseline state prior to the institution of the next treatment in the sequence. This condition was not established in the reviewed studies and is probably impossible to achieve. Crossover studies are extremely sensitive to dropouts, which nullifies many of the supposed benefits of this design. In fact, since in two cases the crossover broke down because of dropouts, only the first period could be analyzed and the treatment groups were unbalanced, with many more patients having received phenylpropanolamine than placebo.

Pitfalls of Small, Independently Performed Trials

Some phenylpropanolamine clinical trials discussed here had too few participants to demonstrate a statistically significant difference. Although small clinical trials, if well-designed and well-conducted, may be able to demonstrate a true difference if it exists, it is also possible for a significant statistical or clinical difference to be missed because of the small number of participants. Increasing the number of subjects in any one trial is not necessarily the only, or even the best, solution to this problem. In many cases, multiple small studies are more valuable than a few large, multicenter ones. Elsewhere in this volume, Blumberg and Morgan present a method for combining and analyzing the data from such studies (see chapter 6). To yield the best results, small studies should involve many investigators and be done at various sites and perhaps even focus on different questions in diverse patient populations. Multiple small studies provide confidence that the data can be generalized from one geographical area to another and from one group of participants to another. Unfortunately, phenylpropanolamine trials often do not take full advantage of these potential benefits. For example, most phenylpropanolamine efficacy studies have been carried out by a small number of investigators working in just a few places.

Failure to Use a Run-In Period

Another common design defect in these studies was the failure to use a run-in period assessing the nonmedication course of participants. This is an important step in understanding the placebo effect associated with entering a study and beginning a diet (Weintraub et al. 1984). In the initial stages of a weight control study, the effect of a change in diet alone (with or without a placebo) is quite marked. Utilizing a diet-only, run-in period to assess how people will do before taking medication may result in two major benefits. First, the initial effect of being in the study may dissipate. Second, the investigator can use the response to a change in diet alone to stratify the population into treatment groups. Such a design would also follow a common "real world" pattern of anorexiant use. Frequently, a period of dietary restriction alone is initially prescribed by physicians or used by people in self-treatment. If following the diet becomes more difficult, medication may then be started.

Inappropriate Medication Schedules

In some of the phenylpropanolamine studies reviewed here, the medication administration schedule was inappropriate. Participants were requested to take the medication 30 minutes prior to breakfast, lunch, and supper. A prebreakfast dose may be illogical for two reasons. First, many people with weight control problems do not eat breakfast, and dieters are often encouraged to eat a morning meal as part of a behavior modification program to improve their eating habits. Thus, reducing an already low morning intake with further appetite suppression is not helpful. Second, due to their busy morning schedules, many people cannot wait 30 minutes after taking the medication to have breakfast. They may eat a rushed, short, unsatisfying meal or even take the medication without ingesting any food, possibly enhancing absorption and causing a rapid increase in blood concentration. Since the interval between the first dose and the second, prelunch dose is short, summed doses of medication may provoke adverse effects. A 10 a.m. and 4 p.m. dosage schedule as used in several of the studies is therefore more appropriate, as is a single time-release preparation taken just after a morning meal. Either of these could be utilized in future studies.

Treatment Group Imbalances

Many of the clinical trials reviewed here are flawed by imbalances in the treatment groups at baseline caused by excessive dependence on simple randomization. Unfortunately, comparability between randomly constituted treatment groups rarely occurs in studies with relatively small numbers of participants drawn from a heterogeneous pool of potential subjects. The resulting imbalances make interpretation of the outcome data difficult, if not impossible. To increase the likelihood that treatment groups would be comparable, investigators could recruit subjects from a more homogeneous population. Alternatively, if that was not desirable or possible, the sample could be stratified on the basis of key characteristics and the randomization and treatment assignment could then be carried out.

Other Problems

Comparing the study protocols to the reports of actual studies reveals that investigators do not always consistently follow the stated protocol. Violations of the study plan result in a variety of problems, such as unbalanced treatment groups, inappropriate participants, and high dropout rates. Investigators must learn the importance of following the protocol and sponsors must ensure that it occurs.

Participant compliance was rarely discussed in the studies analyzed here. In at least one case, data were excluded from the final efficacy analysis because participants had unilaterally lowered the dose of medication. In most instances, however, compliance was neither mentioned nor used in the data analysis.

In only one trial did the investigators vary the phenylpropanolamine treatment dosage in order to explore the dose-response relationship. Unfortunately, I was unable to obtain the data on the various dose sizes from this study and any resulting differences in outcome. Investigators in future phenylpropanolamine trials should consider studying several dose possibilities within the therapeutic range. This will help define a dose-response trend in the same study with similar and appropriate participants.

CONCLUSIONS

The most important conclusion to be drawn from the analysis of the clinical trials discussed in this report is that phenylpropanolamine is an active medication and an effective adjunct in weight control. In the studies summarized here, an average weight loss of approximately 0.5 kg/week (1.1 lb) occurred in phenylpropanolamine-treated participants versus approximately 0.3 kg/week (0.66 lb) in placebo-treated subjects. In the dose range tested, the dose-response relationship between weight loss and phenylpropanolamine daily intake is quite flat. Thus, increasing doses in the clinical trials did not result in markedly increased weight loss.

Yet, as the critics have (or should have) noted, the studies are flawed. However, since clinical trials are always relatively insensitive instruments and investigators frequently have great difficulty in demonstrating any differences, the fact that the findings of these flawed studies are generally consistent strengthens the conclusion that phenylpropanolamine is an effective anorexiant.

The difference in effectiveness between phenylpropanolamine and prescription anorexiants is not so clear. In the three clinical trials comparing phenylpropanolamine and prescription anorexiants discussed here (Altschuler and Conte in Altschuler et al. 1982; Noble 1977), there were no statistically significant differences between treatments. However, failure to demonstrate a difference does not imply that the treatments are identical or interchangeable. This is a common fallacy committed, on occasion, even by drug regulatory agencies (Weintraub 1982b). In the three comparative studies reviewed here, there was a consistent but only slightly greater weight loss with the prescription medications than with phenylpropanolamine. As in the studies of phenylpropanolamine and placebo, the short duration of the comparative clinical trials diminishes differences between treatments, penalizing the more effective ones.

In their review of double-blind clinical trials of anorexiants, Sullivan and Comai (1978) described 15 trials of eight weeks' or less duration in which a prescription anorexiant was compared with placebo. The mean difference in weight loss between active medication and placebo in those studies was 0.33 kg/week, more than 1.5 times greater than the average phenylpropanolamine/placebo difference of approximately 0.2 kg/week found in the comparable studies reviewed here. Of course, in not taking population characteristics and methodological differences into account, such comparisons are left open to bias and potentially significant misinterpretation. To fully compare the effects of phenylpropanolamine with those of prescription anorexiants would require a further series of well-designed, comparative clinical trials.

Critics of the use of phenylpropanolamine and of the clinical trials supporting its efficacy frequently find fault with the modest effect demonstrated. Such criticisms may not be appropriate if actual results are viewed in relation to the typical phenylpropanolamine user's goals. People who purchase phenylpropanolamine generally wish to lose a small amount of weight over a short duration of treatment. Studies indicate they often succeed. Since it is so difficult for many people, expecially women (Conte 1977), to lose weight, even the modest anorexiant effect of phenylpropanolamine has some value.

What cannot be expected of phenylpropanolamine as it is now used is that it enable moderately or severely obese people to lose enough weight to avoid the medical consequences of obesity. It is unlikely that weight loss induced by short-term phenylpropanolamine use will have the positive impact on cardiovascular health, osteoarthritis, cholelithiasis, adult onset diabetes mellitus, or hypertension that some critics seem to demand. The major benefit of phenylpropanolamine is that it can aid efforts to lose small amounts of weight, primarily for cosmetic purposes. However, we should not belittle the value of small weight changes which improve appearance. Important psychosocial and economic benefits can result from these so-called cosmetic weight changes. As Lasagna (1984) has pointed out and as Vener and Krupka report elsewhere in this volume (see chapter 8), weight losses of the magnitude experienced by users of phenylpropanolamine may be as important for them as the avoidance of the medical consequences of obesity is for more significantly overweight people.

Thus, in my opinion and in the view of most purchasers of the medication, phenylpropanolamine is not intended for use by more than moderately overweight people. It has a modest but consistent anorexiant effect across studies, an effect which may, in the proper context, be considered quite valuable.

REFERENCES

Altschuler, S. 1980. Double-blind clinical comparison of the anorectic activity of phenylpropanolamine hydrochloride drops and placebo drops dissolved in coffee/tea in the treatment of outpatients with exogenous obesity. Report on file. New York: Thompson Medical Company.

Altschuler, S. et al. 1982. Three controlled trials of weight loss with phenylpropanolamine. Int J Obes 6:549-56.

Bohensky, F. B. 1973. A single-blind evaluation of the efficacy of Appedrine® (phenylpropanolamine plus caffeine) as a dietary aid. Report on file. New York: Thompson Medical Company.

Bradley, M. H. 1982. Single-blind safety and efficacy evaluation of phenylpropanolamine hydrochloride plus caffeine, phenylpropanolamine alone, and placebo in exogenous obese patients with controlled hypertensive disease. Report on file. New York: Thompson Medical Company.

Conte, A. A. 1978. Double-blind clinical evaluation of the anorectic activity of a diet cube (phenylpropanolamine hydrochloride) compared to a lactose cube dissolved in coffee/tea in the treatment of exogenous obesity. Report on file. New York: Thompson Medical Company.

———. 1977. Double-blind clinical evaluation of the anorectic activity of phenylpropanolamine with caffeine compared to phenylpropanolamine without caffeine in the treatment of patients with exogenous obesity. Report on file. New York: Thompson Medical Company.

Griboff, S. I., R. Berman, and H. I. Silverman. 1975. A double-blind clinical evaluation of a phenylpropanolamine-caffeine-vitamin combination and a placebo in the treatment of exogenous obesity. Current Therapeutic Research 17:535-43.

Health and Human Services, Food and Drug Administration (FDA). 1982. Establishment of a monograph for weight control drug products for over-the-counter human use. FDA docket no. 81N-0022. Federal Register 47:8466-84. February 26.

Hoebel, B. G. et al. 1975a. Appetite suppression by phenylpropanolamine in humans. Obesity and Bariatric Medicine 4:192-97.

Hoebel, B. G. et al. 1975b. Body weight decreased in humans by phenylpropanolamine taken before meals. Obesity and Bariatric Medicine 4:200-206.

Jolly, E. R. 1972. To assess the utility of a phenylpropanolamine-caffeine combination product as an adjunct in a therapeutic program for uncomplicated obesity. Englewood, NJ: Biometrics Company.

Lasagna, L. 1984. Drug interactions involving appetite suppression. In Nervous system, endocrine system, and infusion therapy, edited by J. C. Petrie, 219-23. New York: Elsevier Science.

Lionel, N.D.W. and A. Herxheimer. 1970. Assessing reports of therapeutic trials. Br Med J 3:637-40.

Noble, R. 1977. Double-blind clinical evaluation of the anorectic activity of phenylpropanolamine compared to diethylpropion in obese outpatients. Report on file. New York: Thompson Medical Company.

Noble, R. and S. Kalkhof. 1981. Double-blind comparison of Dietac capsules (sustained release) containing 75 mg phenylpropanolamine with placebo to evaluate its efficacy as an aid in weight reduction. Report on file. Philadelphia: Menley & James Laboratories.

Noble, R. and M. J. Pertschuck. 1981. Multicenter double-blind comparison of Dietac (50 mg phenylpropanolamine plus 200 mg caffeine) versus placebo: an evaluation of safety and efficacy. Report on file. Philadelphia: Menley & James Laboratories.

Noble, R. and N. Respess. 1981. Double-blind comparison of Dietac tablets containing 50 mg phenylpropanolamine with placebo to evaluate its safety efficacy as an aid in weight reduction. Report on file. Philadelphia: Menley & James Laboratories.

Sebok, M. 1977a. Double-blind clinical evaluation of the anorectic activity of Prolamine™ versus placebo in the treatment of outpatients with exogenous obesity. Report on file. New York: Thompson Medical Company.

———. 1977b. Double-blind clinical evaluation of the anorectic activity of Vita Slim™ in comparison with placebo in the treatment of outpatients with exogenous obesity. Report on file. New York: Thompson Medical Company.

Settel, E. 1965. A double-blind study comparing the anorexigenic effect of phenylpropanolamine to placebo in thirty patients. Report on file. New York: Thompson Medical Company.

Sullivan, A. C. and K. Comai. 1978. Pharmacological treatment of obesity. Int J Obes 2:167-89.

Wardell, W. M. and M. Weintraub. 1981. Assessing the literature on therapeutic drugs. Presented (annually) at the postgraduate course in clinical pharmacology, drug development, and regulation, sponsored by the Center for the Study of Drug Development, Rochester, NY.

Weintraub, M. 1982a. How to critically assess clinical drug trials. Drug Therapy 12:131-48.

———. 1982b. The French drug approval process. J Clin Pharmacol 22:213-22.

———. 1979. Clinical trials in rheumatology: asking the relevant question (editorial). J Rhematol 6:365-69.

Weintraub, M. et al. 1984. A double-blind clinical trial in weight control: use of fenfluramine and phentermine alone and in combination. Arch Intern Med 144:1143-48.

Weintraub, M. et al. 1981. Determinants of response to anorexiants. Clin Pharmacol Ther 30:528-33.

Wilcoxon, F. and R. A. Wilcox. 1964. Some rapid approximate statistical procedures. Revision. Pearl River, NY: Lederle Laboratories.

6

COMBINING ANOREXIANT STUDIES FOR ANALYSIS: A STATISTICAL METHOD

Harvey Blumberg and John P. Morgan

INTRODUCTION

Approval of an over-the-counter (OTC) medication by the Food and Drug Administration (FDA) requires that the drug meet "standards of efficacy and safety." Testing whether the product meets those standards is costly and requires considerable involvement, difficulty, and even travail on the part of participating physicians and patients. As a result, most studies are of small sample size and may yield inconclusive results. Ideally, one large cooperative study involving hundreds of patients would be preferable but, if it is not feasible to conduct such a study, combining a number of small, completed studies might provide sufficient power to enable a more definitive conclusion to be reached. But how does one combine studies when, despite their having similar protocols, in each study the idiosyncratic behavior of the investigator and the unique nature of the subject population individualize the experimental results? It is the purpose of this paper to describe a statistical (non-prejudicial) method of combining a number of small studies.

The infatuation with dieting in the United States is well-documented in both the professional literature and the mass media. Appetite suppressants are used frequently to assist dieters in maintaining weight reduction efforts. The

---

Note: The data reported in this chapter are based on statistical revisions made by the Thompson Medical Company in late 1984. Completed cases include only subjects for whom there were complete study data (i.e., who attended each reporting session). Subjects who missed any reporting dates (even if they did complete their studies) were treated as dropouts, not as completed cases.

widespread use of appetite suppressant drugs (anorexiants), some of which are now available over-the-counter, has provoked concern about their efficacy and safety by the FDA, the public at large, and responsible drug companies. Is an anorexiant significantly better than a placebo in promoting weight loss over time? And, more importantly, is the drug reasonably safe to use?

In this report we examine ten independent, previously performed weight reduction studies and combine data from them in order to take advantage of the resulting larger sample size (table 6.1). We hope that combining the data will allow the extrapolation of more definitive conclusions than would be possible if each study were examined separately.

In all ten studies, the anorexiant phenylpropanolamine (PPA), which is found in many OTC diet aids sold in drugstores and food outlets, was tested against either a placebo or another treatment (phenylpropanolamine was combined with caffeine in nine of the studies). The results of some of these studies have previously been published in medical journals (Altschuler et al. 1982; Griboff, Berman, and Silverman 1975).

A NONPARAMETRIC COMPARISON

In six of the ten studies, phenylpropanolamine and a placebo were compared and the resulting weight losses were examined using a nonparametric comparison. An obvious advantage of this nonparametric approach is that the parametric constraints on combining data (e.g., that distributions be normal) are not present, making an across-study comparison undistorted.

The daily dosage of phenylpropanolamine administered in the six studies ranged between 70 and 100 mg. Five of the studies were six weeks in length and one study was four weeks. The combined samples included 169 phenylpropanolamine subjects and 149 placebo subjects who completed the studies. Parametric t-tests comparing the phenylpropanolamine and placebo groups in each study indicated that the initial weights of the two groups in each study were compatible ($p > .40$).

Results

In these studies the weight loss was greater for the subjects on phenylpropanolamine than for those on placebo.

TABLE 6.1

Number of subjects completing unpublished weight loss effectiveness studies

Study	Agents studied*	Number of subjects completing study		
		Total	PPA	Comparison agent
Altschuler† 1980	PPA drops/placebo (both with caffeine)	50	32	18
Conte† 1978	PPA cubes/placebo (both with caffeine)	43	20	23
Sebok 1978	Prolamine™/placebo (both without diet)	56	28	28
Sebok† 1977a	Prolamine™/placebo (both with diet)	49	26	23
Sebok† 1977b	Vita-Slim§/placebo	54	30§	24
Griboff, Berman, and Silverman 1975	Appedrine®/placebo	66	33	33
Conte 1977	PPA alone/PPA with caffeine	49	26§	23‡
Noble† 1977	PPA/diethylpropion	38	23	15
Conte† 1976	Appedrine®/diethylpropion	48	25	23
Altschuler 1977	Dexatrim™/mazindol	55	27	28
	TOTAL	508	293	215

*PPA taken with caffeine (either as part of medication or with beverage) unless otherwise indicated.

†One of six studies combined for parametric analysis.

§PPA without caffeine. ‡PPA with caffeine.

<u>Source</u>: Compiled by the authors.

(This weight loss advantage in favor of phenylpropanolamine was consistent, occurring at the end of two weeks, four weeks, and six weeks). Since each study was independently carried out, the probability of such a result would be .5 for each study. Therefore, the probability that all six studies would result in a weight loss difference in a predicted single direction would be $(.5)^6 = .0156$. This one nonparametric test indicates that phenylpropanolamine consistently outperformed the placebo in producing weight loss. Regardless of the dosage schedule followed, phenylpropanolamine consistently resulted in greater weight loss than did a placebo ($p < .02$). This consistency of performance (six successes out of six trials) speaks well for the anorexiant action of phenylpropanolamine. However, the parametric approaches are also of interest.

PARAMETRIC APPROACHES

Initial Constraints

In order to combine these studies in a technically appropriate and meaningful manner, it is necessary first to demonstrate the baseline equivalence of key parameters--most importantly, the initial weights of the participants. To demonstrate equivalence, it is also necessary that weight assessments should have been performed at the same time intervals, and the quantities of weight lost at those intervals should have been of a similar order. Additionally, to demonstrate safety, comparative appraisals of changes in blood pressure and pulse rates are needed, as are comparisons of patient dropout rates under the different drug conditions.

Within-Study Methodology

Study patients in the ten studies were between 18 and 65 years of age and were from 12% to 50% overweight as determined from the Metropolitan Life Insurance Tables (1959, 1966). All patients were healthy and none showed evidence of having physical conditions that would interfere with the study. Starting weight, blood pressure, and pulse rate were recorded for each subject. The studies were performed under double-blind conditions. Patients were assigned randomly to one of two groups, instructed when to take their medication, and told to report back every two weeks over the course of the study.

The Ten Studies

Each study was a double-blind, matched-group comparison between phenylpropanolamine and another treatment. In the six studies considered above, phenylpropanolamine was matched against a placebo. In three additional studies phenylpropanolamine plus caffeine was matched against an active anorexiant, diethylpropion in two studies and mazindol in another. In the tenth study, phenylpropanolamine alone was compared with phenylpropanolamine in combination with 200 mg of caffeine.

One-way analysis of variance tests were performed to see if the subjects' initial weights were compatible across the tests. This is an essential prerequisite condition for statistically combining the subjects across tests; that is, if the initial weights of subjects in the different studies were not of the same order, then any combination of these groups would create misleading results. Two studies failed to meet this criterion: phenylpropanolamine versus phenylpropanolamine plus caffeine (Conte 1977) and one of the six studies matching phenylpropanolamine with a placebo (Griboff, Berman, and Silverman 1975). The average initial weights of subjects were greater in these two studies than in the other eight. Accordingly, these two studies were eliminated from parametric analysis. Analysis of variance tests were also performed across two-week, four-week, and six-week intervals to ascertain the comparability between studies of weight loss over time since differences here would also invalidate a combined analysis.

Two studies resulted in a different order of weight loss than the other six. In one study matching phenylpropanolamine against a placebo (Sebok 1978), very low levels of weight loss occurred, and the study comparing phenylpropanolamine and mazindol (Altschuler 1977) produced larger than average weight losses (for both anorexiants). Both studies were eliminated from consideration for parametric analysis. The remaining six studies (see table 6.1), with a total of 282 subjects who completed the studies, were then combined.

The subjects were divided into three groups:

<u>Group A</u>: Patients on phenylpropanolamine (n_a = 156);
<u>Group B</u>: Patients on placebo (n_b = 88); and
<u>Group C</u>: Patients on diethylpropion (n_c= 38).

The rationale for combining subjects who had taken the same medication in different studies into the same group is that they did not know which treatment they had been given or which treatment they had been "matched against." There is no reason to suspect that the treatment each subject was matched against influenced his or her behavior. Therefore, subjects in each of the three test conditions were combined regardless of the treatment they had been matched against in their own studies.

Four of the six studies were six weeks in length. The other two studies were each eight weeks long, but data beyond six weeks were omitted from consideration.

Results

Table 6.2 shows that the baseline weights of the phenylpropanolamine subjects and the placebo subjects were very similar, with only a 0.6 lb difference between the initial mean weights (p = .87). Examining weight losses over time shows a steady decrease for subjects on both phenylpropanolamine and placebo, but the cumulative weight loss for subjects on phenylpropanolamine was greater. At the end of two weeks there was a mean difference of 0.82 lb between the phenylpropanolamine and placebo groups. The difference

TABLE 6.2

Mean cumulative weight loss (in lb): phenylpropanolamine (Group A) versus placebo (Group B)

Time	Initial mean weight		t	p
	Group A	Group B		
Baseline	163.3	162.7	0.16	.87

Time	Cumulative mean weight loss		t	p
	Group A	Group B		
End of week 2	3.25	2.43	2.43	.02
End of week 4	4.96	3.67	3.40	.001
End of week 6	5.97	3.97	3.98	.001

Source: Compiled by the authors.

increased to 1.29 lb and 2.00 lb at the end of four and six weeks, respectively. Parametric t-tests showed that the differences in weight loss at the end of two, four, and six weeks were all statistically significant ($p < .001$ at the four- and six-week intervals).

Table 6.3 shows that baseline weights between phenylpropanolamine and diethylpropion were similar with a 3.1 lb difference in mean weight ($p = .56$). More weight was lost by subjects on diethylpropion than by those on phenylpropanolamine. However, these differences did not reach statistical significance, leading us to conclude that there were no differences between the groups. Over time, the percentage difference in weight loss narrowed, with the smallest difference occurring at the end of the sixth week.

TABLE 6.3

Mean cumulative weight loss (in lb): phenylpropanolamine (Group A) versus diethylpropion (Group C)

Time	Initial mean weight		t	p
	Group A	Group C		
Baseline	163.3	160.2	0.59	.56

Time	Cumulative mean weight loss		t	p
	Group A	Group C		
End of week 2	3.25	4.07	1.79	.08
End of week 4	4.96	5.89	1.46	.15
End of week 6	5.97	6.50	0.61	.55

Source: Compiled by the authors.

In table 6.4 we note the differential weight loss in each two-week period separately for each anorexiant and for the placebo group. Under each of the three test conditions, the largest weight loss occurred during the first two weeks. However, there was a slightly better continuation of weight loss over time in the phenylpropanolamine group; i.e., more weight was lost in the final four-week period by subjects in this group than in the others. Early in treatment it is probably easier to lose weight (due to diuresis, and determination), but what occurs in the longer run is particularly important. This suggests the need for longer studies, as yet rarely performed.

TABLE 6.4

Differential weight loss (in lb):
phenylpropanolamine versus diethylpropion versus placebo

Time difference	PPA	Diethylpropion	Placebo
0-2 weeks	3.25	4.07	2.43
2-4 weeks	1.71	1.82	1.24
4-6 weeks	1.01	0.61	0.30

Source: Compiled by the authors.

The ability to sustain motivation is obviously an important underlying factor in weight loss. An appetite suppressant would be of the greatest assistance to those with the strongest motivation (an appetite suppressant does not act like a piece of tape across one's mouth but merely diminishes the "normal" desire to eat). If we define the motivated group as those who lost a minimum of 1 lb/week, or 6 lb overall, we can then compare groups to examine how well the more motivated dieters fared. Table 6.5 indicates that just over half (54.5%) of the subjects on phenylpropanolamine but only 29.5% of the placebo group lost a total of 6 lb or more ($p < .001$) in six weeks.

TABLE 6.5

Patients who lost 6 lb or more: phenylpropanolamine versus placebo

Drug	Proportion losing 6 lb or more	Percentage
PPA	85/156	54.5*
Placebo	26/88	29.5

Source: Compiled by the authors.
*p < .001

Safety Factors

In our examination of "product safety," we included subjects from all ten studies, since the greater the number of subjects observed, the more meaningful would be the results. Four measures of product safety are considered here: systolic and diastolic blood pressures, radial pulse, and the comparative number of subjects who dropped out under each study condition.

Table 6.6 shows that mean changes in diastolic blood pressure were quite small and that the mean blood pressure levels decreased slightly for the phenylpropanolamine, mazindol, and placebo groups. This suggests that in the study settings phenylpropanolamine does not increase diastolic blood pressure.

Changes in systolic blood pressure and in radial pulse rate were similarly analyzed. The results of both analyses were essentially the same as those for diastolic blood pressure shown in table 6.6 (small decreases for phenylpropanolamine, mazindol, and placebo, and a small increase for diethylpropion).

In order to evaluate individual vital sign differences, a count was made of both the number and percentage of subjects, under each treatment condition, who experienced an increase of 15 or more points in any vital sign measurement when they were examined by physicians during the study periods (table 6.7). Each subject had three chances to exhibit a 15-point increase in each vital sign measurement (three examinations after the initial baseline examination). One question to consider is whether the data indicate that

TABLE 6.6

Mean changes in diastolic blood pressure (in mm Hg) over pre-study levels: phenylpropanolamine, diethylpropion, mazindol, and placebo

Time interval	PPA	DEP*	Mazindol	Placebo
Wk 2 - Wk 0	-0.60	2.25	-1.30	0.60
Wk 4 - Wk 0	-1.10	2.10	-2.80	-0.10
Wk 6 - Wk 0	-1.30	0	-2.70	-0.03

*DEP: Diethylpropion.
Source: Compiled by the authors.

TABLE 6.7

Patients showing a 15-point or greater increase in vital sign readings

Drug	n	Number of subjects: Blood pressure, Diastolic	Number of subjects: Blood pressure, Systolic	Number of subjects: Pulse rate	Percentage of subjects: Blood pressure, Diastolic	Percentage of subjects: Blood pressure, Systolic	Percentage of subjects: Pulse rate
PPA	293	10	31	6	3.4	10.6	2.0
DEP*	38	6	8	5	15.8	21.1	13.2
Mazindol	28	0	3	0	0	10.7	0
Placebo	149	9	22	5	6.0	14.8	3.4

*DEP: Diethylpropion.
Source: Compiled by the authors.

any of the drug conditions produced 15-point increases in vital sign measurements in a higher percentage of subjects than did placebo. There is no evidence of this for phenylpropanolamine, since a smaller percentage of phenylpropanolamine subjects than placebo subjects showed such an increase, although these differences do not approach statistical significance. The evidence for mazindol (with a very small n) is similar. In contrast, diethylpropion (with a small n) produced 15-point increases in all vital sign measurements in a greater percentage of subjects than did placebo (2.5 times greater for diastolic blood pressure and four times greater for pulse rate).

Table 6.8 indicates that the highest dropout rate occurred in the diethylpropion group, the second highest in

TABLE 6.8

Comparative dropout rates:
phenylpropanolamine, diethylpropion, mazindol, and placebo

Drug	Total number in studies	Number of dropouts	Number completed	Percentage dropouts
PPA	373	80*	293	21.4*
DEP†	62	24§	38	38.7§
Mazindol	33	5	28	15.2
Placebo	201	52	149	25.9
TOTAL	669	161	508	

*The 21.4% dropout rate for PPA includes three subjects who missed interim reporting times but did complete their studies. If these three subjects are instead considered as having completed the studies, the dropout rate for PPA falls to 20.6% (77/373).

†DEP: Diethylpropion.

§The 38.7% dropout rate for DEP includes six subjects who mised interim reporting times but did complete their studies. If these six subjects are instead considered as having completed the studies, the dropout rate for DEP falls to 29.0% (18/62).

Source: Compiled by the authors.

the placebo group, and the third highest among the phenylpropanolamine subjects. The relatively high dropout rate for subjects on placebo (higher than for two of the three active drugs) indicates that there is no statistical evidence that conditions resulting in subjects dropping out of the studies were drug-related. The dropout pattern also suggests that a major cause of leaving a study may have been failure to experience anorexia. An examination of patient reports indicates that subjects who dropped out complaining of adverse physical reactions were often in the placebo group, suggesting that being in a weight loss program was in itself stressful. There is no evidence that subjects dropped out of a study because of adverse effects associated with an active treatment.

CONCLUSIONS

Combining a number of clinical studies, each of which, by design, contains few subjects, enables conclusions to be drawn which otherwise would not be possible. An increased sample size is a powerful and useful tool in the interpretation of data.

In our study, the efficacy of phenylpropanolamine as an appetite suppressant has been statistically demonstrated. Roughly 50% more weight was lost by the average person taking phenylpropanolamine than by a subject on placebo, a statistically significant difference. It was also found that at the end of six weeks the rate of weight loss had decreased more sharply for dieters on placebo, suggesting that a longer study (perhaps from 12 to 16 weeks) might result in a difference in weight loss between groups greater than the 50% difference found at the end of six weeks. It was also noted that 54.5% of the subjects on phenylpropanolamine lost a minimum of 1 lb/week over the course of the six-week study.

In addition to efficacy, product safety was also analyzed. Examinations of biweekly changes in blood pressure and radial pulse readings showed slight decreases for both the placebo and active medication groups across all subjects. Patient dropout rates were roughly the same for three of the test conditions, with the diethylpropion subjects having the highest dropout rate and the placebo group having a greater percentage of dropouts than the groups on the other two anorexiants. An examination of individuals who experienced a 15-unit or greater increase in blood pressure or radial pulse rate showed that diethylpropion produced a noticeably higher percentage of subjects experiencing such increases, with placebo second highest, followed by phenylpropanolamine and mazindol. Compared to placebo, the phenylpropanolamine and mazindol results were favorable.

The total combined sample size of more than 500 completed cases generates confidence in these demonstrations of product safety.

REFERENCES

Altschuler, S. 1980. Double-blind clinical comparison of the anorectic activity of phenylpropanolamine hydrochloride drops and placebo drops dissolved in coffee/tea in the treatment of outpatients with exogenous obesity. Report on file. New York: Thompson Medical Company.

———. 1977. Double-blind clinical evaluation of the anorectic activity of Dexatrim in comparison with mazindol in the treatment of outpatients who have exogenous obesity. Report on file. New York: Thompson Medical Company.

Altschuler, S. et al. 1982. Three controlled trials of weight loss with phenylpropanolamine. Int J Obes 6:549-56.

Conte, A. A. 1978. Double-blind clinical evaluation of the anorectic activity of a diet cube (phenylpropanolamine hydrochloride) compared to a lactose cube dissolved in coffee/tea in the treatment of exogenous obesity. Report on file. New York: Thompson Medical Company.

———. 1977. Double-blind clinical evaluation of the anorectic activity of phenylpropanolamine with caffeine compared to phenylpropanolamine without caffeine in the treatment of patients with exogenous obesity. Report on file. New York: Thompson Medical Company.

———. 1976. Double-blind clinical evaluation of the anorectic activity of Appedrine in comparison to diethylpropion in the treatment of outpatients with exogenous obesity. Report on file. New York: Thompson Medical Company.

Griboff, S. I., R. Berman, and H. I. Silverman. 1975. A double-blind clinical evaluation of a phenylpropanolamine-caffeine-vitamin combination and a placebo in the treatment of exogenous obesity. Current Therapeutic Research 17:535-43.

Metropolitan Life Insurance Tables. 1966. Statistical Bulletin 47:1.

———. 1959. Statistical Bulletin 40:1.

Noble, R. 1977. Double-blind clinical evaluation of the anorectic activity of phenylpropanolamine compared to diethylpropion in obese outpatients. Report on file. New York: Thompson Medical Company.

Sebok, M. 1978. Double-blind clinical evaluation of the anorectic activity of Prolamine™ versus placebo in the treatment of outpatients with exogenous obesity. Report on file. New York: Thompson Medical Company.

———. 1977a. Double-blind clinical evaluation of the anorectic activity of Prolamine™ versus placebo in the treatment of outpatients with exogenous obesity. Report on file. New York: Thompson Medical Company.

———. 1977b. Double-blind clinical evaluation of the anorectic activity of Vita-Slim™ in comparison with placebo in the treatment of outpatients with exogenous obesity. Report on file. New York: Thompson Medical Company.

7

CURRENT STATUS OF DRUG THERAPY IN OBESITY

George A. Bray

INTRODUCTION

In selecting a treatment for obesity it is necessary, as with all therapies, to balance the underlying risk of the condition itself with the inherent risk of treatment. During the evaluation of an obese patient, the degree and risk of obesity can most usefully be assessed by the body mass index (BMI), defined as weight/(height)^2. When the BMI is between 20 kg/m^2 and 25 kg/m^2, body weight is in the normal range and the only approach to weight loss should be diet with or without exercise. When the BMI is between 25 kg/m^2 and 30 kg/m^2--that is, between the upper limits of normal and 20% above normal--both diet and exercise should be encouraged. Drugs as adjuncts for the treatment of obesity are most appropriate when the BMI approaches or exceeds 30 kg/m^2 (Bray 1982).

The ideal pharmaceutical agent for treatment of obesity ought to have no long- or short-term toxicity, be well-tolerated, allow balancing of body fat to the desired level without impairing lean body mass, have no deleterious metabolic effects, and be inexpensive. Obviously no agent currently available meets these criteria. In this paper I will examine some of the agents now in use as adjuncts in the treatment of obesity.

History of Amphetamine Research

Amphetamine was first synthesized in 1887 by Edeleano, but it was not until 1927 that its psychopharmacological properties were first evaluated (Alles 1928). These include decreased fatigue, wakefulness, alertness, euphoria, and increased energy. Ten years later, during clinical tests of amphetamine as a treatment for depression and narcolepsy, it was noted that patients receiving this drug lost weight (Bahnsen, Jacobson, and Thesleff 1938). Less than a year later, Lesses and Myerson (1938) demonstrated that amphetamine could be used in the treatment of obesity. In subsequent clinical trials amphetamine was shown to be effective in decreasing weight in adults and children (Bray 1976).

It was another ten years before appetite suppression was demonstrated to be the chief mode of action of amphetamine in weight loss (Harris, Ivy, and Searle 1947). In one experiment, eight dogs were trained to eat their entire daily allotment of food in 45 minutes. The quantity of food eaten was carefully weighed. The animals were then treated with doses of amphetamine ranging from 2.5 to 20 mg. When 10 or 20 mg were given one hour before mealtime, food intake was practically abolished. When the drug was given for two weeks, the animals lost up to 26% of their initial body weight.

Studies were also carried out with human beings (Ibid.). In the first experiment, seven obese and two nonobese individuals ate as much as they wanted of three meals each day and their intake was recorded. This procedure was continued over two eight-week periods separated by a four-week vacation. During one of these periods subjects received (±)-amphetamine sulfate (10 mg) before each meal and during the other period a placebo. The administration of amphetamine decreased the intake of food and increased the rate of weight loss compared to placebo. In the final study, subjects were directed to eat the same quantity of food whether they were given amphetamine or placebo. Under these circumstances, amphetamine had no effect on body weight, indicating that the primary action of the drug was to decrease food intake and not to increase energy expenditure.

CHEMISTRY OF THE APPETITE-SUPPRESSING DRUGS

All appetite-suppressing drugs except mazindol are chemical derivatives of phenethylamine. Chemical modifications of the phenyl ring and/or side chain partially separate the appetite-suppressing from the central nervous system (CNS) excitatory effects. Four types of chemical modifications have been useful in distinguishing the cardiovascular and the CNS effects of these drugs from their effects as appetite suppressants.

1. Hydroxylation of the side chain. This reduces the stimulatory effects on the central nervous system more than it reduces the anorexiant properties.

2. Substitution on the alpha-carbon. Placement of a methyl group on the alpha-carbon of the side chain serves to diminish oxidation by monoamine oxidase (MAO). Chemical substitution in this position also contributes to the high affinity of amphetamine for the membranes of the central nervous system and to its ability to decrease the uptake of norepinephrine by these neurons (Bray 1976).

3. N-terminal substitutions. These substitutions serve to reduce the CNS stimulatory effects of the phenethylamine nucleus without destroying its appetite-suppressing properties. For example, cyclization of the amphetamine side chain, as in phenmetrazine and phendimetrazine, preserves anorexiant properties but diminishes the cardiovascular and CNS stimulatory effects.

4. Substitution on the phenyl ring. Substitution of a hydroxyl or methoxyl group on the phenyl ring markedly reduces the anorexiant activity of the compound. Introduction of an electronegative group such as chlorine markedly decreases the CNS stimulatory effects of these compounds, but only moderately reduces their anorexiant properties.

For more details, the reader may wish to consult other reviews (Heil and Ross 1976; Garattini and Samanin 1978; Curtis-Prior 1983).

MECHANISM OF ACTION

Current concepts on the formation, release, and action of central adrenergic neurotransmitters are depicted in figure 7.1, along with potential sites for the effects of amphetamine. This figure is a schematic representation of the terminal axon and receptor neuron of the adrenergic nervous system. Within the axon, tyrosine (TYR) is converted to dihydroxyphenylalanine (DOPA) by hydroxylation of the phenyl ring (1 in figure 7.1). Tyrosine hydroxylase, the enzyme which performs this transformation, limits the rate at which this process can occur. In the presence of the enzyme dopa decarboxylase, DOPA is converted to dopamine (DA), which can be stored in the granule (2 in figure 7.1). Dopamine may also be converted to norepinephrine (NE) by dopamine hydroxylase. The dense granules in which dopamine and/or norepinephrine are stored are located primarily in the nerve ending. The active neurotransmitters are released in small amounts into the nerve ending from the storage granules. This extragranular norepinephrine or dopamine may be oxidized by MAO, reaccumulated by the storage granule, or released into the interneuronal space. Once released from the nerve ending, the norepinephrine can either act on

FIGURE 7.1

Schematic representation
of sites of action of amphetamine

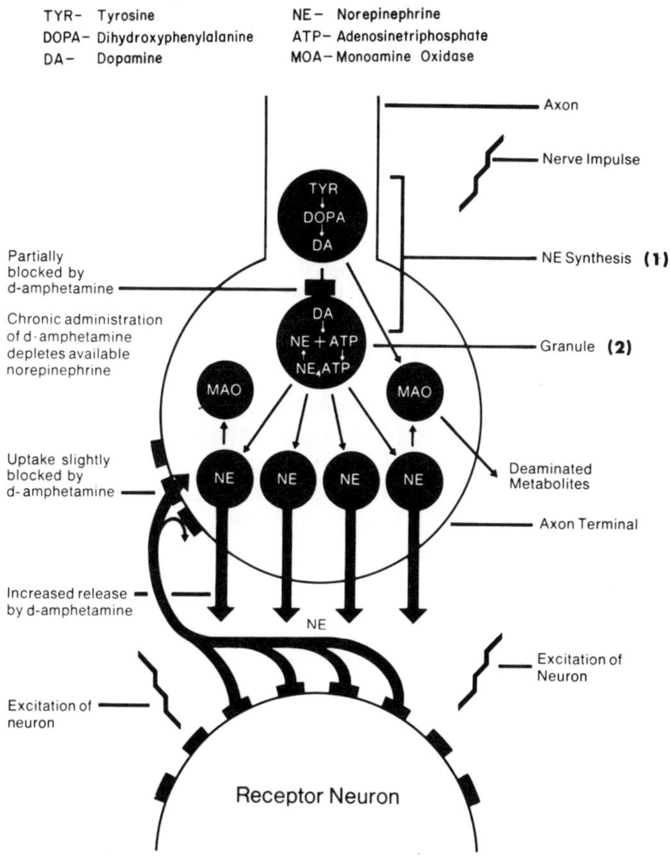

Source: Compiled by the author.

receptors, be O-methylated by an enzyme called catechol-O-methyltransferase (COMT), or be reaccumulated in the cytoplasm of the neuronal axon.

Amphetamine

The effects of amphetamine follow its stereospecific binding to specific receptors in the brain. These receptors bind all the appetite-suppressing drugs and the relative binding affinities for the various drugs are highly correlated with their potencies as anorexiants (Paul et al. 1982). After binding of amphetamine, there is release of norepinephrine, which increases the effective concentration of this compound at the receptor neuron. Other possible sites of action do not appear to be of importance for the primary action of this drug.

Although in high doses amphetamine can release and deplete brain norepinephrine and alter its storage and metabolism, in low doses this does not appear to be an important mechanism of action. Amphetamine increases the turnover of dopamine and norepinephrine and facilitates their release from extragranular sites. (These sites are shown on the left side of figure 7.1.) The anorexia produced by amphetamine can be inhibited by complete blockade of norepinephrine biosynthesis. The anorexiant effect of amphetamine is also specifically blocked by pimozide and other blockers of dopamine receptors. The anorexia induced by amphetamine is enhanced by desmethylimipramine, a drug which blocks the reuptake of norepinephrine by the nerve ending. This suggests that dopamine, rather than norepinephrine, may be the principal neurotransmitter whose effects are facilitated by amphetamine (Blundell and Latham 1980).

Mazindol

The mechanism of action for this drug may differ from that described for amphetamine. The major evidence for this comes from three kinds of experiments which demonstrate differences between mazindol and amphetamine.

First, the effects of mazindol on metabolism of catecholamines in the central nervous system differ from those of amphetamine. Mazindol increases the availability of norepinephrine at the axonal receptor sites largely by inhibiting the usual reaccumulation of norepinephrine by the axonal membrane (figure 7.1). In this respect it differs significantly from the action of amphetamine.

Second, mazindol has an additional effect which amphetamine does not: it abolishes the mouse-killing behavior of killer rats. However, after the septal region of the brain is destroyed with electrolytic lesions, the dose of mazindol required to reduce the mouse-killing behavior of killer rats increases, whereas there is no change in the required dose of methamphetamine or chlorphentermine, two other appetite-suppressing drugs. This suggests that mazindol, in contrast to the other two drugs, has an important action on the septal region of the brain. Further support for an action of mazindol on the septal region is provided by experiments in which changes in the evoked potentials in the hypothalamus were recorded following stimulation of the septum. Norepinephrine potentiates the positive wave form elicited in the hypothalamus by stimulation of the septum, whereas mazindol appears to abolish the effects mediated through the septum.

Third, mazindol may have thermogenic properties in addition to its effects on food intake. It stimulates brown adipose tissue and increases oxygen consumption (Arch 1981). These differences between mazindol and amphetamine suggest different neurophysiological mechanisms for their action.

Fenfluramine

Studies of fenfluramine also suggest a mechanism of action which differs from that for amphetamine or mazindol (Bray and Greenway 1976). Fenfluramine reduces the brain concentration of serotonin and its metabolite, 5-hydroxyindolacetic acid, but has little or no effect on the concentration of norepinephrine or dopamine. Amphetamine, on the other hand, has little effect on serotonin metabolism but has a major influence on brain norepinephrine and dopamine. The action of fenfluramine is also inhibited by drugs which antagonize the action of serotonin. The action of amphetamine, on the other hand, is not affected by such antagonists. The high concentration of hydroxyvanillic acid found in the brain after treatment with either drug indicates increased dopamine metabolism. In contrast to amphetamine, which is thought to release dopamine, fenfluramine may act to block the effect of dopamine at its receptors and thus indirectly increase dopamine metabolism. Logically, fenfluramine antagonizes some of the effects of amphetamine, such as the toxicity of amphetamine to mice when the animals are maintained in groups. Similarly, fenfluramine can antagonize the hyperthermia and vasoconstriction elicited by amphetamine in an isolated mouse artery.

Fenfluramine, given acutely, does not stimulate energy expenditure but, after chronic treatment, energy expenditure may increase. If animals are starved to reduce body weight by 10% to 15% before receiving fenfluramine, they will start to eat when food is made available. Body weight remains lower than in control animals, however, even though food intake is normal. These studies show two things. First, fenfluramine depresses food intake only when body weight is normal, but not when it is below normal. Second, body weight remains lower, although food intake returns to normal (Levitsky, Strupp, and Lupoli 1981). The effects of amphetamine on ingestion of food are characterized by a long initial delay followed by rapid eating in short, infrequent bursts (Blundell 1984). Fenfluramine, on the other hand, produces a marked slowing in the rate of eating with early satiety. Thus amphetamine appears to suppress hunger whereas fenfluramine enhances satiety (Rogers and Blundell 1979). Amphetamine suppresses protein intake, but fenfluramine exerts a greater suppression of carbohydrate intake (Blundell and Rogers 1980; McArthur and Blundell 1983).

In human beings fenfluramine has an effect on the brain electroencephalogram (EEG) which resembles that observed with barbiturates and which differs sharply from that observed with amphetamine (Bray and Greenway 1976).

PHARMACOLOGY OF THE APPETITE-SUPPRESSING DRUGS

Effects on the Central Nervous System

The appetite-suppressing drugs possess many of the pharmacological properties of the naturally occurring adrenergic neurotransmitters, epinephrine and norepinephrine. All the drugs listed in table 7.1 can stimulate the central nervous system and increase locomotor activity, but their relative potency differs greatly. Amphetamine and methamphetamine are the most potent and fenfluramine, chlorphentermine, and phenylpropanolamine (PPA) (not listed in this table because it is not a scheduled drug) the least potent. Indeed, fenfluramine has a mixed stimulant and depressant effect. Benzphetamine and (+)-amphetamine produce the greatest increase in spontaneous activity. Methamphetamine is the most potent stimulator of spontaneous activity and phenmetrazine only slightly less so. At the other extreme are chlorphentermine, diethylpropion, and fenfluramine, which have little effect on spontaneous activity. Chlorphentermine and fenfluramine likewise produce almost no delay in the onset of sleep or reduction in its duration, whereas diethylpropion behaves more like the other drugs. Although both (+) and (-) forms of amphetamine reduce the amount of rapid eye movement (REM) sleep in depressed patients, only (+)-amphetamine delays the onset and shortens the duration of sleep (Gillin et al. 1975). The activation and euphoria associated with (+)-amphetamine are reduced by co-treatment with lithium carbonate (Van Kammen and Murphy 1975). In growing children (+)-amphetamine may be a growth retardant, indicated by the growth rebound when the drug is terminated (Safer, Allen, and Barr 1975); thus, amphetamine should not be administered to growing children.

Cardiovascular Effects

Cardiovascular effects of anorexiants are frequently observed, with increases in heart rate and blood pressure being the most common manifestations. However, the effect on blood pressure can be paradoxical. The acute administration of amphetamine increases the sensitivity of animals to the hypertensive effects of tyramine and norepinephrine. After chronic administration of amphetamine, on the other hand, the hypertensive effect of tyramine is reduced but the hypertensive effect of infused norepinephrine is unchanged. Moreover, individuals who self-administer (+)-amphetamine show no evidence of a sustained increase in blood pressure (Simpson 1979). Tachycardia is produced by many of these drugs but it seldom occurs with mazindol or fenfluramine.

One careful comparative study of several amphetamine-like drugs was conducted at the Addiction Research Center (Martin et al. 1971). In this study the effects of amphetamine, methamphetamine, ephedrine, phenmetrazine, and methylphenidate in human subjects were compared. All drugs produced dose-related increases in both systolic and diastolic blood pressure. Respiratory rate was increased similarly by all the drugs. Their effects on pulse rate were complex. Although all the drugs produced tachycardia, there was an overall negative correlation between pulse rate and the rise in blood pressure when amphetamine, methamphetamine, ephedrine, and phenmetrazine were studied. The relative bradycardia seen during the increased pressor responses was probably of reflex origin. This suggests that the pressor response activates the carotid body sensor and thus inhibits heart rate by stimulating the vagus nerve. These drugs also increased body temperature, dilated the pupils, reduced food intake, and shortened the duration of sleep. Amphetamine and methamphetamine were nearly identical on all parameters studied; phenmetrazine, in contrast, was only one-third to one-fourth as potent as those two drugs on most of the cardiovascular and CNS responses examined.

Metabolic Effects

Some of the appetite-suppressing drugs also have metabolic effects (Dannenburg 1983; Brindley 1983).

Amphetamine, methamphetamine, phenmetrazine, and fenfluramine all increase the concentration of free fatty acids and/or glycerol in plasma. Depletion of catecholamines by prolonged administration of reserpine almost completely abolishes the rise of plasma free fatty acids produced by amphetamine. This suggests that amphetamine acts by releasing endogenous norepinephrine at or near the adipocyte membrane. The effects of fenfluramine have been subjected to intensive investigation (Burland 1976). Fenfluramine has no direct action on isolated adipocytes, yet in vivo it potentiates the release of free fatty acids. At concentrations more than 200 times that of an effective dose of norepinephrine, fenfluramine and methamphetamine have no effect in vitro on the release of free fatty acids from adipocytes. However, methamphetamine and fenfluramine both antagonize the lipolytic effects of norepinephrine in vitro. Fenfluramine also inhibits the lipolysis stimulated by adrenocorticotropic hormone (ACTH), whereas methamphetamine is only a weak antagonist. The release of free fatty acids and glycerol following the addition of cyclic adenosine monophosphate (AMP) to adipose tissue is slightly but significantly reduced by fenfluramine, whereas methamphetamine has no effect on this response. In addition, fenfluramine inhibits the stimulation of lipolysis following the addition of growth hormone plus dexamethasone but does not modify the increased lipolysis observed with adipose tissue from fasting animals.

Another important difference between methamphetamine and fenfluramine is that methamphetamine has no effect on lipolysis after fasting or on the lipolytic effects of growth hormone and dexamethasone in vitro. When methamphetamine and fenfluramine are incubated individually with adipocytes in the presence of radioactively labeled glucose, the incorporation of radioactivity into glyceride/glycerol by adipocytes is unaffected but the incorporation into long chain fatty acids is significantly reduced. Of the anorexiant drugs, only mazindol appears to be without effect on lipid metabolism, which again indicates a possible difference in mechanism of action from that of the other drugs listed in table 7.1.

Fenfluramine and mazindol also influence glucose metabolism. Wichelow and Butterfield (1970) showed that the intra-arterial injection of 0.4 mg/min of fenfluramine increased the glucose uptake and blood flow in the infused arm above that in the control arm. Following two weeks of oral fenfluramine therapy, three obese subjects lost weight and demonstrated increased glucose uptake and utilization by peripheral tissues. Fenfluramine has also been reported to have a hypoglycemic effect in diabetics (Turtle and Burgess 1973), but fenfluramine does not improve glucose tolerance in patients with lipodystrophy (Wilson, Melton, and Clarke 1983). Mazindol and its congener, ciclazindol, produce a dose-related increase in glucose uptake by human gluteus muscle in vitro. This effect is independent of insulin and is not affected by methysergide, which blocks the effect of fenfluramine on glucose uptake (Kirby and Turner 1977).

METABOLISM OF THE APPETITE-SUPPRESSING DRUGS

Absorption

All the commercially available appetite suppressants shown in table 7.1 are bioavailable after oral ingestion. Peak blood concentrations occur one to two hours after ingestion for many of these compounds. The half-time in blood varies from two to more than 30 hours (table 7.1). This variation is undoubtedly influenced by the chemical structure of the compound, as well as by the acidity of the urine. Variations in chemical structure alter lipid solubility relative to amphetamine. Although most appetite suppressants are two to eight times more soluble in fat than amphetamine is, phendimetrazine is 32 times and fenfluramine 67 times more soluble (Dring 1983). Since the pKa of all appetite suppressants is greater than 8.5, excretion of the unchanged form is generally increased when the urine is acidic. This would be expected because the partition between acidic urine and more alkaline body fluids would favor diffusion into the acidic urine. Excretion is generally delayed if the urine is alkaline. The excretion of the unchanged compound in urine varies from a low of 4% to more than 70%.

Metabolic Pathways and Products

The metabolic fate of each of these compounds varies from one species to another, as well as between drugs. At least four metabolic pathways have been defined for these compounds. The first is hydroxylation of the aromatic (phenyl) ring. The second is oxidative deamination of the aminoalkyl group. The third is beta-carbon hydroxylation of the two-carbon side chain, and the fourth is dealkylation of the N-alkyl-phenyl-isopropanolamine side chain. The pathway

TABLE 7.1

Appetite-suppressing drugs

Generic name	Suppliers	Proprietary name	Dosage (mg)
Schedule II*			
(±)-Amphetamine		Benzedrine® and others	5, 10, 15
Methamphetamine	Abbott	Desoxyn® and others	5, 10, 15
Phenmetrazine	Boehringer	Preludin®	25, 50, 75
Schedule III*			
Phendimetrazine	Ayerst	Plegine®	35
Benzphetamine	Upjohn	Didrex®	25, 50
Chlorphentermine	Parke-Davis	Pre-Sate®	65
Clortermine	USV-Pharmaceuticals	Voranil®	50
Schedule IV*			
Diethylpropion	Merrell Riker	Tenuate® Tepanil®	25, 75
Fenfluramine	Robins	Pondimin®	20
Mazindol	Sandoz Wyeth	Sanorex® Mazanor®	1, 2
Phentermine	Beecham Pennwalt	Fastin® Ionamin® (resin)	15, 30

*The Federal Controlled Substances Act of 1970 places the prescription anorexiants into five Schedule categories.

—: Data not available.

Administration (mg)	Peak blood concentration (hrs after p.o. dose)	Half-life in blood (hrs)	% Excreted unchanged in acidic urine
5 to 10 before meals (tid)	1-2	13	55
2.5 or 5 before meals (tid) 10 or 15 in morning	1-2	13	45
25 (bid or tid)	--	--	19
35 before meals	--	4	??
25-50 before meals	1-2	--	??
65 in morning	--	14-38	35
50 in morning	2-5	9	??
25 before meals (tid) 75 in morning	2-4	13.8-30.1	24
20-40 before meals	5	2-5	20
1 before meals; 2 in morning	4	13	22
15 tid 30 in morning	??	7-8	75

Source: Compiled by the author. Data derived from published and unpublished materials, including clinical trial reports, distributed by manufacturers.

for metabolism of amphetamine is shown in figure 7.2. The first step in metabolism is removal of the N-terminal methyl group. This is followed by two alternative pathways, either the oxidation of the amino group to a keto group or the hydroxylation of the phenyl ring.

FIGURE 7.2

Pathways of metabolism of amphetamine

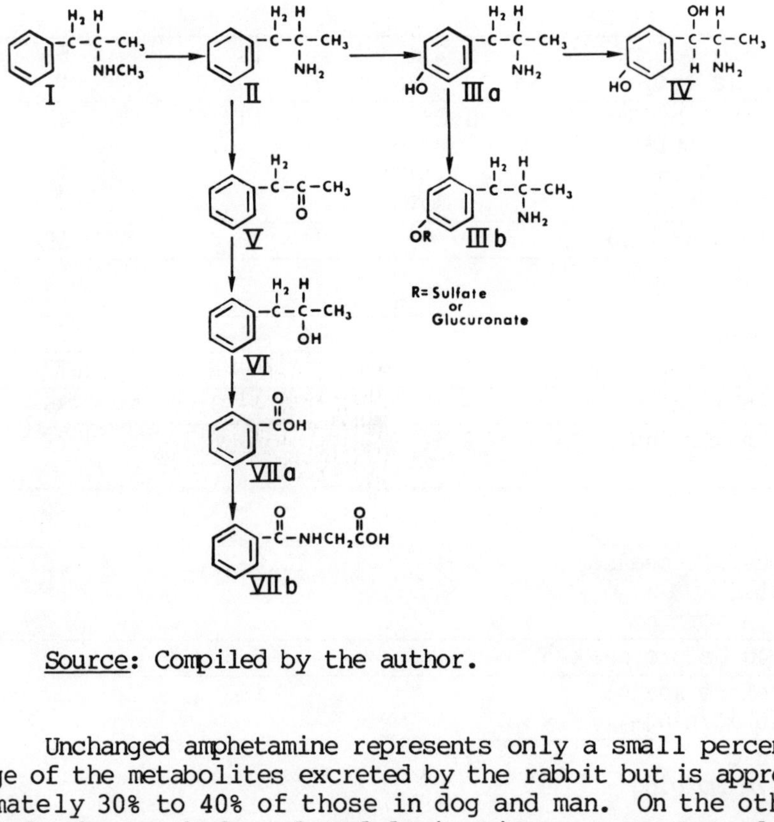

Source: Compiled by the author.

Unchanged amphetamine represents only a small percentage of the metabolites excreted by the rabbit but is approximately 30% to 40% of those in dog and man. On the other hand, the parahydroxylated derivative represents only a small fraction of the metabolites in man. The other major component in human urine is the benzoic acid derivative. In contrast, the benzomethylketone and benzoic acid metabolites make up the major products of metabolism in the rabbit and are also prominent metabolites in the dog. One-fifth of a dose of phenmetrazine is excreted unchanged in human urine, and there are two major metabolic products (Franklin, Dring, and Williams 1977).

CLINICAL USE OF ANOREXIANT DRUGS

In evaluating the clinical usefulness of anorexiant drugs, two questions need to be answered: (1) are they effective, and (2) are they safe? After these two questions are examined, the general principles for use of these agents will be discussed (Douglas and Munro 1982).

Effectiveness

The effectiveness of an anorexiant compound can be established by showing that in a double-blind, randomized trial it is associated with a significantly greater rate of weight loss than a placebo. The most extensive body of data yet assembled on appetite suppessant drugs is provided in a review of U.S. Food and Drug Administration (FDA) evaluations of 105 new drug applications submitted for marketing approval (Scoville 1976). These applications contained 210 double-blind studies of which 145 included two active drugs. The FDA report contained information on 4,543 patients treated with active medications and 3,100 treated with placebo. The dropout rate for those who returned after four weeks of therapy was 18.5% for subjects on placebo and 24.3% for those given active drugs. At the end of study periods lasting three, four, eight, or more weeks, equal percentages of patients receiving placebo and active drugs remained in treatment (49% for placebo versus 47.9% for active drugs). Weight loss averaged 0.25 kg/week (0.56 lb/week) more for subjects receiving active drugs than for those on placebo. The data from one trial of 30 drug-treated and 15 placebo-treated patients (Bray 1976) are shown in figure 7.3. The drug-treated patients lost more weight, and the differences between the groups continued to widen for the entire 20 weeks of the study.

The weight loss effectiveness of the drugs reviewed by the FDA can also be evaluated in terms of the proportion of subjects who lost given amounts of weight per week. A weight loss of at least 0.45 kg/week (1 lb/week) was almost twice as common in patients receiving active drugs (44%) as in those on placebo (26%), as was a weight loss of at least 1.4 kg/week (3 lb/week), achieved by 2% of those on active drugs compared with 1% on placebo. Examining only the weight loss results after four weeks of treatment shows that 68% of the patients on active drugs lost at least 0.45 kg/week compared to 46% on placebo and that 10% of the drug-treated subjects versus only 4% of those receiving placebo lost at least 1.4 kg/week. However, analysis of the data from the 145 studies comparing placebo and two active drugs revealed no significant differences between any of the active drugs. Thus, in clinically effective doses, there was little basis upon which to choose between these compounds in terms of either their weight loss effectiveness or the duration over which this weight loss could be induced. In studies lasting up to 20 weeks in which sufficient numbers of patients were retained, those on any active drug lost significantly more weight than those on placebo.

FIGURE 7.3

Comparison of biphetamine and placebo

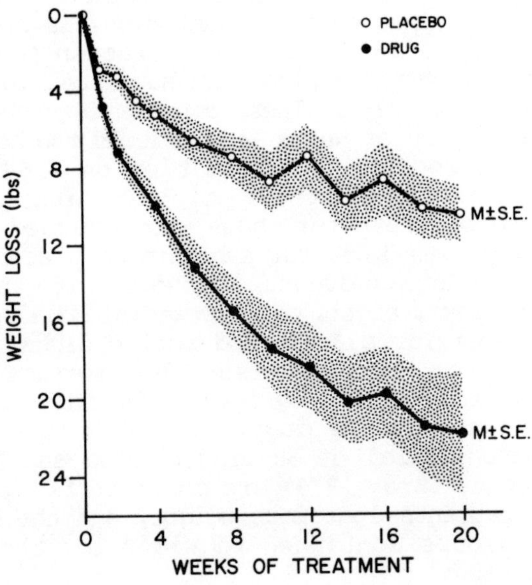

Source: Bray, G. A. 1976. The obese patient. Major problems in internal medicine, vol. 9, 1-450. Philadelphia: W. B. Saunders. Reprinted with permission.

Reports of a number of trials of appetite suppressant drugs lasting from six to 52 weeks have been published since this review by the FDA (Sullivan and Comai 1978; Stunkard 1982). The percentage of patients remaining in these trials has often been above 60%. Data from several of these studies are summarized in table 7.2. Weight loss in these studies persisted for the duration of treatment, which calls

TABLE 7.2

Double-blind clinical trials with appetite-suppressing drugs

Drug	Dosage (mg)	Duration (wks)	Number of subjects		Mean total wt. loss (gain) (kg)		Net weight loss (kg)	Diet restriction (kcal/day)
			Drug	Placebo	Drug	Placebo	(Drug)-(Placebo)	
Schedule II								
Amphetamine	5 tid	12	14	12	4.5	2.4	2.1	—
	5 tid	6	20	21	1.5	0.5	1.0	1,000
	5 tid	12	32	33	6.0	2.6	3.4	1,000
Phenmetrazine	75	6	53	53	1.8	0.6	1.2	None
	75	12	24	0	2.8	n.a.	n.a.	None
	25 bid	6	27	0	2.6	n.a.	n.a.	None
	50	6	28	0	2.0	n.a.	n.a.	None
	25 tid	6	14	12	3.9	1.2	2.7	—
Schedule III								
Clortermine	50	4	7 studies*		0.8–2.2	0.1–1.1	n.a.	None
	50	4	18 studies*		2.2–5.1	1.0–3.7	n.a.	1,000

—: Data not available. n.a.: not applicable.
*There were 2,400 patients on clortermine and 742 on placebo enrolled in these studies.

TABLE 7.2 (continued)

Drug	Dosage (mg)	Duration (wks)	Number of subjects		Mean total wt. loss (gain) (kg)		Net weight loss (kg)	Diet restriction (kcal/day)
			Drug	Placebo	Drug	Placebo	(Drug)-(Placebo)	
Chlorphentermine	65	12	29	0	2.7	n.a.	n.a.	None
Phendimetrazine	105	12	36	35	3.4	0.5	2.9	None
Schedule IV								
Diethylpropion	75	6	28	28	1.9	0.9	1.0	1,200
	75	12	23	21	6.7	4.1	2.6	Restricted
	25 tid	12	41	41	9.1	4.5	4.6	1,000
	75	25	9	4	11.7	1.6	10.1	"Strict"
	25 tid	12	22	19	4.4	1.6	2.8	1,000
	25 tid	12	21	17	6.8	4.4	2.4	1,000
Phentermine	30	16	34	36	9.2	5.2	4.0	9/1b body wt
	30	14	30	29	7.3	1.8	5.5	1,000
	30	6	78	77	3.8	1.5	2.3	1,000
	30	24	34	32	5.3	1.5	3.8	—
Fenfluramine	20 bid	6	44	43	2.4	0.3	2.1	None
	40	6	23	43	1.7	0.3	1.4	None
	20 tid	12	17	0	7.4	n.a.	n.a.	1,000

	60	12	16	0	7.9	n.a.	n.a.	1,000
	20 tid	12	56	58	6.6	2.5	4.1	None
	60	12	60	58	4.7	2.5	2.2	None
Mazindol	2	12	50	43	8.6	5.4	3.2	600
	1 tid	6	18	21	2.3	0.5	1.8	1,000
	1 tid	6	15	12	5.1	1.2	3.9	--
	1 tid	12	32	33	6.4	2.6	3.8	1,000
	1 tid	6	30	30	4.6	1.7	2.9	None
	2	12	15	15	6.9	1.6	5.3	1,200
	2	12	40	20	8.4	1.2	7.3	1,000
	2	12	27	24	8.5	6.5	2.0	1,000
	2	12	19	23	1.4	0.3	1.1	Restricted
	1 tid	8	12	13	5.2	3.8	1.4	1,200
	1 tid	12	12	9	5.2	0.5	4.7	None
	2	12	19	23	5.0	3.6	1.4	5-10/lb body wt
	1	60	11	10	14.8	10.5	4.3	800
	1-3	20	24	24	1.9	(0.7)	2.6	1,200
	1	6	15	15	1.2	(0.5)	1.7	†
	2	12	23	21	5.5	2.3	3.2	50 g carbohydrate

--: Data not available. n.a.: not applicable.

†All patients were under dietary supervision for diabetes mellitus.

Source: Adapted from Sullivan, A. C. and K. Comai. 1978. Pharmacological treatment of obesity. *Int J Obes* 2:167-89. Reprinted with permission.

into question the often stated belief that tolerance develops to these drugs. If tolerance did develop, the drugs would be expected to lose their effectiveness and patients to regain weight.

The results of one long-term trial (figure 7.4) are particularly instructive in this regard (Hudson 1977). The Royal College of General Practitioners conducted a study in which fenfluramine was administered for one year followed by placebo by one year. A weight loss plateau occurred between the eighth and twelfth months, and weight remained 10 to 11 kg (22 to 24 lb) lower for the remainder of the year. When transferred to placebo, patients regained weight. One interpretation of this result is that the drug had "reset" part of the weight control mechanism and that this effect persisted for the entire year. Three clinical findings from this study argue against tolerance. First, subjects regained weight when fenfluramine was discontinued; second, weight loss did not slow for several weeks but eventually reached a new plateau; and third, hunger did not increase during several months of treatment. These observations might provide an argument for chronic use of appetite suppressants in treatment of selected obese patients.

FIGURE 7.4

Long-term trial with fenfluramine

<u>Legend</u>: o treatment with fenfluramine
● placebo

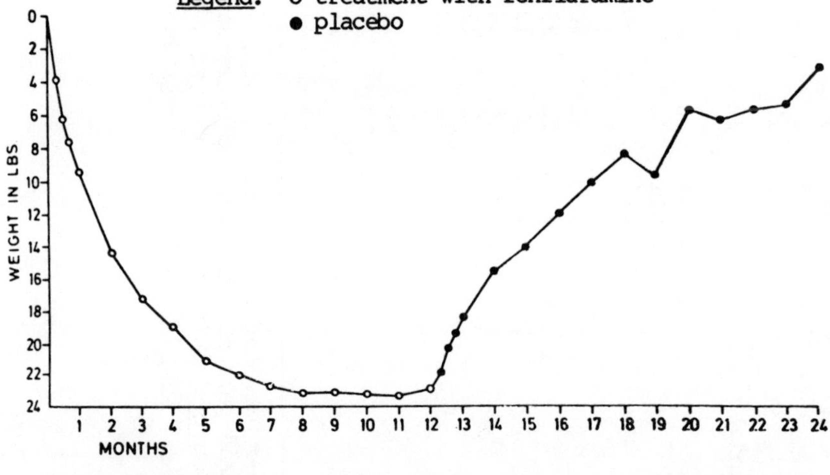

<u>Source</u>: Hudson, K. D. 1972. The anorectic and hypotensive effects of fenfluramine in obesity. <u>J R Coll Gen Pract</u> 27:497. Reprinted with permission.

Safety

The safety of appetite-suppressing drugs has also been the subject of considerable discussion. The possibility of enhanced mortality in patients taking "diet pills" has been brought to public attention in reports presented to a U.S. Senate Committee (Henry 1967; Jelliffe et al. 1969). The agents in question included not only amphetamine, but also thyroid hormone, diuretics, and laxatives. In some patients it appears that potassium loss and the ensuing hypokalemia may have been the major factors leading to death. Asher and Dietz (1972), however, in a review of deaths among patients using amphetamine and thyroid in "reasonable doses," could find no evidence for increased mortality.

An equally serious problem is the potential for drug abuse. Indeed, it is the problem of habituation to and misuse of amphetamine which has led to the professional distaste for this group of drugs. If they were not subject to abuse in our society, there would be far less concern about their use in treating obese patients. Drug abuse has been particularly common with amphetamine, methamphetamine, and phenmetrazine. Claims of drug abuse for other members of this class are much less frequent.

All of the prescription anorexiants are subject to the sanctions of the Federal Controlled Substances Act of 1970. Basically, medicinal products subject to abuse are classified into five schedules based upon accepted medical use and the potential for abuse (table 7.1).

Schedule I lists drugs or other substances with a high potential for abuse and no currently accepted medical use in treatment. Schedule I includes no appetite suppressants and is therefore not further discussed here.

Schedule II includes drugs with a high potential for abuse and a currently acceptable medical use in treatment.

Schedule III includes drugs with less abuse potential than those in Schedule II.

Schedule IV lists drugs with less abuse potential than those in Schedule III.

Schedule V lists drugs with less abuse potential than those in Schedule IV.

The prescriber should avoid the use of Schedule II drugs in the treatment of obesity.

Griffiths, Brady, and Bradfor (1979), using baboons as subjects, have examined the reinforcing properties of intravenous preparations of several anorexiant drugs in relation to their appetite-suppressing effects. Neither phenylpropanolamine nor fenfluramine was shown to exhibit any reinforcing effects. The ratio of anorexiant dose to reinforcing dose, a measure of abuse potential, is shown for several drugs in figure 7.5. At one extreme are diethylpropion and amphetamine; at the other are fenfluramine and phenylpropanolamine. Although the ratio of anorexiant dose to reinforcing dose is of some utility in predicting abuse potential, it does not always correlate with clinical experience. For example, diethylpropion has been widely used as an anorexiant, and episodes of misuse have been few. It is appropriately placed in Schedule IV. However, its anorexiant/reinforcing ratio is greater than that of amphetamine or phenmetrazine, both appropriately classified as Schedule II drugs. The absence of any reinforcing effects of fenfluramine and phenylpropanolamine is almost certainly important. (For further discussion, see Bigelow, chapter 19, this volume.)

FIGURE 7.5

Ratio of anorexiant dose to reinforcing dose of several anorexiant drugs

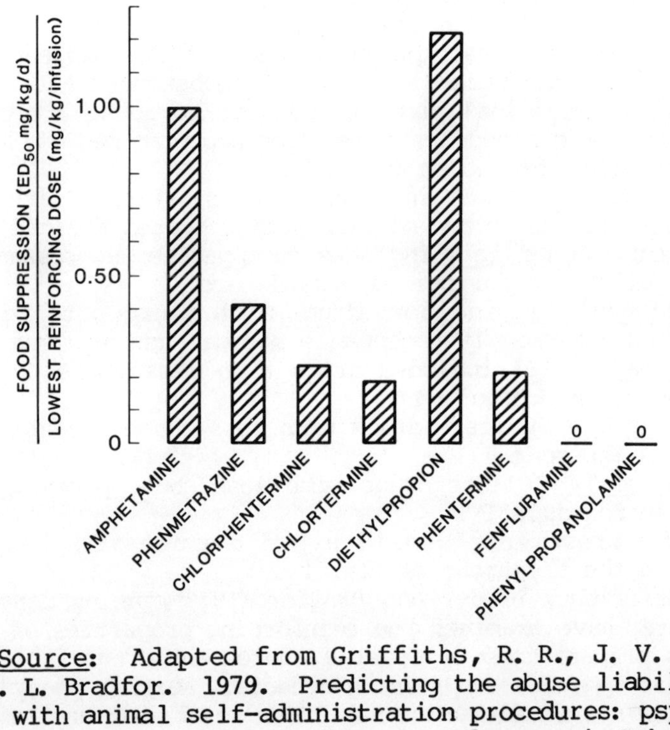

Source: Adapted from Griffiths, R. R., J. V. Brady, and D. L. Bradfor. 1979. Predicting the abuse liability of drugs with animal self-administration procedures: psychomotor stimulants and hallucinogens. Advances in Behavioral Pharmacology 2:201. Reprinted with permission.

In addition to abuse potential, there are a number of side effects associated with use of these drugs. The most common ones are summarized in table 7.3. The data given for each drug are expressed as the ratios of the percentage of drug subjects compared to the percentage of placebo subjects reporting each side effect. In instances in which the side effect was greater on placebo, the ratio is less than 1.0; if more drug subjects than placebo subjects reported the side effect, the ratio is greater than 1.0. The placebo data in the table represent the percentage of placebo subjects reporting each side effect. Since the figures in the table are based only on studies containing enough data to make comparisons possible, they should be considered only as approximations and interpreted with care. According to the studies summarized in the table, the most consistently reported side effects appear to be insomnia, dizziness, and dry mouth. The other effects generally occur less frequently, with the exception of depression and diarrhea, which are reported essentially only with fenfluramine.

General Principles for Use

From the previous discussion, it is clear that these agents can be effective as adjuncts in the treatment of obesity. Their usefulness depends on employing them as part of a total program for the treatment of obesity rather than as the sole form of treatment. Several rules should apply to their use. First, the drug abuse potential of these compounds is highest for those compounds in Schedule II (for a relevant chart of scheduled drugs, see table 7.1.) Therefore, treatment should be initiated with a preparation from Schedule III or IV. If possible, one should also select drugs with the least number of side effects. Fenfluramine should be avoided in patients with depressive tendencies and should not be used in interrupted courses of treatment. In patients with hypertension, mazindol may well be the drug of choice. In patients with diabetes, fenfluramine might be the first choice. For obese patients with or without high blood pressure or diabetes, phentermine in half strength might be combined with half-strength fenfluramine, a combination with few side effects (Weintraub et al. 1984).

With most of these drugs, fenfluramine being the notable exception, the use of intermittent courses of therapy can be as effective as continuous use of the drug (LeRiche and Csima 1967; Garrow 1981). Interrupted courses of therapy usually last for three to six weeks with discontinuation for a period at least half the length of the original period

TABLE 7.3

Side effects of various anorexiant drugs compared with those of placebo

Drugs*	Headache	Insomnia	Nervousness	Dizziness	Weakness or fatigue	Depression
Amphetamine/ Methamphetamine	2.2	6.9	2.1	6.3	0.9	1.2
Phenmetrazine	0.9	6.5	5.5	5.6	1.3	0.4
Phendimetrazine	0	4.6	1.4	6.6	—	0.9
Benzphetamine	—	2.1	7.4	2.2	0	0
Phentermine	—	3.2	—	1.6	—	1.0
Chlorphentermine	1.6	6.2	0.9	3.1	0.8	—
Clortermine	1.7	7.8	1.1	1.2	0.8	—
Diethylpropion	1.2	0.9	1.2	0.7	0.8	—
Mazindol	0.8	4.8	1.3	3.1	0.9	0.4
Fenfluramine	1.15	1.4	0.7	1.0	1.0	3.2
Placebo§	3.4	1.8	3.6	1.0	2.8	1.1

--: Data were not sufficient to make comparisons possible.

*The data given for each drug are expressed as the ratios of the percentage of drug subjects compared to the percentage of placebo subjects reporting each side effect. The placebo data represent the percentage of placebo subjects reporting each side effect.

Rise in blood pressure	Tachycardia	Palpitations	Dry mouth	Nausea	Abdominal discomfort	Constipation	Diarrhea	Edema	Polyuria or frequency
38	30	25	1.6	1.8	0.9	2.7	--	--	1.8†
5	1.7	20	3.8	3.3	0.4	1.6	--	2.3†	0
--	--	--	4.6	--	2.5	1.8	--	--	9.5†
--	--	0.7	1.7	2.0	3.0	--	--	--	--
--	--	--	-0	2.7	--	--	--	--	--
--	--	--	3.7	2.3	--	2.5	--	5.0†	--
--	--	--	3.4	1.1	--	2.5	--	2.6†	--
--	--	--	1.2	3.2	1.3	1.8	--	--	--
0	--	16	3.5	3.4	0.6	0.9	--	--	3.3†
--	--	--	3.0	1.1	--	--	7.2	--	1.5†
0.1	0.3	0.1	3.1	1.4	2.7	3.7	0	1.8	0

†Percentage of patients reporting the symptom.

§Placebo-treated patients also experienced dysuria (0.3%) and chills (0.1%).

Source: Compiled by the author. Data derived from publications referenced in: Bray, G. A. 1976. The obese patient. Major problems in internal medicine, vol. 9:1-450. Philadelphia: W. B. Saunders.

of treatment. Because of the tendency to postdrug depression in some patients, the dosage of fenfluramine should be gradually tapered off as treatment ends. Some of these drugs have been used with apparent effectiveness in children and in pregnant women, but for the present it would be wise not to use these drugs in either group.

CLINICAL PREPARATIONS

There are presently 12 drugs in the appetite suppressant group available in the United States. Eleven of them require a prescription and one, phenylpropanolamine, is available as an over-the-counter preparation. To supplement the following discussion of these drugs, the reader may wish to consult other sources for more details about specific drugs (AMA Drug Evaluation 1983; Samuel and Burland 1976; Silverstone 1983).

Over-the-Counter Drugs

Phenylpropanolamine is the generic name for isomers of norephedrine. In the United States the preparation sold as phenylpropanolamine is the racemic mixture of (+)- and (-)-norephedrine. In Europe, on the other hand, the most commonly used anorexiant form of phenylpropanolamine is (+)-norpseudoephedrine.

The clinical use of phenylpropanolamine for weight loss was first described by Hirsh (1939), but the best early study of its weight loss effects was done by Kalb (1942). He administered (±)-phenylpropanolamine (Propadrine®) in doses of 25 or 45 mg accompanied by an oral anesthetic to 216 and 464 patients, while another group of 1,200 patients received (+)-amphetamine in 10 to 20 mg dosages. The patients receiving Propadrine® or amphetamine demonstrated a decrease in appetite in 40% to 45% of the cases, as compared to a decrease in only 12% of the 100 control patients.

More recently, Hoebel et al. (1975) conducted a double-blind, crossover trial in which phenylpropanolamine (25 mg) or placebo was given three times daily to 70 subjects. During the initial two-week phase of the study, the subjects receiving phenylpropanolamine lost more weight than did those on placebo, although the difference was not statistically significant. In the two-week crossover period, however, the difference in weight loss between the phenylpropanolamine and placebo groups increased, becoming statistically significant. In addition, Hoebel and his colleagues found no difference between the two groups in either ease in going to sleep or feelings of energy. Thus it appears that this drug, which has minimal effects on the central nervous system, may be a useful agent in the treatment of obesity.

Griboff, Berman, and Silverman (1975) compared the effects of phenylpropanolamine (25 mg), combined with caffeine (100 mg) and multivitamins, versus those of a placebo, taken three times daily for five weeks by 77 adult subjects. The median total weight loss was 5 lb (2.27 kg) for those on phenylpropanolamine plus caffeine and 4 lb (1.81 kg) for those on placebo. Only 12% of the placebo-treated group lost 10 lb or more during the five-week study compared to 27% of the drug-treated group.

Altschuler et al. (1982) reported on three studies of phenylpropanolamine/caffeine combinations. In the first study, phenylpropanolamine (35 mg*) and caffeine (140 mg), given twice daily, were compared with placebo for six weeks. The second study compared a preparation of phenylpropanolamine (50 mg) plus caffeine (200 mg) to mazindol (2 mg), given once daily for six weeks. In the third trial, phenylpropanolamine (25 mg) and caffeine (100 mg) were compared with diethylpropion (25 mg), taken three times daily for an eight-week period. In the comparison with placebo the 28 placebo-treated patients lost an average total of 0.94 kg in six weeks, which was significantly less than the weight loss of 2.10 kg for the 28 phenylpropanolamine-treated patients. In the other two trials of phenylpropanolamine compared to established appetite suppressant drugs, there were no significant differences in weight loss between the groups.

In a review of published and unpublished clinical trials with phenylpropanolamine, Weintraub concluded that phenylpropanolamine has a "modest but consistent effect in helping people lose weight" (chapter 5, this volume). He cited FDA data indicating that the average user was a woman under 45 years of age who was less than 4.5 kg above ideal body weight. Two preparations of phenylpropanolamine were used in the studies he surveyed, either phenylpropanolamine alone or in combination with caffeine. The sale of the phenylpropanolamine/caffeine combination is no longer allowed. The phenylpropanolamine preparations were compared with either placebo or active prescription drugs such as mazindol or diethylpropion in trials lasting between two and 12 weeks. Although most of the studies had parallel group designs, a few crossover design studies were also performed.

---

*The published report erroneously listed the dosage administered as 37.5 mg phenylpropanolamine.

In the studies comparing phenylpropanolamine preparations to placebo, subjects receiving phenylpropanolamine lost an average of approximately 0.2 kg/week more than did those on placebo; this finding is consistent with the average 0.25 kg/week weight loss difference between drug- and placebo-treated patients reported in the Scoville (1976) publication discussed earlier in this article. In the comparisons of phenylpropanolamine with either mazindol or diethylpropion described by Weintraub, the rates of reported weight loss were similar.

Because phenylpropanolamine is available over-the-counter, its patterns of use may be quite different from those of prescription drugs. In a survey of students at Michigan State University conducted by Vener and Krupka (see chapter 8, this volume), 45.5% of the women and 5.9% of the men reported having used this drug at least once and 27.3% of the women and 3.5% of the men said they had taken a phenylpropanolamine-containing preparation sometime during the previous year. On a self-perception scale 84.8% of the phenylpropanolamine users rated themselves as being slightly to markedly overweight, while 29.2% thought they were of average weight or slightly underweight.

In one controlled study, Silverman et al. (1980) reported minimal side effects from orally administered phenylpropanolamine. However, there have been a number of reports from Australia (McEwen 1983), Great Britain, Sweden, and the United States of increases in blood pressure associated with phenylpropanolamine consumption. Although most of these cases have occurred after ingestion of higher than recommended doses of phenylpropanolamine, there have been sporadic reports of increased blood pressure after doses as low as 50 mg. The differences between reports of phenylpropanolamine-related hypertensive problems from European and Australian centers and data from the United States may be related to the pharmacologic effects resulting from the different stereoisomers of phenylpropanolamine which are marketed in these areas (see Morgan, chapter 11, this volume).

Several studies have examined the effects of phenylpropanolamine on blood pressure under controlled circumstances. In a review of these studies, Krakoff (chapter 13, this volume) stated that a dose of 75 mg of phenylpropanolamine was reported to be associated with a small but statistically significant increase in blood pressure two to six hours after ingestion. It should be kept in mind, however, that the hypertensive effects of phenylpropanolamine can be enhanced in people who are taking MAO blocking drugs or drugs which inhibit the reuptake of catecholamines into the nerve terminals. It would thus appear prudent to advise individuals with high blood pressure not to use preparations containing phenylpropanolamine.

Prescription Drugs

The remaining 11 appetite suppressants available in the United States are obtainable by prescription only and, because of their potential for abuse and diversion, are scheduled. Most are in Schedules IV and III, but those considered highly subject to abuse are in Schedule II.

Schedule IV

Phentermine (Ionamin®; Fastin®; Adipex®). This compound is available as a resin in 15 or 30 mg capsules and in tablets. Because of its alpha-carbon substitution, phentermine causes less stimulation of the central nervous system than does amphetamine. It can, however, increase blood pressure and produce tachycardia. Insomnia can be a significant side effect with this compound. It was reported by 20% of the patients observed by Steel, Munro, and Duncan (1973); however, the overall average of this side effect indicated in table 7.3 is about 6.0%. Dry mouth may also be a complaint. Because this compound has fewer effects on the central nervous system, it is preferable to the drugs in Schedule II or III.

Diethylpropion (Tenuate®; Tepanil®). This compound is available in 25 mg tablets and 75 mg sustained-release capsules. The introduction of a keto-group on the beta-carbon of the phenethylamine side chain lowers the incidence of side effects due to CNS stimulation. CNS stimulation was observed in less than 1% of 752 patients. Diethylpropion has only minimal effects on blood pressure and respiration, and it rarely alters the electrocardiogram (ECG), even after intravenous injection in patients with hypertension, early congestive failure, coronary artery disease, or angina pectoris. Intermittent courses of therapy are probably the preferred mode of administration. However, continuous therapy for up to 24 weeks has resulted in significantly greater weight loss for diethylpropion-treated subjects than for those receiving placebo (Bray 1976). This drug has been shown to be effective in patients with cardiovascular disease, in those with diabetes mellitus, and in obese children. There have been a few reports of drug abuse. Because of its wide use and relative lack of significant side effects and low tendency to habituation, this is one of the drugs with highest recommendation for use.

Fenfluramine (Pondimin®). This compound is available in 20 mg tablets. It was first used in France and has been studied in trials throughout the world (Burland 1976; Craighead, Stunkard, and O'Brien 1981). It is a unique compound in having a trifluoromethyl substitution on the beta-position of the phenyl ring. This drug differs from the other members of this group in its effects on the central nervous system. In EEG studies, it has been found to act more like a barbiturate than an amphetamine-like drug, producing sedation and slowing of brain waves rather than stimulation. Fenfluramine is almost entirely free of addictive potential. Its major side effects are the diarrhea and depression observed in a significant number of patients. Numerous studies have shown it to be a clinically effective drug in producing more weight loss than observed with placebo. Although it has been suggested that plasma levels of fenfluramine are predictive of weight loss, this has not been confirmed (Pietrusko et al. 1982). It is effective in treating patients with hypertension, as well as obese diabetics and obese children.

Mazindol (Sanorex®, Mazanor®). This compound is available in 1 and 2 mg tablets. Its side effects include mild stimulation of the central nervous system, insomnia, dizziness, and dry mouth. Its tendency to stimulate the cardiovascular system is less than that of phenethylamine derivatives. In a study of the effects of mazindol on overweight diabetics, the insulin requirements of two of the four patients on insulin were reduced when they lost weight, but were unchanged in the other two (Sanders and Beridahl 1976). Although mazindol is listed in Schedule IV, its potential for drug abuse has not been established. In multicenter trials it has been shown to be effective in weight loss (Walker, Ballard, and Gold 1977; Johnson and Hughes 1979; Bandisode and Boshell 1975). The anorexiant efficacy of mazindol has led to its use in research on the effects of weight loss. In one study in which hypertensive patients were treated with mazindol, it was thought that weight loss might result in a reduction in blood pressure, but no blood pressure decrease was found to occur. Weight loss with mazindol is significantly greater than with placebo but there is no obvious difference between this drug and other compounds.

Schedule III

Phendimetrazine (Plegine®). This drug is available in 35 mg tablets. It has two methyl groups on the nitrogen of the ring structure and is metabolized in humans to phenmetrazine. Its effects on the cardiac and respiratory systems in dogs and cats are less prominent than with phenmetrazine. Tachycardia and alterations in the ECG are not produced with phendimetrazine. Although it was one of the earliest drugs on the market, there have been few recent studies of phendimetrazine (Sash 1982), which suggests that it may have been eclipsed by other drugs.

Benzphetamine (Didrex®). This compound is available in 25 mg and 50 mg tablets. Its side effects are generally similar to those observed with amphetamine. In a study by Poindexter (1960), however, benzphetamine and phenmetrazine were found to have fewer side effects than amphetamine. There is little to recommend this compound over those in Schedule IV and probably it produces more euphoria.

Chlorphentermine (Pre-Sate). This drug is available in 65 mg tablets as a sustained-release preparation and was first used in Europe in 1960 and in the United States in 1965. The introduction of chlorine into the phenyl ring reduces the tendency for CNS stimulation. Some patients have actually complained about the lack of CNS stimulation. Its major side effects include dry mouth, nausea, vertigo, and edema. In addition, the restlessness and insomnia noted with many of the compounds discussed above can also be found with this drug. In the early clinical trials, chlorphentermine was shown to produce significant weight loss. Its anorexiant effect is comparable to that observed with amphetamine, phenmetrazine, and diethylpropion. This drug would appear to be the most useful agent in Schedule III, because of its reduced tendency towards CNS stimulation and its documented effectiveness in reducing weight loss.

Clortermine (Voranil). This compound is available in 50 mg tablets and was released by the FDA for use in the United States in 1973. It seems to be similar in most respects to chlorphentermine. It induces significant weight loss and would appear to merit consideration along with chlorphentermine.

Schedule II

Phenmetrazine (Preludin®). This is marketed in tablets of 25 mg and in sustained-action capsules of 50 mg. It stimulates the central nervous system, produces hyperthermia, elevates the blood pressure, and can cause mydriasis and tachycardia; these side effects are less common with the long-acting preparations. One of the most serious potential side effects of this drug is the appearance of a toxic psychosis which is indistinguishable from the psychosis sometimes observed with amphetamine. As with amphetamine and methamphetamine, phenmetrazine has a significant history of drug abuse and may be injected intravenously by misusers. Phenmetrazine has been shown to be effective for weight loss in both adults and children, although to no greater degree than other anorexiant drugs. Because of the frequency of abuse of this compound, it has had only a limited role in the treatment of obesity (Kalb and Mullins 1958).

Dextroamphetamine. This drug has been prescribed alone or with various additives such as prochlorperazine, meprobamate, vitamins, and barbiturates (Rosenberg 1953). The anorexiant dosage ranges from 5 to 30 mg/day (Resnick and Joubert 1967; Silverstone and Stunkard 1968). Insomnia and hyperactivity are present in a high percentage of patients treated with this compound. Because this compound elevates blood pressure and has a significant tendency to be misused (Edison 1971), it is doubtful that it has any present role in the treatment of obesity, even though it is the least expensive of the compounds on the market (Adlersberg and Mayer 1949; Edwards and Swyer 1950; Freed and Mizel 1952; Gelvin and McGavack 1949; Goodman and Housel 1954; Rosenthal and Solomon 1940; Schapiro and Bogran 1960).

Methamphetamine. This compound is available under a variety of trade names in both tablet and injectable form. Its side effects are similar to those observed with amphetamine, but it may have a higher tendency to stimulate the central nervous system. The CNS stimulation and euphoria associated with methamphetamine have led to its widespread abuse. Because of the high frequency of abuse, there would appear to be minimal indication for the use of this compound in treating obese patients.

In summary, among the group of compounds listed in table 7.1, those in Schedule IV merit initial consideration in the treatment of obese patients, although they should be used only as adjuncts in treatment. Among patients with a history of depression or mental illness, phenylpropanolamine, phentermine, mazindol, or diethylpropion might be used, although fenfluramine probably should not be. Among diabetics, fenfluramine might be the drug of choice. For hypertensive patients, phentermine, mazindol, and diethylpropion would appear to be the first choice. The value of intermittent or interrupted courses of therapy should be kept in mind (Munro et al. 1968; Garrow 1981; LeRiche and Csima 1967).

REFERENCES

Adlersberg, D. and E. Mayer. 1949. Results of prolonged medical treatment of obesity with diet alone, diet and thyroid preparations, and diet and amphetamine. J Clin Endocrinol 9:275-84.

Altschuler, S. et al. 1982. Three controlled trials of weight loss with phenylpropanolamine. Int J Obes 6:549-56.

American Medical Association. 1983. AMA Drug Evaluations, 5th ed. Chicago: American Medical Association.

Arch, J.R.S. 1981. The contribution of increased thermogenesis to the effect of anorectic drugs on body composition in mice. Am J Clin Nutr 34:2763-69.

Asher, W. L. and R. E. Dietz. 1972. Effectiveness of weight reduction involving "diet pills". Current Therapeutic Research 14:510-24.

Bahnsen, P., E. Jacobson, and H. Thesleff. 1938. The subjective effect of beta-phenylisopropylaminsulfate on normal adults. Acta Med Scand 97:89-131.

Bandisode, M. S. and B. R. Boshell. 1975. Double-blind clinical evaluation of mazindol in obese diabetics. Current Therapeutic Research 18:816.

Blundell, J. E. 1984. Systems and interactions: an approach to the pharmacology of eating and hunger. Res Publ Assoc New Med Dis 62:39-65.

Blundell, J. E. and C. J. Latham. 1980. Characterisation of adjustments to the structure of feeding behaviour following pharmacological treatment: effects of amphetamine and fenfluramine and the antagonism produced by pimozide and methergoline. Pharmacol Biochem Behav 12:717-22.

Blundell, J. E. and P. J. Rogers. 1980. Effects of anorexic drugs on food intake, food selection and preferences and hunger motivation and subjective experiences. Appetite 1:151-65.

Bray, G. A. 1982. Current concepts: obesity, 4-52. Kalamazoo, MI: The Upjohn Company.

———. 1976. The obese patient. Major problems in internal medicine, vol. 9:1-450. Philadelphia: W. B. Saunders.

Bray, G. A. and F. L. Greenway. 1976. Pharmacological approaches to treating the obese patient. Clin Endocrinol Metab 5:455-79.

Brindley, D. N. 1983. Phenylethylamines and their effect on the synthesis of fatty acids, triacylglycerols and phospholipids. In Biochemical pharmacology of obesity, edited by P. B. Curtis-Prior, 285-308. New York: Elsevier Science.

Burland, W. L. 1976. Review of experience with fenfluramine. In Obesity in perspective. Fogarty International Center for Advanced Studies in the Health Sciences, Series on Preventive Medicine, vol. II, edited by G. A. Bray, 429-40. Washington, D.C.: U.S. Government Printing Office.

Craighead, L. W., A. J. Stunkard, and R. M. O'Brien. 1981. Behavior therapy and pharmacotherapy for obesity. Arch Gen Psychiatry 38:763-68.

Curtis-Prior, P. B., ed. 1983. Biochemical pharmacology of obesity. New York: Elsevier Science.

Dannenburg, W. N. 1983. Metabolic effects of phenylethylamine drugs on glucose and fatty acids in various tissues. In Biochemical pharmacology of obesity, edited by P. B. Curtis-Prior, 264-83. New York: Elsevier Science.

Douglas, J. G. and J. F. Munro. 1982. Drug treatment and obesity. Pharmacol Ther 18:351-73.

Dring, L. G. 1983. Kinetics and metabolism of the phenylethylamine anorectic drugs. In Biochemical pharmacology of obesity, edited by P. B. Curtis-Prior, 221-39. New York: Elsevier Science.

Edeleano, L. 1887. Uber einige derivate der phenylmethacrylsaure und der phenylisobuttersaure. Ber Deutsch Chem Ges 20:616-22.

Edison, G. R. 1971. Amphetamines: a dangerous illusion. Ann Intern Med 74:605-10.

Edwards, D.A.W. and G.I.M. Swyer. 1950. Comparative values of dextroamphetamine sulphate, dried thyroid gland and placebo in the treatment of obesity. Clin Sci 9:115-26.

Franklin, R. B., L. G. Dring, and R. T. Williams. 1977. The metabolism of phenmetrazine in man and laboratory animals. In Drug metabolism and disposition, edited by Ken Leidman, 223-33. Rockville, MD: The American Society for Pharmacology and Experimental Therapeutics.

Freed, S. C. and M. Mizel. 1952. The use of amphetamine combinations for appetite suppression. Ann Intern Med 36:1492-97.

Garattini, S. and R. Samanin, eds. 1978. Central mechanism of anorectic drugs. New York: Raven Press.

Garrow, J. S. 1981. Treat obesity seriously. London: Churchill-Livingstone.

Gelvin, E. P. and T. H. McGavack. 1949. Dexedrine and weight reduction. NY State J Med 49:279-82.

Gillin, J. C. et al. 1975. Differential effects of d- and l-amphetamine on the sleep of depressed patients. Life Sci 17:1233-40.

Goodman, E. L. and E. L. Housel. 1954. The effect of d-amphetamine sulfate in the treatment of the obese hypertensive patient. Am J Med Sci 227:250-54.

Griboff, S. I., R. Berman, and H. I. Silverman. 1975. A double-blind clinical evaluation of a phenylpropanolamine-caffeine-vitamin combination and a placebo in the treatment of exogenous obesity. Current Therapeutic Research 17:535-43.

Griffiths, R. R., J. V. Brady, and D. L. Bradfor. 1979. Predicting the abuse liability of drugs with animal drug self-administration procedures: psychomotor stimulants and hallucinogens. Advances in Behavioral Pharmacology 2:173-208.

Harris, S. C., A. C. Ivy, and L. M. Searle. 1947. The mechanism of amphetamine-induced loss of weight. JAMA 134:1468-75.

Heil, G. and S. Ross. 1976. Chemical agents affecting appetite. In Obesity in perspective. Fogarty International Center for Advanced Studies in the Health Sciences, Series on Preventive Medicine, vol. II, edited by G. A. Bray, 409-18. Washington, D.C.: U.S. Government Printing Office.

Henry, R. C. 1967. Weight reduction pills. JAMA 201: 895-96.

Hirsh, L. S. 1939. Controlling appetite in obesity. J of Medicine (Cincinnati) 20:84-86.

Hoebel, B. G. et al. 1975. Body weight decreased in humans by phenylpropanolamine taken before meals. Obesity and Bariatric Medicine 4:200-206.

Hudson, K. D. 1977. The anorectic and hypotensive effect of fenfluramine in obesity. J R Coll Gen Pract 27:497.

Jelliffe, R. W. et al. 1969. Death from weight-control pills: a case with objective postmortem confirmation. JAMA 208:1843-47.

Johnson, W. G. and J. R. Hughes. 1979. Mazindol: its efficacy and mode of action in generating weight loss. Addict Behav 4:237-44.

Kalb, A. and A. G. Mullins. 1958. Dangers of Preludin. Br Med J 1:1355.

Kalb, S. W. 1942. The effect of amphetamine (benzedrine) sulfate, propadrine and propadrine hydrochloride in combination with sodium delvinal on the appetite of obese patients. J Med Soc N J 39:584-86.

Kirby, M. J. and P. Turner. 1977. The effect of methysergide and other receptor antagonists on fenfluramine-induced glucose uptake in the isolated rat hemidiaphragm. Arch Int Pharmacodyn Ther 225:25-28.

LeRiche, W. H. and A. Csima. 1967. A long-acting appetite suppressant drug studied for 24 weeks in both continuous and sequential admission. Can Med Assoc J 97:1016-20.

Lesses, M. F. and A. Myerson. 1938. Human autonomic pharmacology XVI: Benzedrine sulfate as an aid in the treatment of obesity. N Engl J Med 218:119-24.

Levitsky, D. A., B. J. Strupp, and J. Lupoli. 1981. Tolerance to anorectic drugs: pharmacological or artifactual. Pharmacol Biochem Behav 14:661-67.

Martin, W. R. et al. 1971. Physiologic, subjective and behavioral effects of amphetamine, methamphetamine, ephedrine, phenmetrazine and methylphenidate in man. Clin Pharmacol Ther 12:245-58.

McArthur, R. A. and J. E. Blundell. 1983. Protein and carbohydrate self-selection: modification of the effects of fenfluramine and amphetamine by age and feeding regimen. Appetite 4:113-24.

McEwen, J. 1983. Phenylpropanolamine-associated hypertension after the use of "over-the-counter" appetite suppressant products. Med J Aust 2:71-73.

Munro, J. F. et al. 1968. Comparison of continuous and intermittent anorectic therapy in obesity. Br Med J 1:352-54.

Paul, S. M. et al. 1982. (±)-Amphetamine binding to rat hypothalamus: relation to anorexic potency of phenylethylamines. Science 218:487-89.

Pietrusko, R. et al. 1982. Plasma fenfluramine levels, weight loss and side effects: a failure to find a relationship. Int J Obes 6:567-71.

Poindexter, A. 1960. Appetite suppressant drugs: a controlled clinical comparison of benzphetamine, phenmetrazine, d-amphetamine and placebo. Current Therapeutic Research 2:354-63.

Resnick, M. and L. Joubert. 1967. A double-blind evaluation of an anorexiant, a placebo and diet alone in obese subjects. Can Med Assoc J 97:1011-15.

Rogers, P. J. and J. E. Blundell. 1979. Effect of anorexic drugs on food intake and the micro-structure of eating in human subjects. Psychopharmacology (Berlin) 66:159-65.

Rosenberg, P. 1953. The use of mood ameliorating agents in the treatment of psychogenic obesity. American Practitioner and Digest of Treatment 4:818-20.

Rosenthal, G. and H. A. Solomon. 1940. Benzedrine sulfate in obesity. Endocrinology 26:807-12.

Safer, D. J., R. P. Allen, and E. Barr. 1975. Growth rebound after termination of stimulant drugs. J Pediatr 86:113-16.

Samuel, P. D. and W. L. Burland. 1976. Drug treatment of obesity. In Obesity in perspective. Fogarty International Center for Advanced Studies in the Health Sciences, Series on Preventive Medicine, vol. II, edited by G. A. Bray, 419-28. Washington, D.C.: U.S. Government Printing Office.

Sanders, M. and H. Beridahl. 1976. The effect of an anorectic agent (mazindol) on control of obese diabetics. Med J Aust 63:576-77.

Sash, S. E. 1982. The anorectic effects of Obex-LA (d-phendimetrazine bitartrate) in the treatment of obesity. Current Therapeutic Research 31:181-84.

Schapiro, M. M. and N. Bogran. 1960. Dietless weight loss with benzphetamine (Didrex): a controlled comparison with phenmetrazine and placebo. Current Therapeutic Research 2:333-45.

Scoville, B. A. 1976. Review of amphetamine-like drugs by the Food and Drug Administration. In Obesity in perspective. Fogarty International Center for Advanced Studies in the Health Sciences, Series on Preventive Medicine, vol. II, edited by G. A. Bray, 441-43. Washington, D.C.: U.S. Government Printing Office.

Silverman, H. I. et al. 1980. Lack of side effects from orally administered phenylpropanolamine and phenylpropanolamine with caffeine: a controlled three-phase study. Current Therapeutic Research 28:185-94.

Silverstone, J. T. 1983. Psychopharmacology of hunger and food intake in humans. Pharmacol Ther 19:417-34.

Silverstone, J. T. and A. J. Stunkard. 1968. The anorectic effect of dexamphetamine sulphate. Br J Pharmacol 33:513-22.

Simpson, L. 1979. The effect of behavioral stimulant doses of amphetamine on blood pressure. Arch Gen Psychiat 33:691.

Steel, J. M., J. F. Munro, and L.J.P. Duncan. 1973. A comparative trial of different regimens of fenfluramine and phentermine in obesity. Practitioner 211:232-36.

Stunkard, A. J. 1982. Anorectic agents lower a body weight set point. Life Sci 30:2043-55.

Sullivan, A. C. and K. Comai. 1978. Pharmacological treatment of obesity. Int J Obes 2:167-89.

Turtle, J. R. and J. A. Burgess. 1973. Hypoglycemic action of fenfluramine in diabetes mellitus. Diabetes 22:858-67.

Van Kammen, D. P. and D. L. Murphy. 1975. Attenuation of the euphoriant and activating effects of d- and l-amphetamine by lithium carbonate treatment. Psychopharmacologia 44:215-24.

Walker, B. R., I. M. Ballard, and J. A. Gold. 1977. A multi-center study comparing mazindol and placebo in obese patients. J Int Med Res 5:85-90.

Weintraub, M. et al. 1984. A double-blind clinical trial in weight control: use of fenfluramine and phentermine alone and in combination. Arch Intern Med 144:1143-48.

Wichelow, M. J. and W.J.H. Butterfield. 1970. Effects of fenfluramine on peripheral glucose metabolism in man. In Amphetamines and related compounds. Proc Mario Negri Instit Pharmacol Res, Italy, edited by E. S. Garattini, 611-18. New York: Raven Press.

Wilson, T. A., T. Melton, and W. L. Clarke. 1983. The effect of fenfluramine and caloric restriction on carbohydrate homeostasis in patients with lipodystrophy. Diabetes Care 6:160-65.

8

OVER-THE-COUNTER ANOREXIANTS: USE AND PERCEPTIONS AMONG YOUNG ADULTS

Arthur M. Vener and Lawrence R. Krupka

INTRODUCTION

The use of over-the-counter (OTC) medicinals by adolescents and young adults has not been studied extensively. National drug surveys have been primarily concerned with alcohol and cigarettes, with illicit drugs such as cocaine, heroin, and cannabis, and with illegally diverted drugs such as methaqualone hydrochloride and the barbiturates (O'Donnell et al. 1976; Abelson, Fishburne, and Cisin 1977; Johnston, Bachman, and O'Malley 1977). With possibly two exceptions (Johnston, Bachman, and O'Malley 1977; Krupka and Vener 1983), no survey has obtained data regarding the prevalence of use of OTC stimulants and diet aids.

Employing samples of young adults attending college, we have studied some of the social, psychological, and biological factors associated with the ingestion of such OTC drugs as caffeine (Krupka and Vener 1981; Vener and Krupka 1982) and phenylpropanolamine hydrochloride (PPA) (Krupka and Vener 1983). In one study, we found that college students had inadequate knowledge about proper dieting, calorie utilization, ideal body weight, and the health problems associated with weight gain or loss. We also discovered that biology textbooks do not adequately cover such nutritional topics as the calorie content of foods, caloric expenditure from various physical activities, and the character of or factors involved in obesity, anorexia, and bulimia (Vener and Krupka 1985). Since the discussion of nutrition is incomplete in standard texts and since only half of the high school students enrolled in biology classes will ever take another formal science course (Hurd et al. 1980), it is likely that many college students will never obtain adequate nutritional information.

In the United States and other developed countries, eating disorders such as obesity, anorexia, and bulimia are now not uncommon. If the condition of obesity is defined as being 20% above ideal weight, then a quarter of the United States population can be classified as obese (Cohen 1978). In one study, the prevalence of anorexia nervosa was estimated to be one in 200 for female Caucasians between the ages of 12 and 18 (Alford and Bogle 1982) and, in another, one in 250 (Powers 1980). Of individuals diagnosed as anorexic, 10% to 15% eventually die from this disorder (Alford and Bogle 1982). It has been estimated that bulimia, an eating disorder closely related to anorexia, occurs in approximately 15% to 25% of college women in the United States (Anorexia nervosa and bulimia 1982). An indication of the concern women have regarding weight is our finding that six times more women than men use diet colas such as Tab® (Vener and Krupka 1982).

Seldom does one encounter complimentary remarks regarding those who carry excessive weight (Maddox, Back, and Liederman 1968). Fat children are perceived as being argumentative, forgetful, lazy, untruthful, sloppy, naughty, mean, ugly, dirty, and stupid (Staffieri 1967). We have found that college students are more reluctant to marry the obese than to marry cocaine users, ex-mental patients, shoplifters, the sexually promiscuous, communists, the blind, atheists, marihuana users, and the divorced. More men than women were disinclined to marry the obese (Vener, Krupka, and Gerard 1982). We also discovered that the obese are stigmatized to approximately the same degree as prostitutes and embezzlers. The obese find it difficult to obtain jobs that require attractiveness as a prime criterion of employment, e.g., flight attendant, receptionist, television commentator, hostess, or maître d'hôtel. Appearance seems to be a crucial element in interpersonal relationships. Body configurations help to establish the social identity of strangers when they are first encountered (Goffman 1963). When physical attributes are viewed as extremely discrediting, they stigmatize the individual as having somehow failed or as possessing a serious shortcoming (Cahnman 1968).

To date, only two studies have investigated the prevalence of use of OTC diet pills containing phenylpropanolamine. In 1982 a national probability survey of student drug use found that 42% of high school senior women had consumed such products during their lifetime, 30% within the past year, and 2% had ingested them daily in the past month (Johnston, Bachman, and O'Malley 1982). In our study of 944 college students (18 to 21 years old), we also found that

30% of the women had consumed OTC diet preparations during the year prior to being interviewed (Krupka and Vener 1983).

The active agent in most OTC diet products sold in the United States is phenylpropanolamine, a sympathomimetic amine that shares the pharmacological properties of ephedrine and is approximately equal to it in potency, except that it causes less central nervous system (CNS) stimulation (Innes and Nickerson 1975). Phenylpropanolamine is also commonly used as an orally administered nasal decongestant. The Physicians' Desk Reference (PDR) for 1977 included entries for 56 products containing phenylpropanolamine, only one of which was specifically classified as an anorexiant. By 1984, the number of products containing phenylpropanolamine listed in the PDR had increased to 95, eight of which were indicated for weight control. The 1983 PDR for Nonprescription Drugs listed 75 products containing phenylpropanolamine, including ten specifically designated as anorexiants.

Adverse reactions associated with phenylpropanolamine taken in normal and excess doses and in combination with other drugs have been reported in the literature. These include hypertension, stroke, acute renal failure, rhabdomyolysis, arrhythmias, excitation, psychotic disturbances, and convulsive seizures. Individuals with high blood pressure, heart disease, diabetes, or kidney or thyroid problems are advised either not to use phenylpropanolamine or to use it only with extreme care (Physicians' desk reference 1984). Consumers are also cautioned to avoid its use if they are taking antihypertensive or antidepressive drugs containing monoamine oxidase inhibitors or other medications containing sympathomimetic amines. Pregnant women, nursing mothers, and individuals under the age of 18 are also advised not to use it (Physicians' desk reference 1983). Further, the effectiveness of phenylpropanolamine as an appetite suppressant is controversial. One article has maintained that it has no anorexiant effect at all (Fazekas et al. 1959), another that its effect is primarily placebo-like (Hoebel 1978), while still others have argued that it is very effective (Griboff, Berman, and Silverman 1975; Silverman et al. 1980). In this paper, we will report the findings of our three surveys regarding the patterns of usage and perceived effectiveness of OTC diet products containing phenylpropanolamine.

SURVEYS OF USE BY YOUNG ADULTS OF OTC DRUGS CONTAINING PHENYLPROPANOLAMINE

Methods

Samples

The three surveys reported here were based on different samples of undergraduate students (ages 18 to 21) attending Michigan State University, which has an enrollment of approximately 40,000. Respondents were randomly selected from students in required courses. The sample sizes and study dates of the surveys are listed below:

Survey	Sample size	No. of women	No. of men	Study date
I	944	561	383	Winter 1982
II	425	253	172	Spring 1982
III	1,061	554	507	Winter 1984

Instruments

The instruments used in Surveys I and III were pretested, self-administered questionnaires with both open-ended and closed items. Questions in both surveys elicited information regarding the patterns of use of OTC appetite suppressants containing phenylpropanolamine. Survey III had additional questions designed to obtain more detailed information concerning prevalence and recent use and to corroborate the findings of Survey I. In Survey I those who had used appetite suppressants containing phenylpropanolamine were also asked to judge the effectiveness of the substances. In both surveys, respondents were asked to indicate whether they thought they were very or slightly overweight, of average weight, or slightly or very underweight. Survey III also included questions on preferred methods for weight loss, current medical conditions, and self-esteem.* The instrument employed in Survey II consisted of a checklist of all OTC brand-name drugs containing phenylpropanolamine included in the 1981 *PDR for Nonprescription Drugs*; subjects were asked to indicate which brands they had taken during the previous year.

---

*Abstracted and slightly modified measures of self-esteem were taken from *The antecedents of self-esteem* (Coopersmith 1967).

Results

Prevalence, Recency, and Duration of Use

Table 8.1 shows the low prevalence of usage of OTC diet products containing phenylpropanolamine among men in Surveys I and III. Whereas almost half the women (45.5%) had ingested them sometime during their lives, as few as one out of every 17 men had done so (5.9%). More than one-quarter of the women (27.3%) but only one in 29 men (3.5%) reported having used these substances within the previous year. A relatively small percentage of both men and women reported having consumed these products within the previous 24 hours, with usage by women again being higher (women, 3.1%; men, 0.4%). In all three time frames, women reported nearly an eightfold greater percentage of use. Data analyses of Surveys I and III showed no statistically significant differences between surveys in the prevalence of appetite suppressant consumption by either men or women in the 12 months prior to the interview, with the average for women being 27.3% and for men, 3.5%. Survey I did not investigate either lifetime usage or consumption during the previous 24 hours. Additionally, 24 women (9.5%) reported that they had used OTC diet aids for longer than a three-month period at some interval during their lives. The two men (0.4%) who reported having used the preparations in the last 24 hours also indicated that they had used them longer than the three previous months.

Age at Initial Use

Table 8.2 demonstrates that the average age at which individuals of both genders reported first having used an OTC appetite suppressant containing phenylpropanolamine was 16 years (women, 16.6 years; men, 16.9 years). Of the women, 75% had started using these products before the age of 18, 48% before 17, and 19% before they were 16. Two individuals, a woman and a man, had begun usage at the age of 12.

Self-Perception of Weight and OTC Appetite Suppressant Use

Since only 31 men (3.5%) had used OTC diet aid products in the 12 months prior to the interview, it is difficult to make any statistical generalizations regarding the association between their self-perception of weight and use of

TABLE 8.1

Use of over-the-counter diet products containing phenylpropanolamine, by sex (in percentages)

Time period	Women	Men
Lifetime (Survey III)	45.5 (n = 554)	5.9 (n = 507)
Previous 12 months (Surveys I and III)	27.3 (n = 1,115)	3.5 (n = 890)
Previous 24 hours (Survey III)	3.1 (n = 554)	0.4 (n = 507)

Source: Compiled by the authors.

TABLE 8.2

Age at initial use of over-the-counter diet products containing phenylpropanolamine, by sex (Survey III)

Age	Women (number)	Men (number)
12	1	1
13	5	--
14	13	--
15	30	1
16	71	9
17	69	11
18	41	4
19	16	2
20	4	2
21	2	--
Totals	252	30

Source: Compiled by the authors.

these chemicals. However, it is of interest to note that a majority of the men (19) who had reported usage during the previous 12 months considered themselves as being of average weight or slightly underweight. Eleven perceived themselves as slightly overweight and only one stated that he was very overweight.

Table 8.3 shows that a clear-cut relationship exists between women's usage of OTC anorexiants during the previous 12 months and their self-perception of weight ($p < .001$). Starting with the self-perception of being very overweight, each subsequent self-perception category shows a reduction in usage of the products. Half the women who considered themselves to be very overweight reported using these drugs; approximately one out of three women used them if they thought they were slightly overweight; about one out of five women used them if they perceived themselves as being of average weight; and only one in ten used them if they viewed themselves as slightly underweight. None of the three women who considered themselves to be very underweight reported using the substances.

TABLE 8.3

Use by women of diet products containing phenylpropanolamine during previous 12 months, by self-perception of weight (Surveys I and III)

Weight category	Number in category	Use (%)	Nonuse (%)
Very overweight	72	50.0	50.0
Slightly overweight	523	34.8	65.2
Average weight	442	17.9	82.1
Slightly underweight	75	9.3	90.7
Very underweight	3	0.0	100.0
TOTAL	1,115		

Note: Chi-square test of significance: $p < .001$.
Source: Compiled by the authors.

An association also exists between the amount of weight loss desired and self-perception of weight. Those who perceived themselves as being very overweight wished to lose an average of 37.7 lb; the slightly overweight, 15.2 lb; and those of average weight, 6.6 lb. A relationship was also seen between OTC anorexiant usage and the amount of weight an individual desired to lose in each self-perception category. For example, the very overweight who used these anorexiants wished to lose an average of 42.0 lb, but the very overweight who did not use them wished to lose only 33.3 lb. Among individuals who categorized themselves as slightly underweight, those who used these products wanted to lose an additional 2.0 lb, whereas those who did not use them actually wanted to gain an average of 1.7 lb.

The fact that a much greater percentage of women than men in these surveys used diet pills also could be predicted from the observation that women more frequently perceived themselves to be overweight than did men (table 8.4). More than twice the percentage of women (53.4%) than men (23.3%) considered themselves to be overweight, whereas more men than women thought they were of average weight (men, 51.8%; women, 39.6%) or underweight (men, 24.9%; women, 7.0%).

TABLE 8.4

Self-perception of weight, by sex
(Surveys I and III)
(in percentages)

Self-perception	Women (n = 1,115)	Men (n = 890)	Total (n = 2,005)
Very overweight	6.5	1.0	4.0
Slightly overweight	46.9	22.3	36.0
Average weight	39.6	51.8	45.0
Slightly underweight	6.7	23.7	14.3
Very underweight	0.3	1.2	0.7

<u>Note</u>: Chi-square test of significance: $p < .001$.
<u>Source</u>: Compiled by the authors.

Preferred Methods of Weight Reduction

In general, a greater number of women than men reported that they would utilize any of the seven weight reduction methods listed in table 8.5. However, the rank ordering of preference for these methods was identical for both genders. Exercise was the most preferred and dieting the second most preferred. OTC diet products ranked fourth. In contrast to the high and nearly equal percentages of women (88%) and men (87%) who chose exercise as a preferred method, only 11% of the women and 2% of the men indicated that they would use OTC diet products if they wished to lose weight.

TABLE 8.5

Weight reduction methods preferred by women and men
(Survey III)
(in percentages)

Methods	Women (n = 554)	Men (n = 507)
Exercise	88.3	87.0
Dieting	80.1	60.7
Fasting	16.2	10.8
OTC diet pills	11.4	2.4
Voluntary weight-loss organizations	7.0	1.0
Laxatives	2.3	0.2
Induced vomiting	1.4	0.0

Source: Compiled by the authors.

Perceived Effectiveness and Adverse Reactions

In response to a question asking the 169 women in Survey I who had taken OTC appetite suppressants within the previous 12 months whether these pills had been effective in helping them lose weight, 52.1% reported that they had been ineffective. Although, as can be observed from the data in table 8.6, 47.9% indicated that the diet pills had been effective as an aid in weight loss, more than half (58%) of the subjects nevertheless qualified this when answering an open-ended question that asked them to explain why OTC anorexiants had been either effective or ineffective. These qualifications included the perceptions that the loss of weight had been due primarily to the placebo effect, that the pills had helped them lose weight only for a short period of time (two weeks or less), and that exercise and dieting had been more crucial than the pill in weight loss.

Although Survey I did not include a direct question regarding adverse reactions to OTC diet products, 42 (24.9%) of the 169 women who answered the open-ended question about diet pill effectiveness reported side effects. These 42 included women who rated the products as effective, as well as those who perceived them as ineffective. They listed feelings of being nervous, hyper, shaky, jumpy, tense, bitchy, jittery, high-strung, crazed, short-tempered, clammy, and anxious. Other reported symptoms were feeling sick, having an upset stomach, being dizzy and lightheaded, having a dry mouth, and having difficulty sleeping. In Survey III, 16 (6.3%) of the 252 women who had used OTC anorexiants containing phenylpropanolamine sometime during their lifetimes reported that they had experienced such medical conditions as heart, kidney, or thyroid problems, hypertension, and diabetes. In combined Surveys I and III (n = 1,115), 55.5% of the women who had used OTC diet aid products during the previous year indicated that they would use them again if the need arose. A relationship existed between willingness to use OTC anorexiants again and self-perception of weight. Of the women who perceived themselves as being very overweight, 67% indicated that they would use these substances again, but only 50% of the women who considered themselves slightly overweight would use them again.

Total Phenylpropanolamine Intake

In Survey II, the 253 women and 172 men were asked to indicate on a checklist of brand names all of the OTC products containing phenylpropanolamine (decongestants as well as anorexiants) that they had consumed during the previous year. They were asked to recall whether they had ever taken two, three, or more of these products within a 24-hour period. More than 91% (389) of the respondents indicated

TABLE 8.6

Effectiveness and side effects of diet products containing phenylpropanolamine reported by women users (Survey I) (n = 169)

Perceptions	Number	Percentage
Ineffective as an aid in weight loss	88	52.1
Effective as an aid in weight loss	81	47.9
Loss of weight due to action of drug alone	24	14.2
Loss of weight due to placebo effect	33	19.5
Effectiveness as an aid in weight loss on a temporary basis only	43	25.4
Somewhat effective as an aid in weight loss, but exercise and proper diet more important	22	13.0
Adverse reactions	42	24.9

Source: Compiled by the authors.

that they had used at least one of the OTC products during the previous year. The 1,262 doses of OTC drugs that these respondents had ingested represented an average of 3.2 products per individual. Women reported greater usage than men. Women had used an average of 3.5 products during the year, while the men had used, on average, 2.8. In addition, a larger percentage of women (51.2%) than men (39.0%) who reported having used phenylpropanolamine-containing products recalled that they had ingested two of these drugs within a 24-hour period. Approximately the same percentage of women

(10.6%) as men (10.5%) reported having taken three or more during a 24-hour period. The number of different products used by the respondents ranged from zero to 13.

In contrast to the Survey II question requesting subjects to report on their usage of phenylpropanolamine-containing drugs (anorexiants and decongestants) in 24-hour periods during the previous year, Survey III included a similar question about the 24 hours prior to the interview. Since the Survey III question asked subjects to recall very recent events, it was expected that their memories would be more reliable. Of the 1,061 respondents, 9.4% reported that they had used an OTC drug containing phenylpropanolamine within the last 24 hours. A slightly greater percentage of women (10.5%) than men (8.3%) indicated they had done so. Sixteen of the women and six of the men had used more than one of these substances during the 24 hours prior to the interview.

Self-Esteem and OTC Anorexiant Use

Survey III employed a 20-item scale that measured self-esteem. Items in the scale dealt with such areas as the respondents' relationships with parents, feelings of being in control of their lives, popularity with peers, feelings of success and failure, and desires to change themselves. No statistically significant relationships were found between self-esteem and the use of OTC anorexiants, either on a lifetime or a previous 12-month basis. The data were insufficient to permit generalizations to be made regarding OTC diet drug use in the last 24 hours and self-esteem. No significant trends were discerned even when individual questions measuring self-esteem were analyzed. Further, even when the full range of the self-perception of weight categories was associated with scores on the self-esteem index, no statistically significant relationships were discovered between self-esteem and OTC diet aid use. However, an association was observed in the case of respondents who considered themselves to be very overweight. Individuals in this category who had used diet substances either on a lifetime basis or during the previous 12 months were twice as likely as nonusers to have self-esteem scores which fell in the lower half of the scale. In particular, the very overweight women who used OTC diet pills tended to score very low on questions about their relationships with their parents. They felt that their parents expected too much of them and were "pushing" them too much.

DISCUSSION

Several findings support the overall reliability of the data from these surveys. No significant differences were discerned among the results of our three surveys, executed over a period of two years. Our prevalence data are similar to those of a recent national probability sample of high school seniors (Johnston, Bachman, and O'Malley 1982). Approximately 46% of our sample of undergraduate women students reported having consumed OTC anorexiants containing phenylpropanolamine sometime during their lifetimes, compared to 42% of the high school senior girls in the national survey. With regard to usage of these products within the previous 12 months, we found a prevalence of 27% and the national survey, 30%. We found a prevalence of 3% usage during the 24 hours prior to the interview, and the national survey, 2%.

Several findings have implications for health. Labels on OTC diet products containing phenylpropanolamine indicate that individuals under 18 years of age should not use them without first seeking the advice of a physician. We found that the average age of initial usage was 16, with 75% of the women reporting that they had first ingested these products before the age of 18, 8% between the ages of 12 and 14. Labels on these products also caution that before using them consumers should consult their physicians if they have any evidence of heart disease, hypertension, diabetes, or kidney or thyroid problems. Of the women in Survey III who reported having used these products during their lifetimes, 6% also stated that they had some of these health problems. In all three surveys, when specific inquiries were made, not a single respondent reported consulting a physician prior to taking an OTC diet product, regardless of age or contraindicated health conditions.

Nearly one-quarter of the women in Survey I who had used diet products containing phenylpropanolamine claimed to have had some adverse reactions. Their symptoms were similar to those reported in the literature, mainly related to CNS stimulation. Recall that these side effects were reported even though such information had not been specifically requested. However, caution is necessary in the interpretation of this finding. Many OTC anorexiant products consumed by the respondents also contained up to 200 mg of caffeine. Elsewhere, we have reported this drug's side effects (Krupka and Vener 1981; Vener and Krupka 1982). Since the reported adverse reactions to caffeine and phenylpropanolamine are similar, it is difficult to determine which adverse reactions are caused by which drug. The finding that 91% of the respondents in Survey II reported having used an OTC drug containing phenylpropanolamine (anorexiant or decongestant) during the previous 12 months and that 22% of those in Survey III who had consumed these products in the previous 24 hours had used more than one product represents a potential health hazard involving drug overdose. For example, one woman who wanted to lose weight while suffering from a severe cold had taken one anorexiant and four OTC decongestant products containing phenylpropanolamine within the 24 hours prior to the interview. If she had consumed the maximum manufacturer's recommended dosages, she would have ingested 675 mg of phenylpropanolamine:

Dexatrim Extra Strength™	one 75 mg capsule/ day	75 mg/day
Coricidin D®	two 12.5 mg tablets/ four hours; maximum 12 tablets/24 hours	150 mg/day
Comtrex®	same as Coricidin	150 mg/day
Contac®	one 75 mg tablet/ 12 hours	150 mg/day
Vicks 44D®	37.5 mg/six hours; maximum four doses/ 24 hours	150 mg/day
		675 mg

Even if she had ingested the minimum dosages of these products, her total phenylpropanolamine intake would have been 237.5 mg, 87.5 mg over the recommended Food and Drug Administration allowance for a 24-hour period.

An additional finding that indicates potential health problems is that OTC diet products containing phenylpropanolamine are often consumed for purposes other than weight reduction. Of the men who had consumed these substances in the previous year, 29% had done so without any desire to lose weight; in fact, some of these men actually wished to gain weight. Several of them explicitly stated that they had taken these products for their stimulant effects alone. In contrast, women typically did not report the use of these anorexiants for stimulant purposes. The one exception was a woman on the cross-country track team who felt that her performance level was enhanced by the stimulant effects. In the national survey, 11% of high school senior males reported having used OTC products containing phenylpropanolamine during the previous year (Johnston, Bachman, and O'Malley 1982). Since this percentage is much higher than the 3.5% of male college students found in our surveys, it is our conjecture that a fairly large percentage of high school senior males use these products because they believe they are readily available stimulants.

The drive to achieve or maintain a lean silhouette apparently induced almost one out of every two women in Survey III sometime during their lives, and more than one in four in Surveys I and III during the previous year, to ingest appetite suppressants containing phenylpropanolamine. That over half the women perceived themselves as being overweight to some degree and almost nine out of every ten wished to lose weight attests to how driven they were to remain within culturally accepted limits of the ideal body type. Even when they classified themselves as being of average weight, two-thirds still wished to lose some weight. This striving to lose weight reached its extreme among those who considered themselves to be very overweight. Three respondents in four had consumed OTC diet products sometime during their lifetimes and half had ingested them during the 12 months prior to the interview. The more weight the very overweight felt they needed to lose, the greater was the likelihood that they used OTC anorexiants.

The desire to lose weight is further seen in a commitment to using anorexiants despite uncertainty regarding their efficacy and safety. The vast majority of women (88%) who had used anorexiants reported that they had been useful only on a very short-term basis, had acted as placebos with limited pharmacological action, or had been completely useless as an aid in losing weight. Only 14% felt that the products had been the single reason they had experienced a loss of weight, only 11% chose them as a preferred method of weight reduction, and 25% reported side effects after their use. Despite this, 27% of the women had consumed OTC anorexiants during the year preceding the interview, and over half of these women assured us that they would use them again if the need arose.

That no significant relationship was found between the entire range of self-perception weight categories and self-esteem index scores may indicate that individuals who consider themselves to be only slightly overweight do not feel stigmatized because of it. However, the very overweight women who had used OTC diet control substances sometime in their lives or during the previous 12 months were twice as likely than nonusers to have self-esteem scores in the lower half of the index; this suggests that only in this extreme weight category is the self-esteem of women significantly affected by the stigmatization process.

In conclusion, we believe that drug education programs have not sufficiently emphasized the possible hazards associated with using OTC drugs, including not only aspirin (Krupka et al. 1978) and caffeine (Krupka and Vener 1981; Vener and Krupka 1982; Vener, Krupka, and Climo 1982), but also phenylpropanolamine. Drug education programs should critically examine certain societal values, e.g., that extreme leanness necessarily leads to physical and mental well-being. Finally, alternate weight control methods, other than the use of chemicals, should be explored.

REFERENCES

Abelson, H. I., P. M. Fishburne, and I. H. Cisin. 1977. National survey on drug abuse, 1977: a nationwide study --youth, young adults and older adults. Princeton, NJ: Response Analysis Corporation.

Alford, B. B. and M. L. Bogle. 1982. Nutrition during the life cycle. Englewood Cliffs, NJ: Prentice-Hall.

Anorexia nervosa and bulimia, evaluation and treatment conference brochure. 1982. University of Wisconsin, Milwaukee. Sept. 1-2.

Cahnman, W. J. 1968. The stigma of obesity. Sociological Quarterly 9(Summer):283-99.

Cohen, S. 1978. The volitional disorders. Clin Toxicol 13:633-39.

Coopersmith, S. 1967. The antecedents of self-esteem. San Francisco: W. H. Freeman.

Fazekas, J. F. et al. 1959. Comparative effectiveness of phenylpropanolamine and dextro amphetamine on weight reduction. JAMA 170:1018-21.

Goffman, I. 1963. Stigma. Englewood Cliffs, NJ: Prentice-Hall.

Griboff, S. I., R. Berman, and H. I. Silverman. 1975. A double-blind clinical evaluation of a phenylpropanolamine-caffeine-vitamin combination and a placebo in the treatment of exogenous obesity. Current Therapeutic Research 17:535-43.

Hoebel, B. G. 1978. Three anorectic drugs: similar structures but different effects on brain and behavior. Int J Obes 2:157-66.

Hurd, P. et al. 1980. Biology education in secondary schools of the United States. American Biology Teacher 42:388-410.

Innes, I. R. and M. Nickerson. 1975. Norepinephrine, epinephrine, and the sympathomimetic amines. In The pharmacological basis of therapeutics, 5th ed., edited by L. S. Goodman and A. Gilman. New York: Macmillan.

Johnston, L. D., J. G. Bachman, and P. M. O'Malley. 1982. Student drug use, attitudes, and beliefs: national trends, 1975-1982, National Institute on Drug Abuse research report. Washington, D.C.: U.S. Government Printing Office.

------. 1977. Drug use among American high school students, 1975-1977, National Institute on Drug Abuse research report. Washington, D.C.: U.S. Government Printing Office.

Krupka, L. R. and A. M. Vener. 1983. Over-the-counter appetite suppressants containing phenylpropanolamine hydrochloride (PPA) and the young adult: usage and perceived effectiveness. Journal of Drug Education 13:141-52.

------. 1981. Caffeine knowledge and the young adult. Journal of Drug Education 11:235-44.

Maddox, G. L., K. W. Back, and V. R. Liederman. 1968. Overweight as social deviance and disability. J Health Soc Behav 9:287-98.

O'Donnell, J. A. et al. 1976. Young men and drugs: a nationwide survey. National Institute on Drug Abuse research monograph no. 5. Washington, D.C.: U.S. Government Printing Office.

Physicians' desk reference, 38th ed. 1984. Oradell, NJ: Medical Economics.

------, 37th ed. 1983. Oradell, NJ: Medical Economics.

------, 31st ed. 1977. Oradell, NJ: Medical Economics.

Physicians' desk reference for nonprescription drugs, 4th ed. 1983. Oradell, NJ: Medical Economics.

Powers, P. S. 1980. Obesity: the regulation of weight. Baltimore: Williams and Wilkins.

Silverman, H. I. et al. 1980. Lack of side effects from orally administered phenylpropanolamine and phenylpropanolamine with caffeine: a controlled three-phase study. Current Therapeutic Research 28:185-94.

Staffieri, J. R. 1967. A study of social stereotype of body image in children. J Pers Soc Psych 7:101-4.

Vener, A. M. and L. R. Krupka. 1985. Needed: more attention to weight control knowledge. American Biology Teacher 47:148-53.

------. 1982. Caffeine use and young adult women. Journal of Drug Education 12:273-83.

------, and J. J. Climo. 1982. Drugs (prescription, over-the-counter, social) and the young adult: use and attitudes. Int J Addict 17:399-415.

------, and R. J. Gerard. 1982. Overweight/obese patients: an overview. Practitioner 226:1102-9.

9

THE EMERGENCE OF PHENYLPROPANOLAMINE IN SIMULATED CONTROLLED SUBSTANCES (LOOK-ALIKES) AFTER 1980

John P. Morgan, Karoline S. Puder, and Doreen V. Kagan

INTRODUCTION

The illicit drug market often develops supply shortages. The usual sources--diversion of pharmaceutical material, illicit synthesis, and smuggling--are all subject to abrupt interruption. Depending upon the strength of demand, sellers may resort to substitution, adulteration, or counterfeiting when the supply fails.

After decades of relatively unconstrained availability, the supply of pharmaceutical amphetamine was markedly curtailed in the late 1960s and early 1970s. By 1972, the strictures of the Federal Controlled Substances Act of 1970 were in full force (McGlothlin 1973). The law imposed manufacturing quotas on amphetamine and related chemicals, and this restriction, together with others on storage, ordering, and shipping, gradually stopped the previously easy diversion of amphetamine through wholesalers and retailers.

After 1972, even though the apparent supply of amphetamine had been greatly reduced, speculation about its availability continued. The Drug Abuse Warning Network (DAWN) fueled the notion that use of the drug persisted as a national abuse problem by reporting that there were still many emergency room visits associated with amphetamine use (Health, Education and Welfare 1977). However, DAWN mentions are rarely confirmed by analysis of the drug product or blood or urine assays (Ungerleider et al. 1980).

In a previous study, we reviewed the analysis of samples of illicit drugs purported to be amphetamine and found that the illicit "amphetamine" market was characterized by duplicity and that a number of other chemicals were being sold as amphetamine after being packaged in familiar-looking capsules and tablets (Morgan and Kagan 1978). In this paper, we will report on an extension of our earlier work, an examination of the actual ingredients of bogus amphetamine products. Because of recent publicity about the inclusion of phenylpropanolamine (PPA) in amphetamine fakes, this review will also focus on phenylpropanolamine as an ingredient in "look-alikes."

MATERIALS AND METHODS

We have compiled and studied data gathered from several laboratories that analyze, or in the past have analyzed, illicit drug samples. We have paid particular attention to samples alleged to be amphetamine, i.e., drugs submitted to laboratories as either amphetamine or methamphetamine, including those identified by submitters generically, pharmaceutically (for example Dexamyl®, Biphetamine®), or popularly (for instance, speed, meth, black beauties, whites, crank).

Most of the information from 1972 to 1974 is from an unpublished compilation by Dr. J. Bing Hart of data from street drug analytical laboratories*. Many of these ceased operation in 1974 because of stricter federal laws governing the handling of illicit materials by laboratories. We obtained post-1974 information from PharmChem Laboratories, Inc., Palo Alto, California; the Street Drug Analysis Laboratory, College of Pharmacy, Washington State University in Pullman; On Drugs, Inc., Chicago; the Street Drug Identification Program, LAC-USC Medical Center; and others. Most of these laboratories analyzed drugs for only a portion of the time under consideration and nearly all have now ceased operation. The source of the most regularly reported and reliable data was eliminated in 1984 when PharmChem Laboratories' anonymous analysis program was discontinued (Samples decline: PharmChem discontinues anonymous drug testing 1984).

Each alleged amphetamine sample analyzed by a laboratory was classified according to the month and year of submission, its alleged content, and the results of analysis. All samples containing phenylpropanolamine alone or in combination were carefully noted.

We obtained additional information on the purity of alleged stimulants from U.S. Drug Enforcement Administration (DEA) data on seizures and buys (Fink 1981). Finally, we

---

*Dr. Hart had been interested in street drug analysis and had previously published on this topic (Hart et al. 1971). He collected extensive data from nearly 30 laboratories in 1972-74 and made his compilation available to us.

gathered statistics on the synthetic production of phenylpropanolamine in the United States from an industrial trade publication (U.S. International Trade Commission 1980).

RESULTS

Amphetamine Inauthenticity

Two important categories yielded by the analyses ("only amphetamine" and "any amphetamine") are depicted graphically in figure 9.1. Submissions containing <u>only</u> amphetamine calculated as a percentage of total alleged amphetamine submissions declined significantly from 52% to 5% in the decade 1972-81. An increase in authenticity apparently occurred in 1982 and 1983. The percentage of total submitted samples containing <u>any</u> amphetamine also declined throughout most of the period from 1972 to 1981, from a high of 62% in 1972 to a low of 17% in 1979. This category also exhibited an apparent increase in authenticity in 1982 and 1983.

FIGURE 9.1

The presence of amphetamine in alleged amphetamine samples submitted for analysis to street drug laboratories

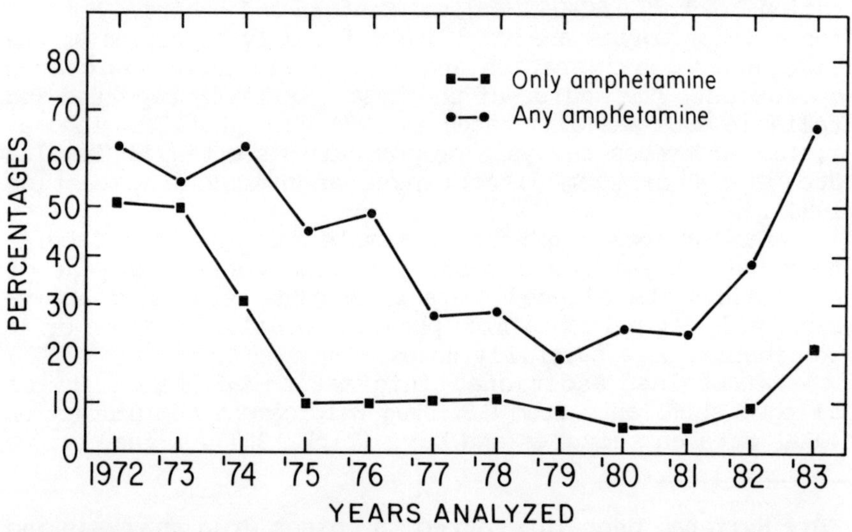

<u>Source</u>: Compiled by the authors. Data derived from combined street drug analysis programs and statistical reports from Dr. J. Bing Hart.

Constituents of Alleged Amphetamine

Table 9.1 lists the total number of alleged amphetamine samples analyzed by the street drug laboratories from 1972 to 1983. Prior to 1981, the total submissions analyzed were greater than 500 in eight of the ten years and the lowest number was 341 in 1979. However, in 1982 and 1983 the number of samples on which we have information fell to 181 and 131, respectively.

TABLE 9.1

Alleged amphetamine samples containing only legally available nonprescription ingredients

Year	Total samples analyzed	Samples containing only ingredients available OTC*	
		Number	Percent
1972	382	50	(13)
1973	981	264	(27)
1974	599	150	(25)
1975	595	256	(43)
1976	1,144	435	(38)
1977	765	420	(55)
1978	891	453	(51)
1979	341	228	(67)
1980	514	269	(52)
1981	503	311	(62)
1982	181	88	(49)
1983	131	29	(22)

*Ingredients include caffeine, ephedrine, pseudeoephedrine, and phenylpropanolamine alone or in combination.

Source: Compiled by the authors. Data derived from combined computations by street drug analysis programs and statistical reports from Dr. J. Bing Hart.

The percentages of analyzed samples containing only legally available, over-the-counter (OTC) ingredients are also listed in table 9.1. These include medicinals such as caffeine, ephedrine, pseudoephedrine, and phenylpropanolamine, alone or in combination. From a low of 13% in 1972, the percentage of samples containing only OTC ingredients climbed to a high of 68% in 1979. Caffeine was by far the most important ingredient in these samples (table 9.2). It

TABLE 9.2

Alleged amphetamine samples containing any caffeine

Year	Total samples analyzed	Samples containing any caffeine*	
		Number	Percent
1972	382	49	(13)
1973	981	206	(21)
1974	599	105	(18)
1975	595	222	(37)
1976	1,144	390	(34)
1977	765	339	(44)
1978	891	358	(40)
1979	341	161	(47)
1980	514	203	(39)
1981	503	286	(57)
1982	181	72	(40)
1983	131	20	(15)

*Samples containing any amphetamine are not included.

Source: Compiled by the authors. Data derived from combined computations by street drug analysis programs and statistical reports from Dr. J. Bing Hart.

appeared alone, in combination with other OTC products, and occasionally with non-OTC drugs. (Samples containing amphetamine were excluded from this count.) Between 1975 and 1982, caffeine was present in an average of 41% of all submitted samples not containing amphetamine.

DEA Seizures and Buys

Table 9.3 provides a further perspective on the universe of illicit sales of purported amphetamine. The DEA, as part of its criminal investigation activities, purchases

TABLE 9.3

Characteristics of "licit" amphetamine lots purchased or seized by the Drug Enforcement Administration, 1973-80

Year	Percentage of lots with unit volume of less than 500 pills	Percentage of lots with no amphetamine	Total lots
1973	61	38	13
1974	83	0	43
1975	70	10	30
1976	88	85	33
1977	84	83	31
1978	100	58	12
1979	65	42	31
1980	100	55	20

Source: Compiled by the authors. Data derived from statistics on seizures, 1981. Provided by Fink, W. G., Assistant Administrator for Intelligence, U.S. Department of Justice, Drug Enforcement Administration, in letter to author (Morgan). May 19.

and seizes drugs in the illicit marketplace. These drugs are then analyzed and categorized. The data in table 9.2 indicate the contents of the diverted materials that were seized and classified on the basis of appearance by the DEA as licit or pharmaceutical amphetamine. From 1973 to 1980, the number of "amphetamine" acquisitions tended to decline as did the number of units included in individual buys or seizures. In both 1976 and 1977, more than 80% of the batches were fakes; that is, of those products seized or purchased as licit amphetamine, more than eight out of ten lots contained no amphetamine. The agency has generally and logically been less active in this market since that time.

Phenylpropanolamine in Look-Alikes

In table 9.4, the 12-year pattern reflecting the percentage of alleged amphetamine samples containing phenylpropanolamine can be seen. The table includes data on submissions that contained phenylpropanolamine alone, phenylpropanolamine in combination with caffeine, and phenylpropanolamine in combination with caffeine and ephedrine (the triple combination).

These figures reveal that phenylpropanolamine became important in the look-alike market only in 1980 and that only the combination with caffeine and ephedrine was prominent. Neither products containing phenylpropanolamine alone nor those with phenylpropanolamine with caffeine, both standard anorexiants, were commonly submitted to these laboratories.

Data on the production of synthetic phenylpropanolamine between 1964 and 1982 by five North American chemical manufacturing firms appear in figure 9.2. This information was obtained from Synthetic Organic Chemicals, a document published by the U.S. International Trade Commission (1980) that includes statistics voluntarily reported by manufacturers. Synthesized phenylpropanolamine is sold to domestic and foreign purchasers for production of OTC and prescription medications or for use as a chemical intermediate in other synthetic reactions. The widespread utilization of phenylpropanolamine is obvious from these compilations. The production of synthetic phenylpropanolamine grew fairly steadily from 1964 to 1978, then rose sharply during the next two years, jumping in 1980 to more than twice the 1978 level, but then fell back to that level by 1982.

TABLE 9.4

The inclusion of phenylpropanolamine in alleged amphetamine samples analyzed by street drug laboratories

Year	Total samples analyzed	PPA alone No.	PPA alone (%)	PPA plus caffeine No.	PPA plus caffeine (%)	PPA, caffeine, and ephedrine No.	PPA, caffeine, and ephedrine (%)
1972	382	1	(0)	0	(0)	0	(0)
1973	981	8	(1)	0	(0)	0	(0)
1974	599	1	(0)	0	(0)	0	(0)
1975	595	0	(0)	1	(0)	0	(0)
1976	1,144	5	(0)	3	(0)	0	(0)
1977	765	2	(0)	9	(1)	0	(0)
1978	891	5	(1)	20	(2)	0	(0)
1979	341	1	(0)	8	(2)	2	(1)
1980	514	8	(2)	3	(1)	120	(23)
1981	503	0	(0)	6	(1)	253	(50)
1982	181	2	(1)	2	(1)	64	(35)
1983	131	1	(1)	0	(0)	8	(6)

Source: Compiled by the authors. Data derived from combined computations by street drug analysis programs and statistical reports from Dr. J. Bing Hart.

FIGURE 9.2

Phenylpropanolamine production
in the United States, 1964-82

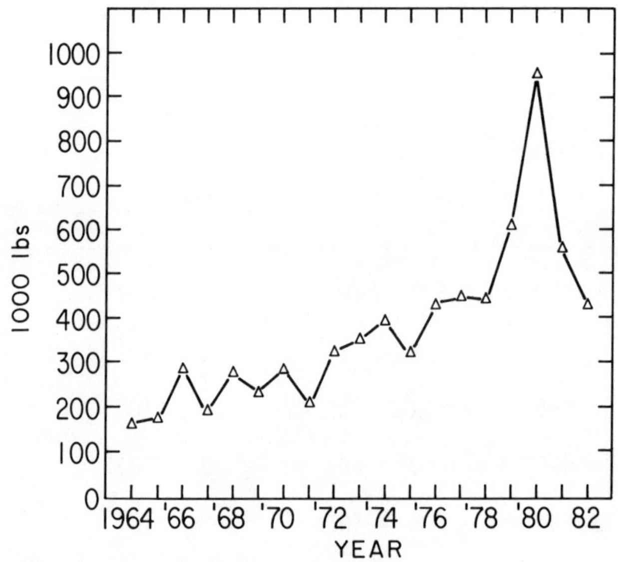

Source: Compiled by the authors. Data derived from United States International Trade Commission. 1980. Synthetic organic chemicals: United States production and sales, 1979, USTIC publication 1099. Washington, D.C.: U.S. Government Printing Office; 1984 telephone conversations with M. Cozel and M. Hioks, United States International Trade Commission.

DISCUSSION

In the 1950s and 1960s, demand for diverted pharmaceutical amphetamine and related stimulant products emerged. Careless and criminal wholesalers and retailers shifted legitimately manufactured products ostensibly bound for the licit market to the illicit marketplace (Morgan 1981).

Various factors, most notably the 1970 Controlled Substances Act (Vodra 1975), curtailed the availability of authentic amphetamine, and the clamor for supply switched to bogus products. As Smith (chapter 20, this volume) has noted:

> A large consumer market for stimulants had been created with its own cultural definitions and identifying characteristics. Supply reduction alone could not resolve the problem. Clearly, the expansion of look-alikes occurred as a consequence of this vacuum.

Bogus Drugs

Out of the confusion, uncertainty, and duplicity of this market, a few clear trends can be discerned. The quantity of authentic amphetamine delivered to the illicit marketplace has fallen steadily and significantly. Although the amount of available data has decreased in recent years as more and more laboratories have discontinued their programs of street drug analysis, the overall trend is nevertheless very convincing. We think that a purchaser of alleged amphetamine today has only a small chance of actually obtaining any real amphetamine.

Diversion

The even more marked reduction in reports of samples containing "only amphetamine" is important, because it serves as the best index of pharmaceutical product diversion. The category of "any amphetamine" includes a variety of illegally compounded products in which bulk amphetamine was mixed with OTC ingredients (for example, combinations of caffeine plus amphetamine were important from 1974 to 1976). The "any amphetamine" category also includes samples of methamphetamine, which is most frequently produced in illicit laboratories. The Controlled Substances Act removed almost all* amphetamine combination products from the market. Therefore, diverted pharmaceutical amphetamine appears chiefly in the "only amphetamine" category, which remained below 11% of all samples submitted from 1975 to 1982.

The apparent increase in authenticity of amphetamine only in 1982 and 1983 is unexplained. Because of the marked

---

*Smith Kline and French continued to market two combination amphetamine products after the Controlled Substances Act was implemented. By legal action they delayed the removal from the market of Dexamyl® (amphetamine and amobarbital) and Eskatrol® (amphetamine and prochlorperazine).

decline in submissions, the increase may not be real. This decline may have occurred in part because publicity about look-alikes became prominent and many individuals may have known or assumed that the products available were fakes (for further discussion of this possibility, see Smith, chapter 20, this volume).

Methamphetamine

The even greater jump in the any amphetamine category in 1982 and 1983 reflects the substantial increase in the percentage of submitted materials that contained illicitly synthesized methamphetamine, usually in bulk powder form. Whether this represents greater output from illicit speed manufacturers or heightened interest in the quality of production is not clear.

OTC Stimulants and Phenylpropanolamine

The products sold as amphetamine today are almost always nonprescription stimulant, bronchodilator, decongestant, or anorexiant products; the three ingredients most frequently contained in them are caffeine, ephedrine, and phenylpropanolamine.

Until 1980, phenylpropanolamine had no importance in the look-alike market. Since it has a reputation as a sympathomimetic with minimal central nervous system stimulatory properties (Aviado 1970), it would not appear to be a likely candidate for inclusion in look-alikes. However, perhaps because of its widespread use in OTC products, particularly anorexiant drugs, and because of its structural resemblance to amphetamine, phenylpropanolamine became a common ingredient after 1980, during the time of greatest expansion of the look-alike market. Its frequent combination with such known stimulants as caffeine and ephedrine does not diminish the evidence indicating that it possesses minimal stimulant properties of its own (see Bigelow, chapter 19, this volume). The legitimate synthetic chemical industry more than doubled its 1978 output of phenylpropanolamine in 1980 almost certainly in order to meet the demand for it generated by look-alike manufacturers and packagers.

Controlling the Look-Alike Industry

The structure of the look-alike industry has not been thoroughly studied or described. However, it is almost certain that a few manufacturers of OTC products purchased legal chemical ingredients and ordered empty capsules resembling previously popular stimulant formats. These manufacturers then supplied a larger number of wholesalers, who marketed the products largely through mail order. On September 30, 1981, the Food and Drug Administration (FDA) raided nine such manufacturers and subsequently charged them with counterfeiting and mislabeling medicinal products. A large volume of tablets and empty capsules and some manufacturing equipment were seized (Golden 1981). In August 1982, the FDA intensified its attack on this market by declaring the triple product to be a new drug, for which significant proof of efficacy and safety would be required before it could be approved for sale (Health and Human Services 1982). Later the agency extended its new drug classification to include any combination of caffeine plus phenethylamine stimulants, such as phenylpropanolamine, ephedrine, or pseudoephedrine. Because of this, the makers of popular anorexiant products are no longer permitted to market phenylpropanolamine/caffeine combinations and have therefore replaced them with phenylpropanolamine alone (Health and Human Services 1983).

The Return of Caffeine

In 1984 and 1985, a few familiar wholesaler names reappeared in advertisements for legal stimulants, some still resembling previously marketed products. One of these ads is shown in illustration 9.1. Apparently all these stimulants are caffeine-alone products. Prior to our data collection, it was known that amphetamine fakes often contained only caffeine (Morgan 1981). The look-alike market may have come full circle in 20 years from caffeine-only back to caffeine-only, and phenylpropanolamine appears to have been removed from its briefly prominent and confusing place in the look-alike market.

ILLUSTRATION 9.1

Recent advertisement for legal stimulants

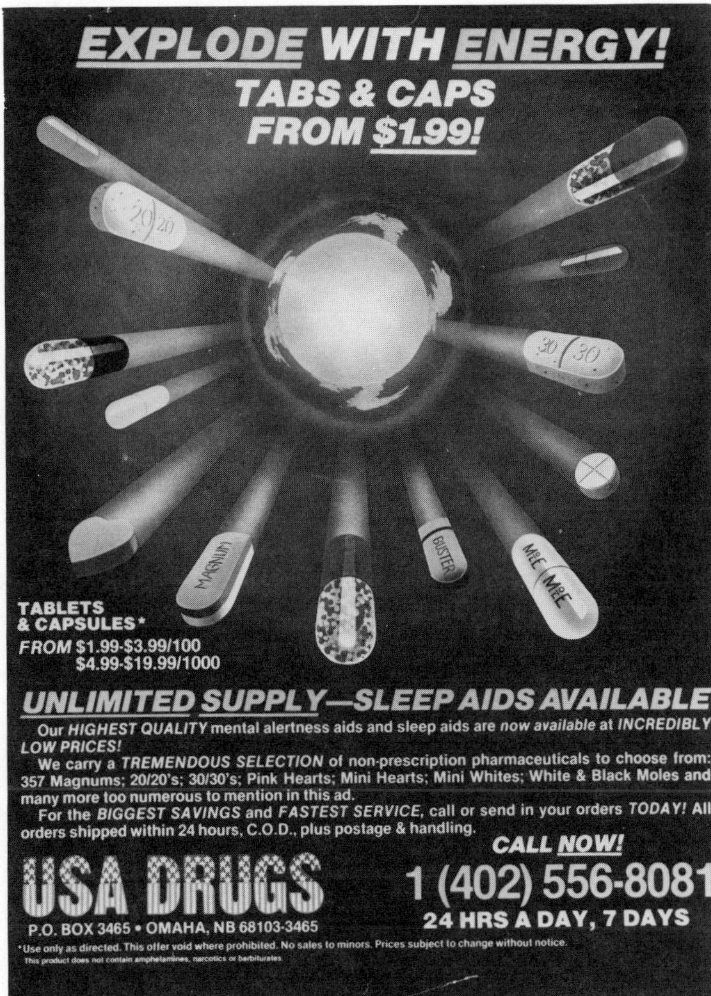

Source: USA Drugs. 1984.

CONCLUSION

Our window on the world of stimulant fakes--our sampling of illicit products sold as amphetamine--is imperfect. Street drug laboratories may have received an unusually large percentage of samples that were known to be inferior or looked funny or had poor effects, since little is known about the individuals who submit samples. Despite this caution, we believe that the data and our interpretations provide a largely correct view of the patterns and character of amphetamine and amphetamine-fake marketing from 1972 to 1983.

REFERENCES

Aviado, D. 1970. Phenylpropanolamine. In _Sympathomimetic drugs_, 240-43. Springfield, IL: Charles C. Thomas.

Fink, W. G. 1981. Seizure data provided by the Assistant Administrator for Intelligence, U.S. Department of Justice, Drug Enforcement Administration, in letter to author (Morgan). May 19.

Golden, L. B. 1981. _Trafficking in look-alikes: an update_. United States Department of Justice. Washington, D.C.: Drug Enforcement Administration. November 2.

Hart, J. B. et al. 1972. Composition of illicit drugs and the use of drug analysis in abuse abatement. _J Psychedelic Drugs_ 5:83-88.

Health and Human Services, Food and Drug Administration (FDA). 1983. Enforcement action under the new drug provisions of the Federal Food, Drug and Cosmetic Act: certain OTC drug products; advisory opinion. FDA docket no. 83A-0339. _Federal Register_ 48:52513-14.

———. 1982. New drug status of OTC combination drug products containing caffeine, phenylpropanolamine and ephedrine. FDA docket no. 82N-0266. _Federal Register_ 47:35344-46.

Health, Education and Welfare, Food and Drug Administration (FDA). 1977. Amphetamines: public hearing. FDA docket no. 77N-0273. _Federal Register_ 42:29827.

McGlothlin, W. H. 1973. Amphetamines, barbiturates, and hallucinogens: an analysis of use, distribution and control. U.S. Department of Justice, Bureau of Narcotics and Dangerous Drugs, contract no. J-70-33. Washington, D.C.: Drug Enforcement Administration.

Morgan, J. P. 1981. Amphetamine. In Substance abuse: clinical problems and perspectives, edited by J. H. Lowinson and P. Ruiz, 167-84. Baltimore, MD: Williams & Wilkins.

Morgan, J. P. and D. Kagan. 1978. Street amphetamine quality and the Controlled Substances Act of 1970. J Psychedelic Drugs 10:303-17.

Samples decline: PharmChem discontinues anonymous drug-testing. 1984. PharmChem Newsletter 13 (May-June):1.

Ungerleider, J. T. et al. 1980. The Drug Abuse Warning Network (DAWN) program: toxicologic verification of 1,008 emergency room mentions. Arch Gen Psychiatry 37:106-9.

United States International Trade Commission. 1980. Synthetic organic chemicals: United States production and sales, 1979. USTIC publication 1099. Washington, D.C.: U.S. Government Printing Office.

Vodra, W. W. 1975. The Controlled Substances Act. Drug Enforcement 2:2.

10

THE RELATIONSHIP BETWEEN PHENYLPROPANOLAMINE AND CAFFEINE

John F. Greden

INTRODUCTION

Phenylpropanolamine (PPA), for decades a seldom discussed but widely used component of decongestants, suddenly has become a controversial drug (Appelt 1983; Bernstein and Diskant 1982; Blum 1981; Dietz 1981). Scientists and critics from various disciplines are engaged in debate about the drug's risk/benefit ratio. Some have even suggested that phenylpropanolamine, currently classified as a Category I drug by the U.S. Food and Drug Administration (FDA), be reclassified as a Category III over-the-counter (OTC) drug (see Wertheimer, chapter 4, this volume for a discussion of the FDA's Categories I, II, and III).

This debate has had little to do with phenylpropanolamine's history as a component of decongestants, but instead developed with the more recent use of phenylpropanolamine as an anorexiant. The debate had its beginnings in 1972, when the FDA's Advisory Review Panel on Over-the-Counter Miscellaneous Internal Drug Products declared that phenylpropanolamine was a "safe and effective" medication for the control of appetite (Health and Human Services 1982b). Following that action, the use of OTC diet aid products containing phenylpropanolamine proliferated (Altschuler et al. 1982). Later, phenylpropanolamine also began to appear in a multitude of "street" stimulants. As the consumption of phenylpropanolamine increased, so did the number of clinical reports of its apparent psychiatric and medical side effects, fueling the claims that the drug had become an agent of abuse (Dietz 1981; Horowitz et al. 1979; Horowitz et al. 1980; Cornelius, Soloff, and Reynolds 1984; Achor and Extein 1981).

Ideally, debates about the risks and benefits of any pharmacological substance should be settled on the basis of scientific data. This has been difficult to do in the case of phenylpropanolamine, however, because much of the available clinical literature comes from uncontrolled studies and is therefore not sufficiently instructive. Most reports describing possible phenylpropanolamine toxicity are anecdotal, consisting of only one or several cases. Often they are based on retrospective reviews of records, without drug screen verification of pharmacological activity or adequate documentation of dosage and duration of use. Furthermore, most recorded instances of phenylpropanolamine toxicity have occurred following use of pharmacological products that also contained other stimulants, usually caffeine and occasionally ephedrine. This fact alone makes it difficult to judge the validity of reports of "phenylpropanolamine" abuse or toxicity, since the adverse reactions could have been due to the other stimulants in the drug combinations.

The existing literature on phenylpropanolamine cannot be interpreted without considering questions about the relationship between phenylpropanolamine and caffeine. Why, for example, was caffeine added to OTC diet aids containing phenylpropanolamine? How are the two agents alike in their effects? How are they different? What are the pharmacological effects of simultaneous ingestion of the two agents? Most importantly, how many of the reported side effects attributed to phenylpropanolamine might have been due to caffeine or to synergistic effects?

CAFFEINE AND PHENYLPROPANOLAMINE: AN OVERVIEW

Caffeine is a trimethylated xanthine (1,3,7-trimethylxanthine) that differs from theobromine and theophylline only in the number of methylated sites (Truitt 1971; Greden 1979). Caffeine's pharmacological structure is different from that of phenylpropanolamine, but both are commonly categorized as pharmacological stimulants. Caffeine originates naturally in 63 species of plants; it is found, for example, in coffee seeds, tea leaves, kola nuts, ilex plants or maté, and cassina (Greden 1979). The drug is available in a multitude of beverages and medications. Common commercial sources of caffeine are listed in table 10.1.

TABLE 10.1

Common sources of caffeine

Source	Approximate dose (mg)
Beverages	
Coffee, brewed	80-140/cup
Coffee, decaffeinated	2-4/cup
Cola drinks	25-55/cup
Tea, bagged	42-100/cup
Tea, instant	50-100/cup
Tea, leaf	30-75/cup
Many OTC cold preparations	30/tablet
Many OTC stimulants	100-200/tablet
Analgesics	
A.P.C.	32/tablet
Anacin®	32.5/tablet
B C tablet	16/tablet
Bromo-Seltzer®	32.5/tablet
Cafergot®	100/tablet
Capron	32/tablet
Comeback	100/tablet
Cope®	32/tablet
Darvon® compound	32/tablet
Dolor®	30/tablet
Easy-Mens	32/tablet
Empirin® compound	32/tablet
Excedrin®	64.8/tablet
Fiorinal®	40/tablet
Goody's headache powder®	32.5/tablet
Maranox	15/tablet
Medache®	32/tablet
Midol®	32/tablet
Migralam™	50/tablet
Nilain	32/tablet
P.A.C.	32/tablet
Pre-Mens	66/tablet
Stanback® powder	32/tablet
Stanback® tablets	16/tablet
Trigesic®	30/tablet
Vanquish	33/tablet

Source: Compiled by the author. Data derived from Greden, J. F. 1981. Caffeine. In Behavior in excess, edited by S. J. Mulé, 164-89. New York: The Free Press; Greden, J. F. 1981. Caffeinism and caffeine withdrawal. In Substance abuse: clinical problems and perspectives, edited by J. H. Lowinson and P. Ruiz, 274-86. Baltimore: Williams & Wilkins.

Historical Parallels between Caffeine and Phenylpropanolamine

The current debate surrounding the use of phenylpropanolamine has distinct similarities to that which has reverberated around the consumption of caffeine throughout its history (Greden 1976). Despite the apparent social acceptance of caffeine, opponents for more than ten centuries have periodically and vociferously attacked it as a potential drug of abuse (Ibid.; Gilbert 1980). In the eighteenth century, the regular coffee consumer was described as:

> A sufferer who is tremulous and loses his self-command; he is subject to fits of agitation and depression; he loses color and has a haggard appearance. . . . The heart also suffers; it palpitates or it intermits. As with other such agents, a renewed dose of the poison gives temporary relief, but at the cost of further misery (Greden 1976; Siegerist 1943, p. 187).

Similar-sounding complaints now are heard about phenylpropanolamine.

Another historical parallel is that phenylpropanolamine has sometimes been equated with other drugs, usually amphetamine, to dramatize its abuse potential (Blum 1981). What is not well-known is that caffeine was once viewed with similar alarm. In 1886, for example, U.S. Surgeon General Hammond conducted self-experiments with cocaine hydrochloride and concluded that the cocaine habit was similar to the habitual use of tea or coffee (Angrist and Sudilovsky 1978). Drinking coffee was also once considered to be as hazardous as opiate use (Greden 1976). These historical similarities may help us place the current debates about all stimulants—including phenylpropanolamine—in proper perspective.

Caffeine and Phenylpropanolamine Anorexiant Combinations

There is no easy answer as to why caffeine was added to phenylpropanolamine in many of the 70 or more diet aid products which appeared after 1972. Several possibilities exist. It has been suggested that caffeine was added in order to counteract the lethargy sometimes induced by dieting. Such a motivation seems questionable and largely unsubstantiated. Or perhaps caffeine was added on the basis of claims, made for centuries, that caffeine itself is an anorexiant. In the eighteenth century, for example, it was stated that "the appetite falls off in the habitual coffee drinker" (Greden 1976; Siegerist 1943). When the first public sale of tea in Britain took place at Garway's Coffee House in London, the brew was promoted as "that excellent and by all physicians approved China drink" (Ukers 1948), said to be of "great avail to men of corpulent bodies and to such as eat much flesh" (Ibid.; Greden 1981a). However, the supposed anorexiant effect of caffeine is also an unlikely reason to include it in diet aid products since, despite such claims, it has never been documented that caffeine effectively induces weight loss. A transient, acute weight loss may be secondary to caffeine's diuretic actions, involving the inhibition of renal tubular absorption of sodium, but long-term, sustained weight loss is unreported. A final possible explanation of the phenylpropanolamine/caffeine combination is that caffeine causes central nervous system (CNS) stimulation, promoting mild euphoria and habituation. Regardless of why caffeine was added to many OTC diet aid products containing phenylpropanolamine, it was done. Thus, caffeine's pharmacological actions must be considered in any thorough attempt to assess the safety of phenylpropanolamine.

In the late 1970s, various combinations of caffeine, phenylpropanolamine, and sometimes ephedrine also began to appear in street products, presumably filling the void created when the availability of amphetamine products decreased. These combinations became known as "look-alike" drugs because they were marketed in capsules designed to resemble the amphetamine products they had replaced. The proliferation and widespread use of look-alikes may account for much of the official concern about the effects of phenylpropanolamine.

Regulation of Products Containing Caffeine and Phenylpropanolamine

As a consequence of the growing debate surrounding the abuse potential of OTC diet aids and look-alikes (Health and Human Services 1982b), the FDA in late 1983 announced its advisory ruling prohibiting OTC drug products labeled as stimulants to contain anything other than caffeine as the active ingredient unless new drug status was sought. It was also required that the following combinations be registered as new drugs: (1) caffeine in combination with ephedrine or pseudoephedrine; (2) phenylpropanolamine in combination with ephedrine or pseudoephedrine; and (3) phenylpropanolamine in combination with caffeine. A transitional period was allowed for the removal from the market of products combining caffeine and phenylpropanolamine, but not the other combinations. The FDA stated that the caffeine/phenylpropanolamine combination was clearly a "new drug" within the meaning of the act, but noted that a panel report to the FDA had recommended that this combination be classified as an "anorectic/stimulant" that was "generally recognized as safe" and effective (Health and Human Services 1982a). No date of enforcement of the ban prohibiting the sale of products containing both caffeine and phenylpropanolamine was announced, although the manufacture of new products was scheduled to cease in 1983.

In considering the effects of this latest FDA action, it is intriguing to note another possible historical parallel between phenylpropanolamine and caffeine. At one time or another, in most of the world, both tea and coffee have been banned by law, but such restrictions have always been ultimately challenged. The following description of the results of such a ban in the sixteenth century is illustrative:

> The coffee [habit] had become so strong, and the use of it so generally agreeable, that people continued, notwithstanding all prohibitions, to drink it in their own houses. The officers of the police, seeing they could not suppress the use of it allowed of the selling it, on paying a tax; and the drinking it provided it was not done openly; so that it was drunk in particular places, with the doors shut, or in the back room of some of the shopkeepers houses. . . . (Ellis 1774, p. 5)

The similarities to currently banned substances are too obvious to require further comment.

The long-term effects of the FDA's ruling await evaluation, but it is unlikely to eliminate combination use of phenylpropanolamine and caffeine even if it is not flouted. Simultaneous ingestion can and does occur via other pathways. Nasal decongestants and cold products have often contained both products. Moreover, even if caffeine and phenylpropanolamine are not combined in the same pharmaceutical product, their simultaneous use by vast numbers of people has occurred and will continue to occur simply because caffeine consumption is so prevalent in the United States. Thus, the majority of phenylpropanolamine users are likely also to be consuming caffeine daily.

To elaborate, several billion kilograms of caffeine are consumed annually in the United States, when all forms (tea, coffee, soft drinks, cold tablets, analgesics, and stimulants) are considered. More than 60% of all persons in the United States above the age of ten consume some caffeine. Over 80% of adults report coffee use, and the majority now report drinking tea. More than 20% of all adults consume more than 500 mg of caffeine a day, a pharmacologically significant dose above which symptoms of caffeinism are likely to occur. Thus, on a statistical basis, any individual who takes a phenylpropanolamine-containing product is probably using caffeine concurrently.

PHARMACOLOGICAL CONSIDERATIONS

Caffeine and phenylpropanolamine are both classified as stimulants. Both agents exhibit dose-related CNS stimulatory effects (Weiner 1980; Greden 1979). Both alter adrenergic function, directly or indirectly.

Caffeine's CNS effects may be attributable to: (1) a significant increase in norepinephrine excretion; (2) sensitization of central catecholamine postsynaptic receptors, including those of dopamine; (3) possible alterations of cyclic adenosine 3',5'-monophosphate (cyclic AMP) and cyclic guanosine 3',5'-monophosphate (cyclic GMP); (4) a possible modification of calcium's neuromodulating effects; (5) possible alterations of turnover and receptor binding for acetylcholine and serotonin; and (6) inhibition of the CNS effects of adenosine or other endogenous purines and possible competitive antagonism of naturally occurring benzodiazepine receptors (Greden 1981b). Caffeine has received renewed attention from investigators and many pharmacological studies of its CNS actions are under way, but the relative importance of each of these potential mechanisms is still unknown.

Nor are the CNS actions of phenylpropanolamine completely understood. The stimulatory actions of phenylpropanolamine may result from the direct stimulation of receptors as well as changes in the release and turnover of norepinephrine. Phenylpropanolamine is also reported to have indirect alpha-adrenergic activity with lesser beta activity. This combination means that if there is simultaneous postsynaptic and presynaptic alpha-adrenergic stimulation, it may induce concurrent postural hypotension and hypertension.

Whether the metabolisms of phenylpropanolamine and caffeine are altered when they are administered together is little understood. The pharmacokinetic and other interactions between the drugs have been inadequately studied.

A largely ignored but intriguing pharmacological question is whether the simultaneous use of phenylpropanolamine and aspirin (acetylsalicyclic acid) might have deleterious consequences. The combination may be dangerous because aspirin is a prostaglandin inhibitor, and prostaglandins may alter the negative feedback loop which regulates the release of catecholamines at sympathetic nerve endings. If the aspirin in analgesic products sufficiently inhibits prostaglandins, the stimulatory effects of caffeine and phenylpropanolamine in releasing catecholamines might be even greater than expected. This prospect has epidemiologic importance, because people with colds often take both OTC cough/cold preparations (many of which contain phenylpropanolamine, either alone or combined with caffeine) and aspirin or combination analgesics containing both aspirin and caffeine.

TOXICITY CONSIDERATIONS

The clinical features of caffeinism have been described in recent reviews (Greden 1981a, 1981b; Gilbert 1980). The toxic effects of caffeine are dose-related extensions of its expected pharmacological actions. In general, the clinical symptoms of caffeinism occur in several different constellations: (1) manifestations of anxiety; (2) psychophysiological effects; (3) sleep disruptions; and (4) signs of withdrawal. Other possible problems include depression, the accentuation of stress or exacerbation of psychosis, the complication of preexisting medical conditions such as renal or cardiac disease, and drug interactions.

The toxicity profile of phenylpropanolamine is similar to that of caffeine and is clearly dose-related. The available literature strongly suggests that phenylpropanolamine is quite safe taken in dosages within the accepted range and that phenylpropanolamine/caffeine combinations have few side effects when ingested in recommended doses (Silverman et al. 1980). As with caffeine, however, when phenylpropanolamine is taken in higher doses or in conjunction with other medications, extensions of its expected pharmacological actions are likely.

The frequency of clinically significant reactions to products containing phenylpropanolamine and caffeine is not fully known. However, from 1975 to 1980, the frequency of claimed phenylpropanolamine involvement in poison control center case reports increased tenfold (Bernstein and Diskant 1982).

Table 10.2 summarizes some of the common toxic effects attributed to phenylpropanolamine, caffeine, and their combinations. The similarities between them are evident.

TABLE 10.2

Reported adverse clinical reactions from ingestion of phenylpropanolamine, caffeine, and combinations

Reactions	PPA	Caffeine	PPA/caffeine combinations
Psychiatric			
Agitation	+	+	+
Anxiety	+	+	+
Hallucinations	+	+	+
Mania	+	?	+
Nervousness	+	+	+
Paranoia	+	+	+
Psychosis	+	+	+
Neurologic			
Blurred vision	+	+	+
Confusion	?	?	+
Disorientation	+	+	+
Dizziness	+	+	+
Headaches	+	+	+
Insomnia	+	+	+
Intercerebral hemorrhage	+	–	+
Seizures	+	+	+
Slurred speech	–	–	+
Cardiovascular			
Arrhythmias	+	+	+
Hypertensive crisis (often in interaction with other drugs)	+	+	+
Increased blood pressure	+	+	+
Tachycardia	+	+	+
Respiratory			
Chest pain	+	?	+
Dyspnea	+	+	+
Gastrointestinal			
Diarrhea	?	+	?
Epigastric pain	?	+	+
Hematemesis	?	+	+
Nausea/vomiting	+	+	+
Death	+	+	+

+: reported -: not reported
?: implied but not well-documented

Source: Compiled by the author. Data derived from Greden, J. F. 1981. Caffeine. In Behavior in excess, edited by S. J. Mulé, 164-89. New York: The Free Press; Greden, J. F. 1981. Caffeinism and caffeine withdrawal. In Substance abuse: clinical problems and perspectives, edited by J. H. Lowinson and P. Ruiz, 274-86. Baltimore: Williams & Wilkins.

Withdrawal Manifestations

Caffeine withdrawal is a well-documented phenomenon. Among habitual heavy users, an abstinence even as brief as 12 to 18 hours may produce clinically significant manifestations. The most common symptoms include headache, drowsiness, lethargy, rhinorrhea, irritability, nervousness, and vague feelings of depression. There has been relatively little study of withdrawal symptoms associated with phenylpropanolamine and, in fact, high-dose, prolonged use has not been investigated.

Drug Interactions

Both caffeine and phenylpropanolamine have the potential to interact with other medications, often in comparable fashion. Two of these drug interactions merit mention. First, both agents can produce severe hypertensive crises when combined with monoamine oxidase (MAO) inhibitors. Second, it has been reported that caffeine and other methyl xanthines increase the cardiotoxic potential of beta-adrenergic agonists such as isoproterenol, inducing a higher incidence of cardiac arrhythmias. These two side effects have special importance, since a number of the deaths apparently due to products containing phenylpropanolamine and caffeine appear to have stemmed from cardiovascular pathophysiology (Chouinard, Ghadirian, and Jones 1978; Bernstein and Diskant 1982). Future investigators must consider whether combinations of phenylpropanolamine and caffeine may have a greater potential to induce cardiac arrhythmias than either drug taken alone.

Is the abuse potential of the phenylpropanolamine/caffeine combination higher than that of either product used alone? The answer is not known. In considering whether the combination might meet accepted criteria for drugs subject to habituation, we can examine the following list. According to an Expert Committee of the World Health Organization (Angrist and Sudilovsky 1978), high-dose nonmedical stimulant use is characterized by:

1. A desire or need to continue taking the drug;
2. Consumption of increasing amounts to obtain greater excitatory and euphoric effects or to combat fatigue, accompanied by the development of some degree of tolerance;
3. Psychic dependence on the effects of the drug; and

4. General absence of physical dependence so that discontinuation of the drug does not lead to a withdrawal syndrome.

Clinical evidence suggests that caffeine meets the first three requirements and, despite some claims to the contrary, that it may also induce a characteristic withdrawal syndrome when chronic use is discontinued (Greden 1981b; Goldstein and Kazen 1969). It has not yet been determined whether phenylpropanolamine satisfies these criteria. Nor is it known whether the combination of phenylpropanolamine and caffeine accelerates or accentuates the pattern. Perhaps the effects are additive.

Clinical Diagnosis of Phenylpropanolamine/Caffeine Toxicity

Reactions to phenylpropanolamine/caffeine combinations do not appear to be characterized by any unique features. Instead, the pattern of side effects is simply a version of the well-known profile associated with low-potency stimulants. Thus, a diagnosis of possible phenylpropanolamine/caffeine toxicity will depend primarily upon a thorough history being taken. The clinician must ask about all drug ingestion patterns.

High-risk subjects for phenylpropanolamine/caffeine interactions are likely to include those with obesity, concerns about weight, preoccupations with social functioning and appearance, and patterns of periodic dieting. Even if these patients admit dieting, however, they often do not spontaneously reveal that they use products containing phenylpropanolamine. They should be asked questions, possibly in the form of questionnaires, about their use of both phenylpropanolamine and caffeine.

For clinical research purposes, if diagnosis is to be confirmed and our understanding of the symptomatology of reactions to phenylpropanolamine is to improve, a plasma or urine drug screen should be conducted. A word of caution, however: the enzyme-multiplied immunoassay technique (EMIT) used in many drug analysis laboratories does not differentiate between phenylpropanolamine and amphetamine. Thus, the omission of phenylpropanolamine from drug reports does not prove that the drug was not present. Tests for phenylpropanolamine must be specifically ordered, and thin-layer chromatography and gas chromatography must be used to confirm its presence (Tan and Salvador 1983). A problem that further contributes to incomplete diagnosis is that clinicians rarely request drug screens for caffeine. Indeed, even if requested, many laboratories would be unable to test for this ubiquitous agent. To confirm apparent toxic reactions, an A-B-A ("start-stop-start") trial can be conducted if it is clinically safe to do so.

SUMMARY AND FUTURE DIRECTIONS

In summary, there are several points that can be made about the relationship between phenylpropanolamine and caffeine.

First, neither caffeine nor phenylpropanolamine is an innocuous drug; clinical case reports are common enough and have sufficient pharmacologic validity to suggest that phenylpropanolamine and caffeine--singly or in combination-- may induce occasional adverse reactions. Some of these can be significant but rarely are they life-threatening. The severity of such reactions appears to be proportional to the amount ingested and the duration of use. In addition, chronic use and habituation may occur.

Second, our scientific database is inadequate and confusing. Further study is needed, especially to determine if drug interactions between the two agents occur.

Third, regulatory decisions about phenylpropanolamine cannot be made with confidence on the basis of currently available reports that describe reactions in people who ingested combination products. Pharmacologic common sense dictates that side effects which occur under such circumstances cannot be accurately attributed to phenylpropanolamine without further study.

Fourth, it is unlikely that the FDA's ban of products containing combinations of phenylpropanolamine, ephedrine, and caffeine will solve the problem of potential drug interactions between phenylpropanolamine and caffeine. There are numerous commercial sources of caffeine, and it will continue to be widely consumed by phenylpropanolamine users. The simultaneous ingestion of the two products in separate medications will also still take place. Thus, continued scientific interest in the drug interaction problem should be encouraged, with dissemination of warnings to consumers if warranted.

Fifth, dose-response curves need to be developed, with special emphasis on monitoring CNS and cardiovascular variables, for phenylpropanolamine alone and combined with caffeine.

Sixth, consideration might be given in the future to eliminating caffeine from OTC analgesics, since they constitute a common source of the caffeine in drug interactions and there is little good evidence for caffeine's analgesic utility.

REFERENCES

Achor, M. B. and I. Extein. 1981. Diet aids, mania, and affective illness. Am J Psychiatry 138:392.

Altschuler, S. et al. 1982. Three controlled trials of weight loss with phenylpropanolamine. Int J Obes 6:549-56.

Angrist, B. and A. Sudilovsky. 1978. Central nervous system stimulants: historical aspects and clinical effects. In Handbook of psychopharmacology: stimulants, vol. 2, edited by L. L. Iverson, S. D. Iverson, and S. H. Snyder, 99-166. New York: Plenum.

Appelt, G. D. 1983. The safety of phenylpropanolamine. J Clin Psychopharmacol 3:332-33.

Bernstein, E. and B. M. Diskant. 1982. Phenylpropanolamine: a potentially hazardous drug. Ann Emerg Med 11:311-15.

Blum, A. 1981. Phenylpropanolamine: an over-the-counter amphetamine? JAMA 245:1346-47.

Chouinard, G., A. M. Ghadirian, and B. D. Jones. 1978. Death attributed to ventricular arrhythmia induced by thioridazine in combination with a single Contac C capsule. Can Med Assoc J 119:729-31.

Cornelius, J. R., P. H. Soloff, and C. F. Reynolds III. 1984. Paranoia, homicidal behavior, and seizures associated with phenylpropanolamine. Am J Psychiatry 141:120-21.

Dietz, A. J. 1981. Amphetamine-like reactions to phenylpropanolamine. JAMA 245:601-2.

Ellis, J. 1774. An historical account of coffee. London: Edward and Charles Dilly.

Gilbert, R. M. 1980. Caffeine as a drug of abuse. In Research advances in alcohol and drug problems, vol. 3, edited by R. J. Gibbons et al., 127-68. New York: Wiley.

Goldstein, A. and S. Kazen. 1969. Psychotropic effects of caffeine in man. Clin Pharmacol Ther 10:477-88.

Greden, J. F. 1981a. Caffeine. In Behavior in excess, edited by S. J. Mulé, 164-89. New York: The Free Press.

———. 1981b. Caffeinism and caffeine withdrawal. In Substance abuse: clinical problems and perspectives, edited by J. H. Lowinson and P. Ruiz, 274-86. Baltimore, MD: Williams & Wilkins.

———. 1979. Coffee, tea, and you. The Sciences 19:6-11.

———. 1976. The tea controversy in colonial America. JAMA 236:63-66.

Health and Human Services, Food and Drug Administration (FDA). 1982a. Establishment of a monograph for weight control drug products for over-the-counter human use. FDA docket no. 81N-0022. Federal Register 47:8466-84. February 26.

Health and Human Services, Food and Drug Administration (FDA). 1982b. New drug status of OTC combination drug products containing caffeine, phenylpropanolamine, and ephedrine. FDA docket no. 82N-0266. Federal Register 47:35344-46. August 13.

Horowitz, J. D. et al. 1980. Hypertensive responses induced by phenylpropanolamine in anorectic and decongestant preparations. Lancet 1:60-61.

Horowitz, J. D. et al. 1979. Hypertension and postural hypotension induced by phenylpropanolamine (Trimolets). Med J Aust 1:175-76.

Mikkelsen, E. J. 1978. Caffeine and schizophrenia. J Clin Psychiatry 3:732-36.

Siegerist, H. E. 1943. Literary controversy over tea in 18th century England. Bull Hist Med 13:185-89.

Silverman, H. I. et al. 1980. Lack of side effects from orally administered phenylpropanolamine and phenylpropanolamine with caffeine: a controlled three-phase study. Current Therapeutic Research 28:185-94.

Tan, H. S. and G. C. Salvador. 1983. Assay of mixtures of phenylpropanolamine hydrochloride and caffeine in appetite suppressant formulations by high performance liquid chromatography. J Chromatogr 261:111-16.

Truitt, E. B., Jr. 1971. The xanthines. In Drill's pharmacology in medicine, 4th ed., edited by J. R. DiPalma, 533-56. New York: McGraw-Hill.

Ukers, W. H. 1948. The romance of coffee. New York: The Tea and Coffee Trade Journal Company.

Weiner, N. 1980. Norepinephrine, epinephrine, and the sympathomimetic amines. In The pharmacological basis of therapeutics, 6th ed., edited by L. S. Goodman and A. Gilman, 142-43. New York: Macmillan.

11

NOREPHEDRINE AND NORPSEUDOEPHEDRINE: PHARMACOLOGICALLY AND CLINICALLY DISTINCT ISOMERS OF PHENYLPROPANOLAMINE

John P. Morgan

INTRODUCTION

Phenylisopropylamine compounds (figure 11.1) have been extremely important in medical and pharmaceutical science. An understanding of their effects, character, and relative clinical utility is of obvious importance. There are certain characteristics they share in common: they are active after oral ingestion; they are sympathomimetic but are not metabolized by endogenous enzymes that degrade endogenous sympathetic agents; and they are largely indirectly acting. Because of their related structures and qualitatively similar physiological effects, we are prone to group them in our thinking and to focus on their nondistinctiveness. On closer inspection, however, we find that they do have marked differences. Amphetamine has pronounced central nervous system (CNS) stimulating properties not shared by all others (Schulte et al. 1941). Norephedrine has minimal bronchodilating properties (Cameron and Tainter 1936); ephedrine is very irritating when applied locally to the nasal mucosa (Black 1937). Further, we must carefully consider isomeric differences. (-)-Amphetamine has more cardiovascular activity than (+)-amphetamine (Caldwell and Sever 1974). Pseudoephedrine has less CNS activity than ephedrine (Haefely, Bartholini, and Pletscher 1976). Such distinctions may be usefully exploited to achieve desired therapeutic effects or to diminish unwanted ones.

Despite this historical approach focusing on distinctions between similar chemicals, confusion about the possible abuse of similar molecules persists. There is even a tendency to blur distinctions when evaluating lists of chemicals for abuse potential as if a report of abuse by one person were equal to abuse by hundreds. Hence, this review is directed at examining the historical and pharmacological distinctions between two extremely similar compounds, phenylpropanolamine (PPA) (norephedrine) and norpseudoephedrine (cathine).

FIGURE 11.1

Phenylisopropylamine compounds

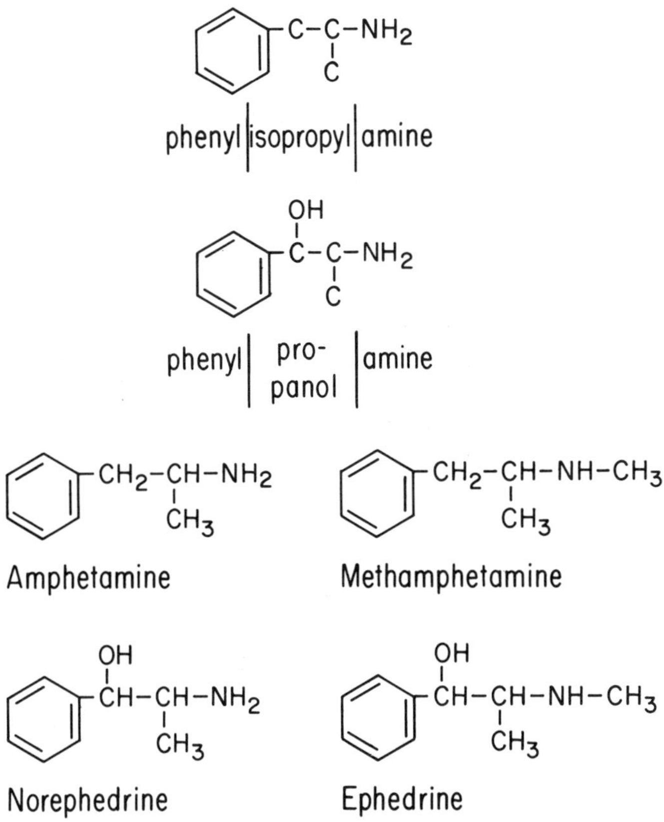

Source: Compiled by the author.

STEREOCHEMICAL CONVENTIONS

Most compounds discussed in this report have different isomeric forms.* Optically active forms that rotate a beam of polarized light clockwise are preceded by (+)-, as in (+)-ephedrine; those that rotate a beam of light counterclockwise are preceded by (-)-, as in (-)-amphetamine. Very often, the lower-case letters "d" (dextrorotatory) and "l" (leverotatory) were and are used for these distinctions. Confusion abounds, however, because some writers use an upper-case "D" or "L". These do not refer to a direction of light rotation but to an absolute configurational relationship to some standard substance (usually a three- or four-carbon sugar). Therefore, some compounds are D(+) but others may be D(-).

Equal mixtures of optically active isomers are not themselves optically active. Such products are called racemic mixtures and are best labeled (±)-, but are often labeled d,l-. Optical isomers which are mirror images of one another are called enantiomorphs; those that do not yield superimposable images are diastereomers. A carbon linked to four distinct groups (once labeled "asymmetric") is properly called a chiral carbon. The presence of a chiral carbon signals the presence of isomers. Despite similar configurations and similar physiochemical attributes, isomers may have markedly different effects. A recent review of chiral drug action makes this very clear (Simonyi 1984).

NOREPHEDRINE AND NORPSEUDOEPHEDRINE

Norephedrine, the n-demethylated congener of ephedrine, was isolated in a synthetic mixture as early as 1910. Its pharmacological actions were compared to those of ephedrine and found similar as early as 1917 (Chen and Schmidt 1930). The synthetic reactions yielding norephedrine produced (as synthetic reactions essentially always do) a racemic mixture equally composed of optically active isomers of the compound. A patent application for (±)-norephedrine (Mydriatine®) was filed in 1921 (Chen and Schmidt 1930). The development in 1930 of a cost-effective synthetic method for

---

*A very readable review of the definitions and nomenclature of stereochemistry is given in: Gunstone, F. D. 1975. Guidebook to stereochemistry. New York: Longman. Particularly useful are pages 21-34.

producing (±)-norephedrine preceded the first testing of it in humans in 1931 (Levy and Tiffeneau 1931). It entered clinical medicine as a nasal decongestant in the United States in 1936. The name norephedrine was generally replaced by the more descriptive name phenylpropanolamine, which acknowledges its three structural subcomponents.

Simplified line drawings (figures 11.2 and 11.3) reveal that both the alpha- and beta-carbons are chiral—they each bind to four distinct structural groups. Therefore, norephedrine (or phenylpropanolamine) has four distinct spatial arrangements and four distinct stereoisomers. Any of these forms or any mixtures of them might be called "phenylpropanolamine." Usually the product so named has been a racemic mixture of (+)- and (-)-norephedrine enantiomers.

FIGURE 11.2

Configurational characteristics of norephedrine isomers

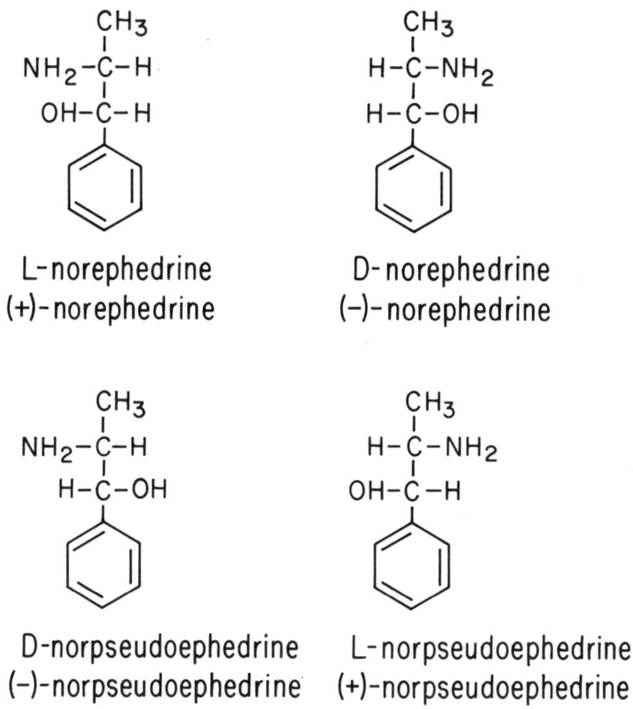

Source: Compiled by the author.

FIGURE 11.3

Chiral structure and variations of norephedrine isomers

*chiral carbons

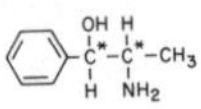

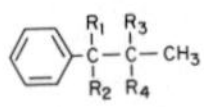

	$\underline{R_1}$	$\underline{R_2}$	$\underline{R_3}$	$\underline{R_4}$
D-norephedrine	H	OH	H	NH_2
L-norpseudoephedrine	OH	H	H	NH_2
L-norephedrine	OH	H	NH_2	H
D-norpseudoephedrine	H	OH	NH_2	H

Source: Compiled by the author.

Another confusion of nomenclature may occur here. The apposition of two chiral carbons leads to the possible presence of four isomers. In the line drawings, it is clear that isomers in which the "major" functional groups (NH_2, OH) are represented on different sides of the two-carbon skeleton are called "pseudo" forms; hence, norpseudoephedrine. In yet another convention, these forms were once labeled "threo," while norephedrines were labeled "erythro," after similar configurations of the sugars threose and erythrose.

(+)-Norpseudoephedrine is a clinically important isomeric "phenylpropanolamine." (+)-Norpseudoephedrine is a naturally occurring plant material. It was first described after isolation from the ephedra species in 1924 (Smith 1928). In 1930 it was isolated from "khat" (Catha edulis), a plant whose leaves are chewed for their psychoactive and stimulant effects (Lugman and Danowski 1976). For many years it was assumed that (+)-norpseudoephedrine [(+)-cathine] was responsible for the plant's psychoactivity (figure 11.4). Such speculations were supported by a number of studies indicating that khat had both stimulant and anorexiant effects (van Rossum and Simons 1966; Zelger and Carlini 1980; Knoll 1980). However, the low concentration of (+)-norpseudoephedrine in fresh khat provoked recent careful analyses of the pharmacology and chemistry of Catha edulis.

In brief summary, fresh khat contains a related phenylalkylamine ketone, (-)-alpha-aminopropiophenone, in relatively high concentrations (Szendrei 1980). This product, now known as cathinone, has been tested in a number of species and has greater stimulant and reinforcing properties than does cathine (Zelger, Schorno, and Carlini 1980). It is probably the chief source of khat's psychoactivity and is the parent compound of cathine, which is a metabolic product of cathinone both in the plant and in man (Braenden 1980).

FIGURE 11.4

Constituents of khat

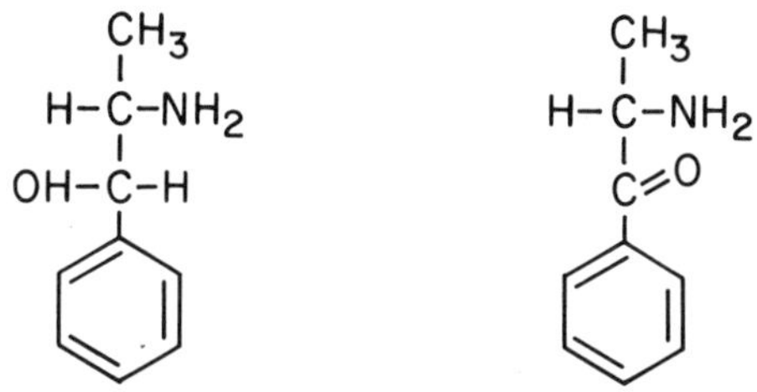

(+)-cathine [(+)-norpseudo-ephedrine]

(-)-cathinone [(-)-alpha-amino-propiophenone]

Source: Compiled by the author.

COMPARISONS OF NOREPHEDRINE AND NORPSEUDOEPHEDRINE

Confusion about and a nonchalant approach to the distinctions between these products emerged early in their history. In 1929 (+)-norpseudoephedrine isolated from ephedra vulgaris was first studied in humans (Chen and Henricksen 1929). It was found to cause mydriasis and to produce notable pressor effects in man after a single 50 mg dose. Two subsequent studies of synthetic ($\pm$)-norephedrine cited this earlier study of (+)-norpseudoephedrine and compared the products as if they were identical (Loman, Rinkel, and Myerson 1939; Lorhan and Mosser 1947). Loman and his co-workers in 1939 even published some quantitative data from the 1929 study which had not appeared in the original report:

> Chen and his co-workers administered the drug orally in 50 mg. doses to two individuals and noted rises of 16 and 30 mm. Hg, respectively, in the systolic blood pressure. (Loman, Rinkel, and Myerson 1939, p. 90)

This type of confusion has been once again reactivated (Gianini and Castellani 1982). A recent report described a case of psychosis in a North African student resident in the United States. The authors learned that the patient had chewed a few khat leaves before he was admitted to the hospital, and a urine toxicology screen revealed the presence of "phenylpropanolamine." The authors decided that these findings supported the notion that this was the first khat psychosis reported in the United States. This is inconsistent with the knowledge that khat psychosis is rare or absent in Yemen, where hundreds of leaves are chewed at a sitting. Further, even if the authors did accurately identify norpseudoephedrine, this does not prove their contention, because most urinary norpseudoephedrine is present as a metabolite of pseudoephedrine (Lo, Land, and Bye 1981).

THREE COMPARATIVE PHARMACOLOGICAL STUDIES

In 1967, a single study compared the effects of all the optical isomers of norephedrine, ephedrine, and amphetamine in rats (Fairchild and Alles 1967). The authors synthesized all the isomers and included experimental verification of their optical activity. Assigning a score of 1.0 to (+)-amphetamine, the compound that caused the most locomotor activity in rats, generated the following order of stimulant effects:

(+)-amphetamine	1.0
(-)-amphetamine	.25
(+)-norpseudoephedrine	.10
(-)-ephedrine	.04
(-)-norpseudoephedrine	.02
(-)-norephedrine	*
(+)-norephedrine	*
(-)-pseudoephedrine	*
(+)-pseudoephedrine	*
(+)-ephedrine	*

Fairchild and Alles (Ibid.) cited earlier studies indicating that in the stimulation of human subjects (+)-norpseudoephedrine was more potent than caffeine but less potent than (+)-methamphetamine and that racemic (±)-norpseudoephedrine was a stronger CNS stimulant than (±)-ephedrine (Hofman, Opitz, and Schelle 1955).

---

*Stimulation only at lethal or near-lethal doses.

These studies were consistent with the known status of (±)-norephedrine. It has consistently been shown to possess negligible stimulant properties in comparison to (+)-amphetamine and (-)-ephedrine. More recent studies have confirmed these impressions. (±)-Norephedrine will not act as a reinforcing agent in primates in self-injection experiments although most anorexiant phenethylamines will (Griffiths, Brachy, and Snell 1978), as will cathinone (Schuster and Johanson 1980).

There are two, more recent experiments in which specific norephedrine isomers were again compared. These also attest to the distinctions between similar compounds. In a complicated series of experiments in genetically obese and normal mice eating at liberty and in meal-fed rats, Arch and his co-workers compared a series of ephedrine isomers and related congeners (Arch, Ainsworth, and Cawthorne 1982). Assessments were made of weight gain patterns and energy expenditure (related indirectly to oxygen utilization). Many distinctions were found. (+)-Norpseudoephedrine was very active in early suppression of weight gain, but only (±)-norephedrine acted to depress weight over the entire 28-day study. (+)-Norpseudoephedrine was more active than (+)-norephedrine in increasing energy expenditure in obese mice. (+)-Norpseudoephedrine was more active than the other products in causing diminished lipid content in normal mice, although an equivalent effect was produced by (-)-ephedrine and (+)-pseudoephedrine in obese mice.

In another study directed at assessing the norepinephrine-potentiating effect of various sympathomimetic amines, optical isomers differed dramatically (Swamy et al. 1969). Among 25 alpha-methylated drugs and isomers, (+)-norpseudoephedrine ranked third, (-)-norephedrine was sixth, and (+)-norephedrine was 21st in augmenting norepinephrine-caused contractions of rat vas deferens. However, (-)-norephedrine ranked above (fourth) (+)-norpseudoephedrine (11th) and both ranked well above (+)-norephedrine in augmenting a norepinephrine-augmented rate increase in isolated rat atria.

CURRENT USES AND STATUS

(±)-Norephedrine is widely available in the United States, both as a cough/cold product and as an appetite suppressant. Consumption in recent years has reached literally billions of doses. Despite recent controversy surrounding its use as an over-the-counter (OTC) diet aid, there are no clinical studies indicating that it has a significant stimulant effect on the human central nervous system at clinical or even moderately elevated doses.

(+)-Norpseudoephedrine is not available for medicinal use in the United States, but it is widely used in Europe as a nonprescription anorexiant. It is available as a 25 mg capsule (Mirapront®, Fugoa®, Minusin®) or in a 30 mg preparation with vitamins (Recatol®). It is also marketed in a mixture of 15 mg with caffeine, herbs, vitamins, and nikethamide as Antiadipositum X-112. There is evidence in the European medical literature of human habituation and abuse of (+)-norpseudoephedrine (Renfordt and Wirtz 1980).

"TRIMOLETS" AND PHENYLPROPANOLAMINE

Beginning in 1978, a series of six articles reported pressor effects in humans utilizing a phenylpropanolamine-containing Australian diet aid, "Trimolets" (Frewin, Leonello, and Frewin 1978; Horowitz et al. 1979; King 1979; Lee, Beilin, and Vandongen 1979; Horowitz et al. 1980; McEwen 1983). Although most were case reports, two studies contained controlled evaluations of the pressor effects of this product.

The study by Horowitz et al. (1980) has been widely discussed because it depicts a drug with different effects than many studies with (±)-phenylpropanolamine, past and present. After a single dose of Trimolets, normal subjects experienced a statistically significant increase in systolic and diastolic blood pressure, with 12 of 37 subjects attaining a diastolic pressure greater than 100 mg Hg. Trimolets subjects reported significantly more subjective symptoms than the control group. Although many of these subjective reports may have been related to the elevation in blood pressure, some (dizziness, headache, tremors, palpitations, chest tightness, tinnitus, "hot" feelings) might have reflected stimulant drug effects. This study was instrumental in removing phenylpropanolamine anorexiant products from the OTC market in Australia and is often cited by those such as Blum (1981) who wish to effect the same removal in the United States. It is now obvious that the actual content of Trimolets was never clear.

In the 1980 Horowitz et al. paper, "Trimolets" is identified as "containing 85 mg of phenylpropanolamine per capsule." There is no further information offerred. Subsequently a number of familiarly confusing findings have emerged.

The Trimolets packages were generally labeled "one-per-day," yet it is now clear that none of the products so named were timed-disintegration or controlled-release but were all immediate-release. Two of the Australian papers describing

ILLUSTRATION 11.1

Versions of Trimolets available in Australia

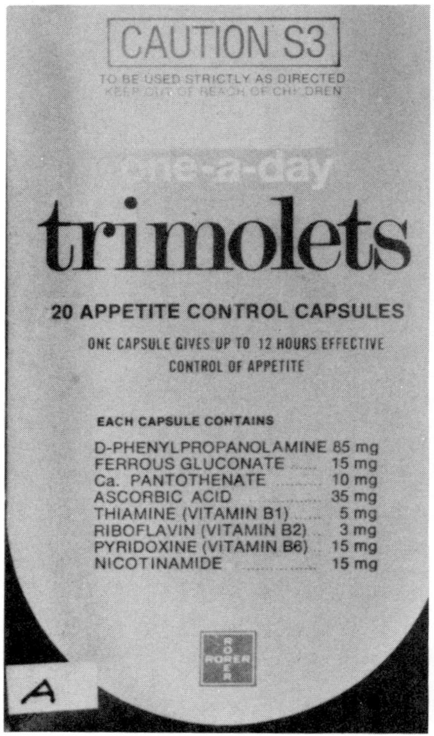

(a)

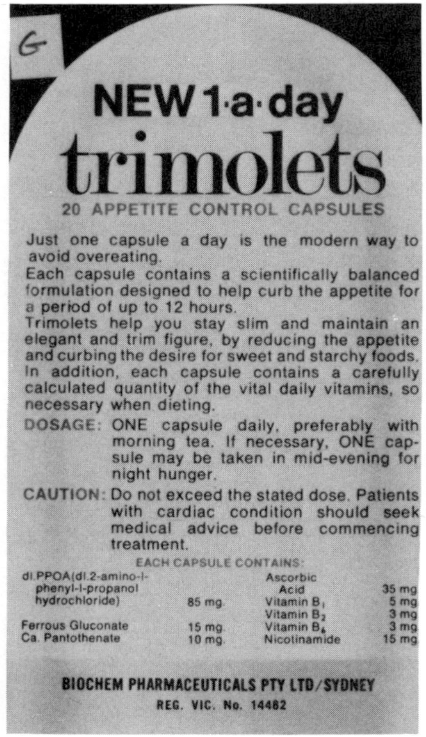

(b)

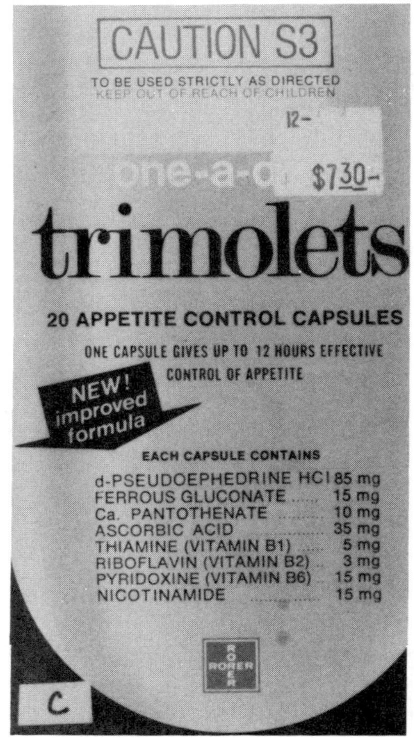

(c)

Source: Supplied by the author.

adverse reactions referred to nonracemic products. Lee, Beilin, and Vandongen (1979) described Trimolets as "D-phenylpropanolamine" and Frewin, Leonello, and Frewin (1978) called it "d-phenylpropanolamine." Recently I obtained a number of package versions of the OTC product Trimolets through the Proprietary Association of Australia, Mr. Thomas Kemney of the Thompson Medical Company, and Sachey and Sachey Advertising Agency of Sydney. I also talked with Mr. David Cole (1984) of the Rorer Company, which marketed Trimolets in Australia at the time of the 1980 Horowitz et al. study. Briefly, the packages were labeled:

1. "D-phenylpropanolamine 85 mg" (illustration 11.1a) ("phenylpropanolamine HCl 85 mg," inner foil);
2. "dl.PPOA (dl.2-amino-1-phenyl-1-propanol hydrochloride) 85 mg" (illustration 11.1b) ("phenylpropanolamine HCl 85 mg," inner foil); and
3. "d-Pseudoephedrine HCl 85 mg" (illustration 11.1c) ("dl-Pseudoephedrine HCl 85 mg," inner foil).

The Rorer Company reported to me that the Trimolets product was nonracemic d-pseudoephedrine and a later letter from the president of Rorer identified the product as "d-phenylpropanolamine."

The Proprietary Association of Australia also recorded the Australian importation of "D-norpseudoephedrine" by a Trimolets distributor in 1972-73. In Europe, norpseudoephedrine is often referred to as phenylpropanolamine.

Dr. W. J. Louis (1984) confirmed that the Trimolets used in the Horowitz et al. study (1979) was purchased at a retail outlet and had not been assayed.

The use of an immediate-release 85 mg preparation may be important. The immediate-release products available in the United States did not exceed 50 mg. However, the most important issue of the Australian Trimolets is the chiral confusion. Trimolets may have been (±)-norephedrine, pseudoephedrine, or norpseudoephedrine. It seems very likely that it was a nonracemic dextrorotatory form of one of the above at least some of the time. Because of the subjective symptoms noted in the 1980 Horowitz et al. study, I suspect that the product was most likely the most centrally active version of the above, (+)-norpseudoephedrine. This probably explains why U.S. reports (Saltzman, Dolan, and Doyne 1983; Ekins and Spoerke 1983) generally have found (±)-phenylpropanolamine to be the relatively safe drug it was thought to be since its introduction in 1936.

REFERENCES

Arch, J.R.S., A. T. Ainsworth, and M. A. Cawthorne. 1982. Thermogenic and anorectic effects of ephedrine and congeners in mice and rats. Life Sci 30:1817-26.

Black, J. H. 1937. The control of allergic manifestations by phenyl-propanol-amine (Propadrine) hydrochloride. Journal--Lancet 57:101-2.

Blum, A. 1981. Phenylpropanolamine: an over-the-counter amphetamine? JAMA 245:1346-47.

Braenden, O. J. 1980. Research on the chemical composition of khat. In Problems of drug dependence, 1979, edited by L. S. Harris, 320-21. National Institute on Drug Abuse research monograph no. 27. Washington, D.C.: U.S. Government Printing Office.

Caldwell, J. and P. A. Sever. 1974. The biochemical pharmacology of abused drugs: I. Amphetamine, cocaine and LSD. Clin Pharmacol Ther 16:625-38.

Cameron, W. M. and M. L. Tainter. 1936. Comparative actions of sympathomimetic compounds: bronchodilator action in bronchial spasm induced by histamine. J Pharmacol Exp Ther 57:152-69.

Chen, K. K. and C. F. Schmidt. 1930. Ephedrine and related substances. Medicine 9:1-117.

Chen, K. K., C. K. Wu, and E. Henricksen. 1929. Relationship between the pharmacological action and the chemical constitution and configuration of the optical isomers of ephedrine and related compounds. J Pharmacol Exp Ther 36:363-400.

Cole, D. 1984. Telephone conversation with author. September.

Ekins, B. R. and D. G. Spoerke. 1983. An estimation of the toxicity of nonprescription diet aids from seventy exposure cases. Vet Hum Toxicol 25:81-85.

Fairchild, M. D. and G. A. Alles. 1967. The central locomotor stimulatory activity and acute toxicity of the ephedrine and norephedrine isomers in mice. J Pharmacol Exp Ther 158:135-39.

Frewin, D. B., P. P. Leonello, and M. E. Frewin. 1978. Hypertension after ingestion of Trimolets. Med J Aust 2:497-98.

Giannini, A. J. and S. Castellani. 1982. A manic-like psychosis due to khat (Catha edulis Forsk.). J Toxicol Clin Toxicol 19:455-59.

Griffiths, R. R., J. V. Brady, and J. D. Snell. 1978. Relationship between anorectic and reinforcing properties of appetite suppressant drugs: implications for assessment of abuse liability. Biol Psychiatry 13:283-90.

Haefely, W., G. Bartholini, and A. Pletscher. 1976. Monoaminergic drugs: general pharmacology. Pharmacol Ther (B) 2:185-218.

Hofmann, H., K. Opitz, and H. J. Schnelle. 1955. Die wirkung des norpseudoephedrins. Arzneimittel Forschung 5:367-70.

Horowitz, J. D. et al. 1980. Hypertensive responses induced by phenylpropanolamine in anorectic and decongestant preparations. Lancet 1:60-61.

Horowitz, J. D. et al. 1979. Hypertension and postural hypotension induced by phenylpropanolamine (Trimolets). Med J Aust 1:175-76.

King, J. 1979. Hypertension and cerebral hemorrhage after Trimolets ingestion. Med J Aust 2:258.

Knoll, J. 1979. Studies on the central effects of (-)-cathinone. In Problems of drug dependence, 1979, edited by L. S. Harris, 322-23. National Institute on Drug Abuse research monograph no. 27. Washington, D.C.: U.S. Government Printing Office.

Lee, K. Y., L. J. Beilin, and R. Vandongen. 1979. Severe hypertension after ingestion of an appetite suppressant (phenylpropanolamine) with indomethacin. Lancet 1:1110-11.

Levy, J. and M. Tiffeneau. 1931. Sur les proprites cardiovasculaires de la norephedrine. C R Soc Biol 106:548-51.

Lo, L. Y., G. Land, and A. Bye. 1981. Sensitive assay for pseudoephedrine and its metabolite norpseudoephedrine in plasma and urine using gas-liquid chromatography with electro-capture detection. J Chromatogr 222:297-302.

Loman, J., M. Rinkel, and A. Myerson. 1939. Comparative effects of amphetamine sulfate (benzedrine sulfate), paredrine, and propadrine on the blood pressure. Am Heart J 18:89-93.

Lorhan, P. H. and D. Mosser. 1947. Phenylpropanolamine hydrochloride: a vasopressor drug for maintaining blood pressure during spinal anesthesia. Ann Surg 125:171-76.

Louis, W. J. 1984. Personal interview with author.

Lugman, W. and T. S. Danowski. 1976. The use of khat (Catha edulis) in Yemen: social and medical observations. Ann Intern Med 85:246-49.

McEwen, J. 1983. Phenylpropanolamine-associated hypertension after the use of "over-the-counter" appetite suppressant products. Med J Aust 2:71-73.

Renfordt, E. and W. Wirtz. 1980. Mifbrauch von d-norpseudoephedrine appetitzuglern. Der Nervenarzt 51:691-93.

Saltzman, M. B., M. M. Dolan, and N. Doyne. 1983. Comparison of effects of two dosage regimens of phenylpropanolamine on blood pressure and plasma levels in normal subjects under steady state conditions. Drug Intell Clin Pharm 17:746-50.

Schulte, J. W. et al. 1941. Further study of central stimulation from sympathomimetic amines. J Pharmacol Exp Ther 71:62-74.

Schuster, C. R. and C. E. Johanson. 1979. Behavioral studies of cathinone in monkeys and rats. In Problems of drug dependence, 1979, edited by L. S. Harris, 324-25. National Institute on Drug Abuse research monograph no. 27. Washington, D.C.: U.S. Government Printing Office.

Simonyi, M. 1984. On chiral drug action. Med Res Rev 4:339-442.

Smith, S. 1928. Nor-d-"pseudo"-ephedrine, an alkaloid from ephedra species. J Chem Soc 51-53.

Swamy, V. C. et al. 1969. Steric aspects of adrenergic drugs: XIII. Norepinephrine potentiating effects of isomers of sympathomimetic amine in rat vas deferens and atria. Arch Int Pharmacodyn Ther 182:24-31.

Szendrei, K. 1979. The chemistry of khat. Bull Narc 32:5-36.

van Rossum, J. M. and F. Simons. 1966. Locomotor activity and anorexigenic action. Psychopharmacologia 14:248.

Zelger, J. L. and E. A. Carlini. 1980. Anorexigenic effects of two amines obtained from Catha edulis Forsk. (khat) in rats. Pharmacol Biochem Behav 12:701-5.

Zelger, J. L., H. X. Schorno, and E. A. Carlini. 1980. Behavioral effects of cathinone, an amine obtained from Catha edulis Forsk.: comparisons with amphetamine, norpseudoephedrine, apomorphine, and nomifensine. Bull Narc 32:67-82.

II

ISSUES OF TOXICITY

A. WHAT IS PHENYLPROPANOLAMINE'S LIABILITY REGARDING CARDIOVASCULAR TOXICITY?

12

HYPERTENSIVE RESPONSES TO PHENYLPROPANOLAMINE

William J. Louis and John D. Horowitz

INTRODUCTION

Phenylpropanolamine (PPA) is a sympathomimetic drug (structurally related to ephedrine) which is widely used as a component in over-the-counter (OTC) nasal decongestants and anorexiant medications. Hypertensive responses have been reported after ingestion of single doses of phenylpropanolamine in previously normotensive subjects (Cuthbert, Greenberg, and Morley 1969; Frewin, Leonello, and Frewin 1978) and in patients with special sensitivity to adrenergic pressor agents. In Australia phenylpropanolamine is available in a wide range of preparations in unit doses ranging from 15 to 100 mg (table 12.1). Recently there have been moves to reduce dosages of all phenylpropanolamine-containing preparations to a maximum of 25 mg, but this recommendation has not yet been fully implemented.

The active ingredient in most of these products is phenylpropanolamine hydrochloride (or dl-norephedrine hydrochloride), which consists of four stereoisomers. There is little published information on the relative cardiovascular properties and anorexiant effects of the individual isomers. In the pithed rat the pressor effects ratio of (-)- to (+)-norephedrine was 1.0:68 (Patil, LaPidus, and Tye 1970). As far as we can establish, racemic phenylpropanolamine has been used in the manufacture of all preparations currently marketed in Australia.

CASE REPORTS

We became interested in the occurrence potential of hypertensive responses to phenylpropanolamine because of two medical cases seen at the Austin Hospital in Heidelberg,

TABLE 12.1

Products containing phenylpropanolamine marketed in Australia, October 1979

Preparation	PPA/ unit dose (mg)	Dosage recommendations (doses/day)
Appetite suppressant		
A.S.T.	20	3
Dietgard™	75	1
Slim-Rite	75	2
Soulls Slimming Tabs	25	2-4
Spindell	27.5	2
Statavar	25	3
Trimtabs™	60	1
Trimolets	50*	1-2
Nasal decongestant		
Contac 500	50	2
Dimetapp elixir	5	3-4
Dimetapp tablets L.A.	15	3-4
Elixamine	15	6
Eskornade	50	2
Neopiphen	16	6
Ornex spansules	18	12
Sinugard	20	3
Sinutabs®	25	6
Sinutabs® with codeine	35	6-12
Sinutabs S.A.	100	1-2
Triaminic®	50	3
Triogesic	12.5	6
Tuss-Ornade® capsules	50	2

*Reduced from 85 mg in early 1979.

Source: Compiled by the authors. Data derived from Kallis, S. G. and P. Passmore. 1979. Australian proprietary preparations containing phenylpropanolamine. Med J Aust 2:425-26.

Victoria, Australia. The first case (Horowitz et al. 1979) involved a 17-year-old girl who for three weeks had been taking twice daily an OTC anorexiant product, Trimolets, which at that time contained 85 mg phenylpropanolamine per capsule. Then, in an attempt to increase the product's anorexiant effect, she took six capsules at one time. Three hours later, she developed a severe bifrontal headache and nausea. Her local doctor, who examined her, found her supine blood pressure to be 200/130 mm Hg. She was admitted to the hospital. Subsequently the patient developed dizziness with postural hypotension, which persisted for 48 hours. All clinical investigations, including serum catecholamine estimations, were within normal limits. Three weeks later she was rechallenged with one capsule (85 mg) of phenylpropanolamine, which after 90 minutes produced a rise in blood pressure to 175/120 mm Hg.

The second case involved a 68-year-old man with a long history of hypertension which had been stabilized with a thiazide diuretic and methyldopa. This patient routinely measured his blood pressure at home and noted an increase after he had taken Sinutab S.A., a nasal decongestant containing 100 mg phenylpropanolamine and 325 mg acetaminophen per tablet. When he was examined at Austin Hospital, his blood pressure was 220/130 mm Hg supine and 160/110 mm Hg standing. Two days after he discontinued the use of this product, his blood pressure had returned to 140/90 mm Hg supine and 145/95 mm Hg standing.

AUSTRALIAN ADVERSE DRUG REACTION REPORTS

These two cases suggest that phenylpropanolamine may induce hypertension in normotensive individuals who possess a special sensitivity to it, such as women on contraceptive pills, as well as in those who have a preexistent hypertensive condition. A review of cases reported since 1973 to the Adverse Drug Reactions Advisory Committee (ADRAC), the Australian adverse drug reaction monitoring body, indicates this occurrence is not rare. Some of these cases have recently been described in detail by McEwen (1983). Sixteen reported occurrences of hypertension in previously normotensive individuals were associated with daily phenylpropanolamine dosages between 50 and 170 mg. Except for one man, all the patients were women; all were between 17 and 54 years of age. Trimolets, the preparation taken by the first patient described above, was involved in 11 of the 16 reports (table 12.2). Symptoms included headaches, nausea, vomiting, dizziness, and chest pain. Two patients developed hypertensive cerebrovascular hemorrhages; one patient died (King 1979). From 1973 to 1983 seven more reports of phenylpropanolamine-associated headaches, nausea, and dizziness, without hypertension, were also filed.

TABLE 12.2

Preparations containing phenylpropanolamine implicated in hypertensive responses among previously normotensive individuals, 1973-83

Preparation	PPA content (mg)	Number of reports
Trimolets	85	10
Dietgard™	75	2
Trimtabs™	60	2
Orthoxicol®	60	1
Trimolets (new formulation)	50	1

Source: Compiled by the authors. Data derived from Department of Health of Australia, unpublished cumulative reports of ADRAC, 1973-83. Filed. Canberra, Australia: Department of Health.

Four reports illustrate the potential adverse drug interactions that can occur between phenylpropanolamine and other medications (table 12.3). Three of these cases involved an interaction between phenylpropanolamine and the monoamine oxidase inhibitor phenelzine. In case four (Lee, Beilin, and Vandongen 1979), 25 mg of indomethacin induced hypertensive responses in a patient taking Trimolets. In four additional cases (table 12.4), phenylpropanolamine containing at least 50 mg per unit dose was implicated in the aggravation of preexistent hypertensive conditions. These cases also illustrate the drug interactions possible between phenylpropanolamine and medications used to treat

TABLE 12.3

Four reported cases of hypertension induced by drug interactions with phenylpropanolamine, 1973-83

Case	Age	PPA dosage/ tablet (mg)	Interacting drug
1	58	25	Phenelzine
2	30	85	Phenelzine
3	55	85	Phenelzine
4	27	85	Indomethacin

Source: Compiled by the authors. Data derived from Department of Health of Australia, unpublished cumulative reports of ADRAC, 1973-83. Filed. Canberra, Australia: Department of Health.

TABLE 12.4

Four reported cases of hypertension aggravated by phenylpropanolamine, 1973-83

Case	Age	PPA dosage/ tablet (mg)	Other medication	Peak blood pressure (mm Hg)
1	37	50	Bethanidine	180/110
2	50	100	Methyldopa	?
3	49	75	Chlorothiazide	240/120
4	62	100	Methyldopa	220/130

Source: Compiled by the authors. Data derived from Department of Health of Australia, unpublished cumulative reports of ADRAC, 1973-83. Filed. Canberra, Australia: Department of Health.

hypertension. Two of these four patients were being treated with methyldopa, the same medication taken by the second patient, the 64-year-old man, described previously.

EXPERIMENTAL STUDIES

We performed three controlled studies at Austin Hospital to determine the extent to which hypertensive responses induced by phenylpropanolamine-containing preparations might be predictable in previously normotensive subjects.

Crossover Study

Six normotensive medical students ages 22 to 24 years participated in a double-blind, crossover trial comparing Trimolets (85 mg phenylpropanolamine) and identical placebo capsules, taken once daily. After phenylpropanolamine ingestion, all six volunteers experienced an increase in both systolic and diastolic blood pressure, which peaked after three hours and stayed abnormally high throughout the six hours of the study (table 12.5). The diastolic blood pressure of two subjects reached levels greater than 110 mm Hg. Five of the six participants developed malaise, headache, or tightness of the chest on Trimolets, while no symptoms occurred under placebo administration. Less marked but statistically significant rises in the subjects' standing blood pressure levels occurred, indicating a postural hypotensive drug effect.

Double-Blind Randomized Studies

Two separate double-blind studies were conducted, using 141 medical student volunteer participants between the ages of 21 and 28. The studies measured the drug-induced blood pressure effects of two brand-name products containing phenylpropanolamine, Trimolets (85 mg) and Contac 500 (50 mg plus 0.2 mg belladonna alkaloids), against matching placebo. Drug study groups were randomly assigned. Before deciding whether to take part in the study, subjects were informed of the possible effects of the drug. Those with heart disease, hypertension, asthma, diabetes mellitus, or who were concurrently being treated with antidepressant or sympathomimetic drugs were excluded from participation.

TABLE 12.5

Results of phenylpropanolamine crossover study of six normotensive medical students

Physical findings	Measurements (mm Hg)* Initial	3 hours post-ingestion	p
Systolic blood pressure (mm Hg)			
Phenylpropanolamine	129 ± 4	151 ± 7	< .01
Placebo	127 ± 4	115 ± 6	
Diastolic blood pressure (mm Hg)			
Phenylpropanolamine	83 ± 3	100 ± 6	< .05
Placebo	83 ± 3	78 ± 3	
Heart rate (beats/minute)			
Phenylpropanolamine	71 ± 5	55 ± 3	< .05

*Mean value ± standard error of the mean.

Source: Compiled by the authors. Data derived from statistical reports and from Horowitz, J. D. et al. 1979. Hypertension and postural hypotension induced by phenylpropanolamine (Trimolets). Med J Aust 1:175-76.

Trimolets

In the first study, 37 subjects took Trimolets, compared to 35 given placebo. Within one hour after ingestion, the supine diastolic blood pressure levels of all Trimolets subjects rose from an initial value of 70 ± 1 mm Hg to 94 ± 3 mm Hg versus 74 ± 1 mm Hg to 77 ± 2 mm Hg on placebo medication ($p < .001$). The supine diastolic blood pressure of Trimolets subjects peaked (68-142 mm Hg) between 1.5 and three hours after ingestion. In 12 of the 37 Trimolets subjects and one of the 35 placebo subjects, the peak supine diastolic blood pressure was greater than 100 mm Hg.

The symptoms that 20 of the 37 Trimolets subjects reported experiencing are summarized in table 12.6. One placebo subject also reported a feeling of nausea. It is important to note that the appearance of symptoms corresponded closely with individual increases in blood pressure.

TABLE 12.6

Symptoms experienced by 20 study subjects after ingestion of Trimolets (85 mg)

Symptoms	Number of reports
Tingling in head	6
Dizziness	5
Postural dizziness	4
Palpitations	5
Chest tightness	3
Headache	6
Rash	3
Tremor	2
Nausea	2
Lassitude	1
Tinnitus	1

Source: Compiled by the authors. Data derived from statistical reports and from Horowitz, J. D. et al. 1980. Hypertensive responses induced by phenylpropanolamine in anorectic and decongestant preparations. Lancet 1:60-61.

Contac 500

Study groups in the second study consisted of 34 subjects on Contac 500 and 35 given placebo. Within 90-180 minutes after ingestion, the supine diastolic blood pressure of the Contac 500 group rose from 78 $\pm$ 2 mm Hg to 83 $\pm$ 2 mm Hg, whereas the mean value of the placebo group did not rise above the initial value of 77 $\pm$ 2 mm Hg ($p < .05$). In four subjects on Contac 500, the peak supine diastolic blood pressure exceeded 100 mm Hg, while in none of the placebo subjects did this same elevation occur. One Contac 500 subject had a maximum supine blood pressure level of 145/110 mm Hg. No symptoms were reported by subjects in either group.

DISCUSSION

Evidence from reported cases and our own controlled studies confirms for us that ingestion of phenylpropanolamine may sometimes be associated with severe blood pressure increases in previously normal subjects. There is also a strong suggestion that a dose-response relationship exists, with most cases of spontaneous hypertension occurring after ingestion of more than 50 mg of phenylpropanolamine. A comparison of the drug effects of Contac 500 (50 mg phenylpropanolamine) and Trimolets (85 mg) further supports the existence of a dose-response relationship; only four of the 35 subjects on Contac 500 developed a peak supine diastolic blood pressure level greater than 100 mm Hg, in contrast to 12 of the 37 subjects receiving Trimolets. The frequency of hypertensive responses to Trimolets may in part reflect rapid bioavailability of phenylpropanolamine, at least with this particular preparation. Therefore, a possible safety measure against serious hypertension might be to limit phenylpropanolamine use to controlled-release products or to single, low dosages not exceeding 50 mg.

Other hypertensive responses may be associated with the ingestion of high doses of phenylpropanolamine. Over half the subjects treated with Trimolets in our study developed symptoms, including chest pain and palpitations. Additional evidence suggests that phenylpropanolamine-induced hypertension may result in cerebrovascular hemorrhage, myocardial injury (Pentel, Mikell, and Zavoral 1982), and cardiac arrhythmias.

Further serious problems may arise with potential drug interactions between phenylpropanolamine and monoamine oxidase inhibitors (Cuthbert, Greenberg, and Morley 1969), antihypertensive medications (McLaren 1976), oral contraceptives (Horowitz et al. 1980), and aspirin-like drugs (Lee, Beilin, and Vandongen 1979). Since these are commonly prescribed drugs, potential drug-drug interactions present a particular threat when at the same time phenylpropanolamine-containing products are easily obtainable as OTC preparations. Furthermore, even when specific dosage instructions accompany OTC preparations, patients may take higher than recommended doses out of enthusiasm to achieve a greater anorexiant effect. The case cited earlier (Horowitz et al. 1979) illustrates how easily this problem can arise in weight reduction regimens. Such crises occur often enough to raise concern about the ready availability of OTC products containing phenylpropanolamine.

A further matter which needs to be considered is whether the lower-dose phenylpropanolamine preparations are still therapeutic. Even if they are, their use should only be ancillary to sensible dieting. For example, in a 40-week crossover comparison of the anorexiant drug mazindol and placebo (Miach et al. 1976), patients on active medication found weight loss difficult to maintain and apparently relaxed the dietary restrictions imposed when they had entered the clinical trial. In the crossover phase, many patients rapidly regained weight on placebo.

Such evidence suggests that use of anorexiant agents, even if "safe," may be an ineffective form of therapy unless combined with long-term changes in diet and life style.

REFERENCES

Cuthbert, M. F., M. P. Greenberg, and S. W. Morley. 1969. Cough and cold remedies: a potential danger to patients on monoamine oxidase inhibitors. Br Med J 1:404-6.

Frewin, D. B., P. P. Leonello, and M. E. Frewin. 1978. Hypertension after ingestion of Trimolets. Med J Aust 2:497-98.

Horowitz, J. D. et al. 1980. Hypertensive responses induced by phenylpropanolamine in anorectic and decongestant preparations. Lancet 1:60-61.

Horowitz, J. D. et al. 1979. Hypertension and postural hypotension induced by phenylpropanolamine (Trimolets). Med J Aust 1:175-76.

Kallis, S. G. and P. Passmore. 1979. Australian proprietary preparations containing phenylpropanolamine. Med J Aust 2:425-26.

King, J. 1979. Hypertension and cerebral haemorrhage after Trimolets ingestion. Med J Aust 2:258.

Lee, K. Y., L. J. Beilin, and R. Vandongen. 1979. Severe hypertension after ingestion of an appetite suppressant (phenylpropanolamine) with indomethacin. Lancet 1:1110-11.

McEwen, J. 1983. Phenylpropanolamine-associated hypertension after the use of "over-the-counter" appetite-suppressant products. Med J Aust 2:71-73.

McLaren, E. H. 1976. Severe hypertension produced by interaction of phenylpropanolamine with methyldopa and oxprenolol. Br Med J 2:283-84.

Miach, P. J. et al. 1976. Double-blind cross-over evaluation of mazindol in the treatment of obese hypertensive patients. Med J Aust 2:378-80.

Ostern, S. and W. H. Dodson. 1965. Hypertension following Ornade ingestion. Letter. JAMA 194:472.

Patil, P. N., J. B. LaPidus, and A. Tye. 1970. Steric aspects of adrenergic drugs. J Pharm Sci 59:1205-34.

Pentel, P. R., F. L. Mikell, and J. H. Zavoral. 1982. Myocardial injury after phenylpropanolamine ingestion. Br Heart J 47:51-54.

ACKNOWLEDGMENT

We gratefully acknowledge the assistance of Drs. J. McEwen and M. L. Mashford of ADRAC for obtaining data regarding phenylpropanolamine adverse reactions in Australia.

13

REVIEW OF RECENT STUDIES ON THE EFFECT OF PHENYLPROPANOLAMINE ON SYSTEMIC ARTERIAL BLOOD PRESSURE IN HUMAN SUBJECTS

Lawrence R. Krakoff

INTRODUCTION

I have been asked to review several recent studies assessing the effect of phenylpropanolamine (PPA) upon systemic arterial pressure. These studies reflect concern that the well-known adrenergic agonist effects of phenylpropanolamine be thoroughly defined so that the potential risk of the agent can be quantified. My review proceeds from the perspective of cardiovascular health and the well-defined epidemiologic risk factors that are pertinent to it. First, there is a continuous relationship between either systolic or diastolic arterial pressure and future cardiovascular risk as indicated in the extensive epidemiologic survey conducted by the High Blood Pressure Detection and Follow-up Group (Hypertension Detection and Follow-up Program Cooperative Group 1977). Second, although being overweight, per se, is not clearly an independent risk factor for cardiovascular disease, its causative relationships to hypertension, hyperlipidemia, and diabetes underscore the therapeutic significance of weight reduction (Bray 1983). For those concerned with the prevention of cardiovascular disease, the reasons to lose weight are to reduce blood pressure, lower serum low-density lipoprotein (LDL) cholesterol, improve glucose tolerance, and perhaps, when combined with other behavioral changes, to increase both the state of conditioning and the serum high-density lipoprotein (HDL) cholesterol.

It has already been established that some, perhaps all, therapeutic interventions result in a tradeoff of risk factors. Use of thiazide or chlorthalidone diuretics may lower blood pressure, but increase serum total and LDL cholesterol. One effect may cancel the other in altering risk status for the future (Ames and Hill 1976; Grimm et al. 1981). With this as background, the effect of phenylpropanolamine

TABLE 13.1

Studies of the effects of phenylpropanolamine on systemic arterial blood pressure

	Investigator/ location	Design	Treatments	Number of subjects
A.	I. Liebson et al. (1982b) Behavioral Pharmacology Research Unit Johns Hopkins School of Med. Baltimore	Parallel 3 groups	Placebo 25 mg t.i.d. 75 mg SR	150
B.	I. Liebson et al. (1982a) Behavioral Pharmacology Research Unit Johns Hopkins School of Med. Baltimore	Crossover 2 groups	Placebo to 75 mg SR 75 mg SR to placebo	59
C.	R. Noble (1983) Cathedral Hill Obesity Clinic San Francisco	Stratified Parallel group	Placebo 25 mg t.i.d. 75 mg SR	216
D.	P. Robertson (1983) Dept. of Medicine University of Washington Seattle	Stratified Parallel group	Placebo 25 mg t.i.d. 75 mg SR	224
E.	M. H. Bradley (1982) Miami	Single-blind One-way crossover	25 mg + caffeine 100 mg to placebo to 75 mg SR	10

SR: Sustained-release.
<u>Source</u>: Compiled by the author.

upon systemic arterial pressure was evaluated in five recently conducted, but unpublished, studies.

The Thompson Medical Company, which supported these five separate studies, has provided me with the results. The investigators, location of study sites, study design, and number of subjects are given in table 13.1. In four of the studies, only normotensive overweight subjects were evaluated. In the fifth, a small number of overweight hypertensives whose blood pressure was controlled by diuretic therapy were assessed. Each study will be analyzed separately in the section to follow.

REVIEW OF SPECIFIC STUDIES

Study A. Parallel Group Study by Liebson et al.

One hundred fifty healthy, normal subjects were enrolled in a parallel group design with three groups (Liebson et al. 1982b). One group received a 75 mg sustained-release form of phenylpropanolamine followed by two placebo tablets four hours apart. The second group received 25 mg phenylpropanolamine three times daily and the third group received three placebo tablets. Blood pressure and heart rate in supine, seated, and standing positions were monitored before and one-half hour, one hour, two, four, six, eight, ten, and 12 hours after the initial dose. Figure 13.1 indicates that both systolic and diastolic blood pressures in the seated position were highest in the 75 mg sustained-release phenylpropanolamine group. However, statistical analysis fails to reveal a significant difference in blood pressure due to treatment at any time or in any condition.

Study B. Crossover Study by Liebson et al.

Fifty-nine healthy subjects received a 75 mg sustained-release phenylpropanolamine tablet and a placebo two days apart, allowing one day for wash-out (Liebson et al. 1982a). One group took the placebo first; the other took the 75 mg sustained-release phenylpropanolamine tablet first. Blood pressure and heart rate were monitored over 12 hours according to the same schedule followed in Study A. In this study the 75 mg sustained-release phenylpropanolamine dosage was associated with a small but statistically significant increase from baseline in systolic and diastolic blood pressure in the sitting position from two to 12 hours after ingestion. The greatest changes were evident two and four hours after the initial dose, as shown in figure 13.2. In

FIGURE 13.1

Effects of phenylpropanolamine and placebo
on blood pressure:
parallel group study by Liebson et al.

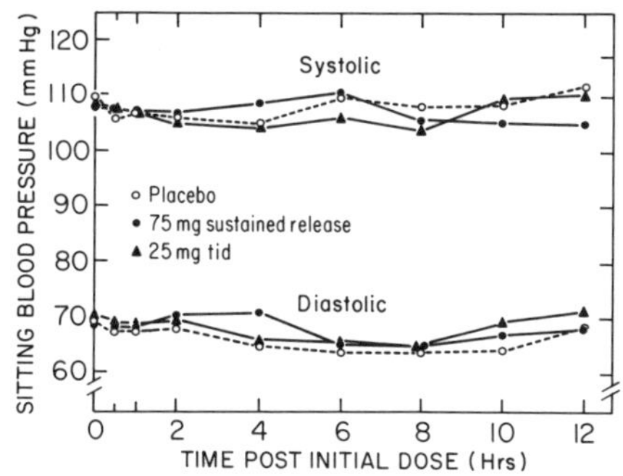

Source: Liebson, I. et al. 1982. An evaluation of the acute effects of phenylpropanolamine in normal volunteers: parallel design. Unpublished manuscript: appendix F-1. Baltimore: Johns Hopkins University School of Medicine. Printed with permission.

FIGURE 13.2

Effects of phenylpropanolamine and placebo
on blood pressure:
crossover study by Liebson et al.

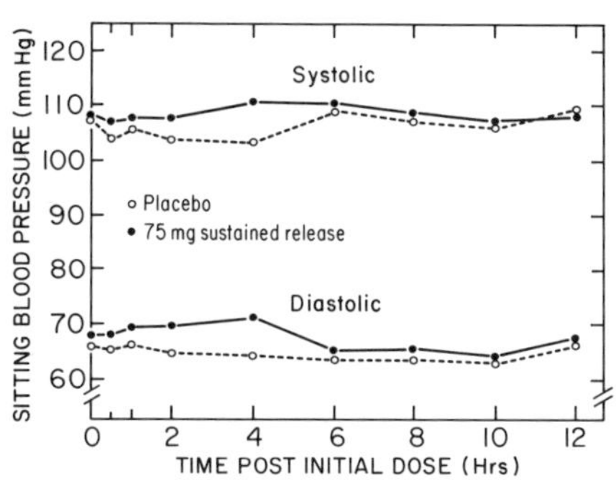

Source: Liebson, I. et al. 1982. An evaluation of the acute effects of phenylpropanolamine in normal volunteers: crossover design. Unpublished manuscript: appendix C-1. Baltimore: Johns Hopkins University School of Medicine. Printed with permission.

TABLE 13.2

Blood pressure following administration of phenylpropanolamine, phenylpropanolamine with caffeine, and placebo (n = 10)

Measurement*	Baseline		½ hour after medication	
	Range	(Mean)	Range	(Mean)
Weeks 1-2 (25 mg PPA, 100 mg caffeine, t.i.d.)				
Standing pulse	54-88	(73.0)	58-88	(75.2)
Supine pulse	54-92	(73.3)	52-84	(69.6)
Standing diastolic	74-92	(84.2)	70-94	(87.0)
Supine diastolic	70-94	(83.4)	68-96	(85.0)
Standing systolic	116-142	(130.6)	126-152	(135.6)
Supine systolic	114-170	(133.5)	118-172	(136.0)
Weeks 3-4 (placebo)				
Standing pulse	64-96	(76.4)	64-96	(78.4)
Supine pulse	56-88	(72.5)	56-92	(72.6)
Standing diastolic	70-94	(82.0)	58-94	(81.0)
Supine diastolic	60-90	(80.0)	50-94	(79.6)
Standing systolic	100-166	(125.2)	86-144	(120.4)
Supine systolic	108-164	(127.8)	104-172	(125.8)
Weeks 5-6 (75 mg PPA, q.d.)				
Standing pulse	56-88	(75.8)	58-96	(73.4)
Supine pulse	56-84	(73.6)	56-88	(70.0)
Standing diastolic	70-90	(82.2)	70-90	(82.4)
Supine diastolic	62-90	(81.2)	70-90	(83.0)
Standing systolic	114-144	(126.2)	100-146	(129.0)
Supine systolic	112-150	(132.4)	110-146	(135.4)

*Blood pressure given in mm Hg; pulse rate given in beats/min.

†Statistically significant differences ($p < .05$).

1 hour after medication		2 hours after medication		4 hours after medication	
Range	(Mean)	Range	(Mean)	Range	(Mean)
60-96	(76.8)	56-100	(84.2)†	56-96	(80.6)
52-88	(68.4)	72-96	(76.4)	64-96	(76.0)
80-100	(88.4)†	70-94	(85.9)	74-94	(85.6)
84-100	(88.0)†	80-98	(87.5)	70-98	(87.8)
110-150	(134.2)	110-160	(137.2)†	110-150	(134.0)
138-190	(145.4)†	130-170	(143.2)†	114-160	(142.4)†
58-100	(78.8)	72-100	(82.0)†	60-96	(79.0)
54-96	(71.0)	54-88	(74.8)	50-88	(73.6)
62-100	(82.8)	54-92	(77.0)	58-90	(77.8)
76-94	(82.4)	56-90	(78.8)	60-92	(78.6)
90-158	(119.0)	92-160	(116.6)†	96-160	(121.4)
100-152	(123.4)	90-158	(124.8)	108-160	(126.4)
68-96	(81.0)	76-120	(88.7)†	70-100	(81.3)
60-96	(75.1)	64-124	(83.6)	60-100	(78.9)
80-94	(85.8)	74-90	(81.8)	70-90	(82.7)
76-96	(86.2)	76-90	(85.3)	70-98	(85.6)
110-152	(137.8)†	118-142	(127.6)	110-150	(131.8)
106-160	(139.6)	128-140	(137.4)	108-146	(136.0)

Source: Bradley, M. H. 1982. Single-blind safety and efficacy evaluation of phenylpropanolamine hydrochloride plus caffeine, phenylpropanolamine alone, and placebo in exogenous obese patients with controlled hypertensive disease. Unpublished manuscript: 5. Miami. Printed with permission.

general the differences between the 75 mg sustained-release phenylpropanolamine and placebo groups were small; the differences in systolic and diastolic blood pressure means (supine, seated, and standing positions) between the two groups were all between 2 and 3 mm Hg.

Study C. Parallel Group Study by Noble

This study of 216 subjects (Noble 1983) and the one discussed next were part of a cooperative effort undertaken by two different study centers. Subjects were separated into normal weight and mildly, moderately, and severely overweight groups. Subjects in each category were randomly assigned to three treatment schedules for one day of study: 25 mg phenylpropanolamine three times a day, 75 mg sustained-release phenylpropanolamine once daily, or placebo, according to the same design followed in Study A. The weight classification did have an effect upon arterial pressure with higher diastolic pressures observed in heavier weight categories. Phenylpropanolamine drug treatments with either 25 mg three times daily or 75 mg sustained-release once daily did not result in significantly detectable alterations in blood pressure in any weight category.

Study D. Parallel Group Study by Robertson

At another center, Robertson (1983) enrolled 224 subjects who were stratified and grouped according to the design described in Study C. As in the previous study, heavier weight categories were associated with overall higher blood pressures. However, in this study the 75 mg sustained-release phenylpropanolamine treatment did result in a significant increase in supine diastolic pressure compared to either placebo or the 25 mg phenylpropanolamine tablet given three times a day (4.5 mm Hg mean difference for 75 mg sustained-release phenylpropanolamine versus placebo). This effect was most marked two to four hours after the initial dose, as indicated in figure 13.3.

Upon examination of the raw data provided in the reports of this study, it is evident that a few subjects who received 75 mg sustained-release phenylpropanolamine had greater increases in blood pressure. For example, two hours after ingestion of the drug, subject #230, a 41-year-old woman weighing 250 lb, had an increase in supine systolic pressure from 129 mm Hg to 160 mm Hg and an increase in supine diastolic blood pressure from 66 mm Hg to 96 mm Hg.

After four hours, her blood pressure was 140/90 mm Hg. Subject #182, a 62-year-old woman weighing 200 lb, had a baseline blood pressure of 136/88 mm Hg in the supine position; two hours after administration, her blood pressure was 140/96 mm Hg. Subject #162, a 59-year-old man weighing 184 lb, had an increase in supine blood pressure from 145/80 mm Hg before drug treatment to 160/90 mm Hg four hours after drug treatment. While many other subjects had lesser changes in arterial pressure when given 75 mg sustained-release phenylpropanolamine, the results of this study are similar to the changes observed by Horowitz et al. (1980) in finding a high degree of variability in the blood pressure response to another substance containing phenylpropanolamine (85 mg).

FIGURE 13.3

Effects of phenylpropanolamine and placebo on blood pressure: parallel group study by Robertson

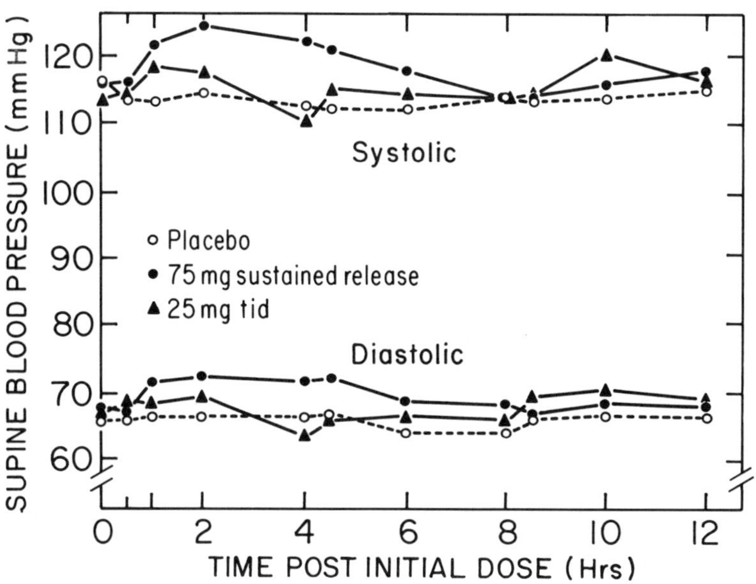

Source: Robertson, P. 1983. A multisite evaluation of the acute effects of phenylpropanolamine in normal volunteers. Unpublished manuscript: appendix IV-2. Seattle: University of Washington Department of Medicine. Printed with permission.

Study E. Crossover Study by Bradley

Twelve overweight, mildly hypertensive patients whose blood pressure was controlled by thiazide diuretic therapy were enrolled for this six-week trial (Bradley 1982). Ten completed the study. In a single-blind, one-way crossover design, subjects received phenylpropanolamine (25 mg) plus caffeine (100 mg) three times a day for the first two-week period. During the second two weeks they were given placebo tablets twice daily. For the final two-week period 75 mg sustained-release phenylpropanolamine tablets were given once daily. Blood pressure, weight, and other measurements were made at weekly intervals. At the end of every two-week segment, serial pulse and blood pressure determinations in supine and standing positions were made before and one-half hour, one hour, two, and four hours after the first dose.

Changes in heart rate and blood pressure detected in these serial studies are indicated in table 13.2 and figure 13.4. A few of these changes were statistically significant. The majority of the changes were apparent at the end of the second week, one to two hours after the 25 mg phenylpropanolamine tablet had been taken (table 13.2). Compared to the fall in systolic blood pressure in both supine and standing positions after placebo (weeks 3-4), there was a clear-cut tendency for the supine systolic blood pressure to rise after 25 mg phenylpropanolamine plus 100 mg caffeine (weeks 1-2) and a slight trend after 75 mg sustained-release phenylpropanolamine (weeks 5-6) (figure 13.4). No statistically significant main treatment effects upon either blood pressure or heart rate were observed during the six weeks of the study.

INTERPRETATION

The results of these studies do not reveal an entirely consistent pattern despite the number of subjects who were evaluated. Perhaps the inherent variability of arterial pressure and the poor precision of traditional clinical methods for noninvasive measurement of arterial pressure obscured uniform findings of small differences. Little detail is provided in these studies regarding the method for measurement of arterial pressure except to state that the procedures recommended by the American Heart Association for routine clinical management (Kirkendall et al. 1980) were followed. Neither random zero devices nor automated mechanisms were used. There was no description of the training or standardization of personnel who made the blood pressure determinations.

FIGURE 13.4

Effects of phenylpropanolamine,
phenylpropanolamine with caffeine, and placebo
on blood pressure and pulse rate:
crossover study by Bradley

(a) Weeks 1-2

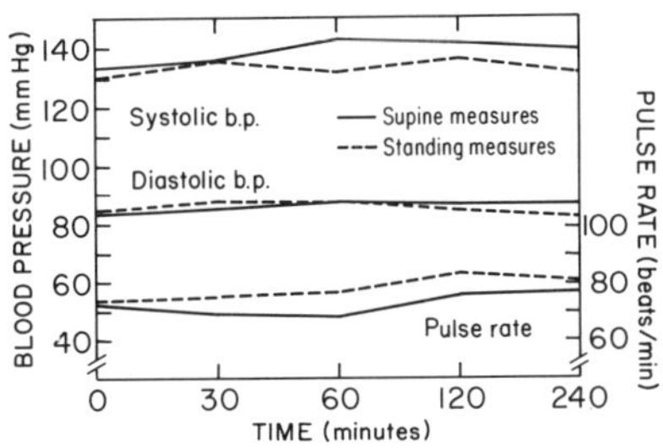

(b) Weeks 3-4

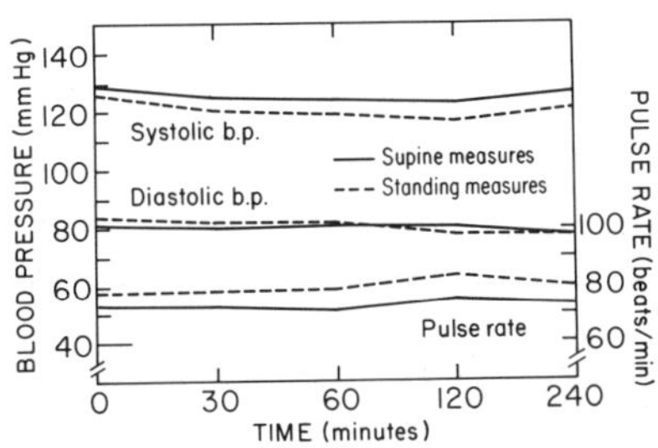

(c) Weeks 5-6

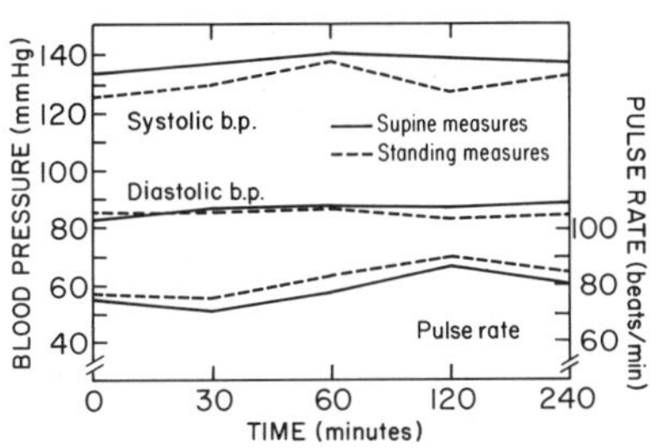

Source: Bradley, M. H. 1982. Single-blind safety and efficacy evaluation of phenylpropanolamine hydrochloride plus caffeine, phenylpropanolamine alone, and placebo in exogenous obese patients with controlled hypertensive disease. Unpublished manuscript: 5. Miami. Printed with permission.

In comparing studies, one can conclude that whereas several did find that phenylpropanolamine caused small mean increases in blood pressure, more consistently for the 75 mg sustained-release preparation two to four hours after administration, none found a reduction in blood pressure after either phenylpropanolamine preparation. In the one crossover study, in which intersubject variance should have been reduced, the effect of 75 mg sustained-release phenylpropanolamine in raising blood pressure was most apparent and of greatest magnitude. The data may also be reviewed from another perspective by asking whether a small number of individuals may not exhibit idiosyncratic excessive elevation of blood pressure when exposed to phenylpropanolamine; a few subjects in the study by Robertson (1983) displayed this pattern. Predisposition to an excessive increase in blood pressure due to phenylpropanolamine may be augmented by nonsteroidal anti-inflammatory agents inhibiting vasodilator prostaglandin synthesis as suggested in one report (Lee, Beilin, and Vandongen 1979).

On the basis of the studies reviewed here, it is apparent that most normal subjects do not have a detectable elevation of arterial pressure due to phenylpropanolamine given 25 mg three times a day or as a 75 mg sustained-release preparation. Why, then, should any attention be given to the effects of phenylpropanolamine upon arterial pressure? First, the epidemiologic significance of small and transient increases in arterial pressure, observed in a few studies of phenylpropanolamine, remains undefined. There is no evidence that small, short-term increases in blood pressure caused by this drug lead to an increased long-term risk of cardiovascular disease. Consideration should be given, however, to the effect of small increases in blood pressure that may mislead physicians into a false diagnosis of chronic hypertension. It is all too common for patients to be told on the basis of a single blood pressure determination that they have hypertension and for unnecessary treatment to be initiated. In addition, the impact of labeling individuals as hypertensive may alter their behavior or self-perception (Haynes et al. 1978). All those screening for hypertension should exclude use of phenylpropanolamine as a possible cause for blood pressure elevation and re-evaluate patients often enough for an accurate diagnosis to be made.

The major concern is that significant hypertensive reactions may occur on an idiosyncratic basis in a small number of subjects. These reactions may well be undetected unless appropriate monitoring takes place. Unless subjects with this predisposition are exposed to nonsteroidal anti-inflammatory agents (e.g., indomethacin), such elevations of blood pressure may never be clinically manifest. Nonetheless, it seems prudent that patients with hypertension or other disorders of the cardiovascular system be made especially aware of this possibility and that subjects predisposed to cardiovascular disease on the basis of known risk factors be advised by their physicians regarding all meaningful preventive therapy.

With regard to those who are hypertensive and overweight, there is now excellent evidence that successful weight reduction programs employing diet alone can effectively reduce arterial pressure (Reisin et al. 1978; Tuck et al. 1981). The safety or effectiveness of phenylpropanolamine within the hypertensive population has not yet been established. There is reason to doubt that this agent ever causes the long-term reduction in weight necessary for improvement in risk status (Phenylpropanolamine for weight reduction 1984). Thus, from the perspective of long-term cardiovascular health, use of phenylpropanolamine offers no apparent benefit but carries some potential for increased risk. Physicians and those tempted to use phenylpropanolamine-containing preparations for weight reduction should be made fully aware of these considerations.

REFERENCES

Ames, R. P. and P. Hill. 1976. Increase in serum lipids during treatment of hypertension with chlorthalidone. Lancet 1:721-23.

Bradley, M. H. 1982. Single-blind safety and efficacy evaluation of phenylpropanolamine hydrochloride plus caffeine, phenylpropanolamine alone, and placebo in exogenous obese patients with controlled hypertensive disease. Unpublished manuscript. Miami.

Bray, G. A. 1983. Obesity. In Prevention of coronary heart disease: practical management of the risk factors, edited by N. M. Kaplan and J. Stamler, 75-77. Philadelphia: W. B. Saunders.

Grimm, R. H. et al. 1981. Effects of thiazide diuretics on plasma lipids and lipoproteins in mildly hypertensive patients. Ann Intern Med 94:7-11.

Haynes, R. B. et al. 1978. Increased absenteeism from work after detection and labeling of hypertensive patients. N Engl J Med 299:741-44.

Horowitz, J. D. et al. 1980. Hypertensive responses induced by phenylpropanolamine in anorectic and decongestant preparations. Lancet 1:60-61.

Hypertension Detection and Follow-up Program, Cooperative Group. 1977. The hypertension detection and follow-up program: a progress report. Circ Res (Supp I) 40:I-106-9.

Kirkendall, W. M. et al. 1980. Recommendations for human blood pressure determination by sphygmomanometers. Report of the Postgraduate Education Committee, American Heart Association.

Lee, K. Y., L. J. Beilin, and R. Vandongen. 1979. Severe hypertension after ingestion of an appetite suppressant (phenylpropanolamine) with indomethacin. Lancet 1:1110-11.

Liebson, I. et al. 1982a. An evaluation of the acute effects of phenylpropanolamine in normal volunteers: crossover design. Unpublished manuscript. Baltimore: Johns Hopkins University School of Medicine.

------. 1982b. An evaluation of the acute effects of phenylpropanolamine in normal volunteers: parallel design. Unpublished manuscript. Baltimore: Johns Hopkins University School of Medicine.

Noble, R. 1983. A multisite evaluation of the acute effects of phenylpropanolamine in normal volunteers. Unpublished manuscript. San Francisco: Cathedral Hill Obesity Clinic.

Phenylpropanolamine for weight reduction. 1984. Med Lett Drugs Ther 26:55-56.

Reisin, E. et al. 1978. Effect of weight loss without salt restriction on the reduction of blood pressure in overweight hypertensive patients. N Engl J Med 298:1-6.

Robertson, P. 1983. A multisite evaluation of the acute effects of phenylpropanolamine in normal volunteers. Unpublished manuscript. Seattle: University of Washington Department of Medicine.

Tuck, M. L. et al. 1981. The effect of weight reduction on blood pressure, plasma renin activity, and plasma aldosterone levels in obese patients. N Engl J Med 304:930-33.

14

PHENYLPROPANOLAMINE AND CEREBROVASCULAR TOXICITY IN RODENTS

Shirley M. Mueller

INTRODUCTION

Until the 1970s phenylpropanolamine (PPA) was marketed primarily in nasal decongestants. Five to six years ago, however, phenylpropanolamine began to appear in diet pills and "street" stimulants, products that had previously contained amphetamine as the major ingredient. Although amphetamine had been legally available only by prescription, the phenylpropanolamine-containing diet pills and street drug "look-alikes" were not controlled by prescription. This ready availability of phenylpropanolamine led to its widespread usage. As public exposure to phenylpropanolamine increased, many complications began to be reported, the most severe being stroke, although most stroke cases involved ingestion of drug combinations rather than phenylpropanolamine alone (Bernstein and Diskant 1982; Center for Science in the Public Interest 1984; Elliott and Whyte 1981; Johnson, Etter, and Reeves 1983; King 1979).

Phenylpropanolamine in combination with caffeine has frequently been found in street look-alike pills (Bernstein and Diskant 1982; Mueller and Solow 1982; Mueller 1983) and in diet preparations (Health and Human Services 1982). However, since November 18, 1983, diet aids containing combinations of phenylpropanolamine and caffeine have been classified as a "new drug" by the Food and Drug Administration (FDA) and their sale (except of products already on store shelves) has been banned (Health and Human Services 1983). This did not eliminate the consumption of phenylpropanolamine/caffeine combinations, however, since users can combine phenylpropanolamine products with beverages and other substances containing caffeine at their discretion.

The experiments described below were performed to determine if a combination of phenylpropanolamine and caffeine in an amount corresponding to a greater than recommended human dose could lead to stroke or an elevation in blood pressure in normotensive and hypertensive rats. Animal subjects were used for these experiments so that environmental conditions could be carefully controlled. (Retrospective case studies of humans do not permit this luxury.) Some of the described studies were done in conjunction with Susan Asdell and Dr. Jans Muller, a neuropathologist, and have been previously reported (Mueller, Muller, and Asdell 1984).

METHODS

The Advisory Review Panel on Over-the-Counter Miscellaneous Internal Drug Products of the FDA (Health and Human Services 1982) has concluded that phenylpropanolamine is safe in doses approximately equivalent to 1 mg/kg. The ratio of caffeine to phenylpropanolamine in combination products has often been 4:1; thus, a usual human dose of caffeine in combination with phenylpropanolamine can be estimated as approximately 4 mg/kg. In these experiments, six times these recommended levels were used in each drug administration: 24 mg/kg caffeine combined with 6 mg/kg phenylpropanolamine. This phenylpropanolamine/caffeine combination is referred to as "drug" in the remainder of the paper.

Three different animal strains were studied: normotensive Sprague-Dawley rats, spontaneously hypertensive rats, and stroke-prone, spontaneously hypertensive rats. The stroke-prone, spontaneously hypertensive rats were administered a 1% sodium chloride solution as drinking water in order to promote elevation of blood pressure. All animals were between six and eight months of age. Within each of the three animal groups approximately one-half were treated with drug intraperitoneally while the remaining rats were treated with a 0.9% sodium chloride solution intraperitoneally. The intraperitoneal route of administration was chosen because in our laboratory it appears to be more reliable than the oral route. Preliminary studies performed with Dr. Phillip Shea of the Indiana University Department of Psychiatry have indicated that blood levels of phenylpropanolamine 90 minutes after intraperitoneal injection are almost identical to those found after oral administration [intraperitoneal, 378 $\pm$ 35 ng/ml (mean $\pm$ standard error), n = 2; oral, 442 $\pm$ 128 ng/ml, n = 3] but are more consistent. Caffeine is known to be very well-absorbed after oral administration (Goodman, Goodman, and Gilman 1980) so blood levels of caffeine after intraperitoneal or oral administration should be similar. Both a chronic study and an acute study were carried out and will be described separately.

Chronic Study

The assessment measure for the chronic study was histological evidence for stroke. Intraperitoneal drug or sodium chloride was administered two times a day for five days. The animals were starved as though they were dieting except for one hour following the second drug injection each day. Three to seven days after the last drug or saline injection, the brain vasculature was perfused via a cannula through the heart. First, 0.9% sodium chloride was used for perfusion for three minutes to remove existing intravascular blood. This was followed with a 10% buffered formalin perfusion for three minutes for proper fixation of the tissue. The rat brains were allowed to fix in situ for approximately three hours before removal and placement in a 10% buffered Formalin fixative. This careful procedure is optimal for histologic identification of brain pathology (Zeman and Innes 1963). The brains were prepared for hematoxylin and eosin histologic sections in the routine manner and read by a neuropathologist unaware of whether the animals had received the drug or sodium chloride treatment (Mueller, Muller, and Asdell 1984).

Acute Study

The end point of the acute study was the determination of awake blood pressure. Before 10 a.m., the animal was anesthetized with a short-acting barbiturate (Brevital®). The femoral artery was catheterized and the catheter was exteriorized at the back of the neck. The animal recovered from the sedation within approximately 30 minutes. The same day, after 1 p.m., awake blood pressures were recorded before and two hours after a single intraperitoneal injection of sodium chloride or drug (Ibid.).

Table 14.1 shows the number of subjects and the results in each study.

TABLE 14.1

Blood pressure changes and strokes induced in rats by the administration of phenylpropanolamine/caffeine combinations

Rat strain	Chronic study				Acute study			
	Number of animals		Number with evidence of stroke		Number of animals		Change in blood pressure (mm Hg)	
	Drug	Saline	Drug	Saline	Drug	Saline	Drug	Saline
Normotensive	5	5	0	0	6	4	43 ± 7	4 ± 4
Spontaneously hypertensive	11	11	2	0	7	6	22 ± 2	3 ± 3
Stroke-prone, spontaneously hypertensive	6	6	1	0	2	2	72 ± 1	-9 ± 4

Source: Compiled by the author.

RESULTS

Chronic Study

None of the histological examinations of the normotensive animals treated with drug (n = 5) or sodium chloride (n = 5) showed evidence of stroke. However, three of the 17 drug-treated, hypertensive rats demonstrated histologic evidence of stroke: two of the 11 spontaneously hypertensive rats showed subarachnoid hemorrhages and one of the six stroke-prone, spontaneously hypertensive rats showed intracerebral and intraventricular hemorrhage. This was in marked contrast to the 17 saline-treated hypertensive control animals, not one of which showed evidence of stroke.

Of the six drug-treated, stroke-prone, spontaneously hypertensive rats, two died prior to the end of the experiment. One animal died after two drug injections on the first day. Gross inspection revealed evidence of extensive hemorrhage into the flank region bilaterally, and acute tubular necrosis was noted during histologic examination of the kidneys. Another rat died about 20 minutes after the third drug injection on the second day. Histological examination of the brain revealed intracerebral and intraventricular hemorrhage.

Acute Study

In the acute blood pressure experiment, the blood pressure increase over baseline attained after a single drug injection was 43 $\pm$ 7 mm Hg in the normotensive animals (n = 6), 22 $\pm$ 2 mm Hg in the spontaneously hypertensive rats (n = 7), and 72 $\pm$ 1 mm Hg in the two stroke-prone rats. Saline-treated controls showed a negligible change in blood pressure. The post-injection blood pressure in all three drug-treated groups was significantly higher than the control, pre-injection blood pressure and the increase in blood pressure was significantly greater than that shown by the saline-treated controls ($p < .001$).

DISCUSSION

The results of these experiments indicate that repetitive administration of a combination of phenylpropanolamine and caffeine at six times the suggested human dose per weight can lead to cerebral hemorrhage in hypertensive rats. In addition, a single drug administration led to an acute increase in blood pressure in both normotensive and hypertensive animals.

It should be noted that, although cerebral hemorrhage was not observed in the drug-treated normotensive rats in this study, the possibility cannot be excluded that secondary abnormalities were produced by the phenylpropanolamine/caffeine combination. Since only a small number of drug-treated normotensive animals (n = 5) were studied, the incidence of cerebral hemorrhage would have had to have been substantial to detect this complication. In addition, histologic changes occur only when physiologic function is markedly abnormal. More sensitive techniques of monitoring physiologic changes in vivo might reveal effects not detectable using the present procedure.

There are several comments that should be made concerning the experimental approach. First, the histologic examinations were performed in blinded fashion so that bias could not contribute to the interpretation of the histologic data. Second, sodium chloride-injected controls were used in every experiment so that methodological problems would not be expected to contribute to the results. Third, the drug dose administered was greater than that normally ingested. This higher dose was chosen in order to optimize the chance of finding a reaction to the phenylpropanolamine/caffeine combination while using a small number of animals. Furthermore, though high, this is not an uncommon self-administered dose in humans. Fourth, the drug was given intraperitoneally rather than orally. This was done because intraperitoneal injection was a more reliable route of administration in our laboratory. In addition, in a very small preliminary study, the blood levels between the two routes of administration were similar after 90 minutes.

When the phenylpropanolamine dose was increased six times, the caffeine dose was also increased six times to 24 mg/kg. The possibility should be considered that this dose of caffeine was independently responsible for the hemorrhagic stroke noted in three of the drug-treated, hypertensive rats. This is unlikely for two reasons: (1) hemorrhagic stroke has not been reported as occurring in conjunction with caffeine overdose (Curatolo and Robertson 1983; Rall 1980); and (2) the dose of caffeine that causes death in normotensive rodents (230 mg/kg) (Sattin 1971) is about nine times the dose used in these experiments; it is unlikely that the lethal dose for hypertensive rats would be only one-ninth that found for normotensive animals. Thus, it appears that hypertensive rats are sensitive to phenylpropanolamine/caffeine combinations and experience adverse reactions to them. Recently Schlemmer et al. (1984) noted that the lethal dose of phenylpropanolamine in rats is decreased when it is combined with caffeine. Potentiation of adverse effects of phenylpropanolamine by caffeine could have contributed to the stroke morbidity and mortality found in this experiment.

Another possible explanation of the results of these studies is related to the fact that phenylpropanolamine is metabolized differently in rats than in humans. In rats, 30% of phenylpropanolamine is metabolized to 4-hydroxy-norephedrine (Smith and Dring 1970). In humans, very little phenylpropanolamine is metabolized; at least 90% is excreted unchanged. Although 4-hydroxy-norephedrine could be a more potent vasoconstrictor than phenylpropanolamine, preliminary results from our laboratory indicate that the observed effects of phenylpropanolamine are not due to 4-hydroxy-norephedrine (Snoddy, Mueller, and Black 1985).

A crucial question concerns the applicability of the results of these experiments to human beings. There are two major factors to be considered. First, although the drug combination studied in these experiments, phenylpropanolamine and caffeine, is no longer approved for sale, the combination may still be ingested because caffeine is readily available. Thus, a consumer with poor judgment may take five or six phenylpropanolamine-containing diet pills (Mueller, Graham, and Duggan 1985), some No-Doz®, and cola or coffee and, unknowingly, be at considerable risk.

Second, how does our finding that hypertensive rats appear particularly sensitive to the adverse effects of phenylpropanolamine/caffeine combinations apply to human beings? These animal results suggest that there may be subgroups of humans, including hypertensive individuals, who are potentially susceptible to the adverse effects of phenylpropanolamine combined with caffeine. Since a large percentage of the hypertensive population are not aware that they have hypertension (Health, Education and Welfare 1979) and since hypertension is more common among overweight individuals, who are the most likely to take diet pills (Berchtold et al. 1979; Kannel et al 1967), the "at risk" group may be large.

REFERENCES

Berchtold, P. et al. 1981. Epidemiology of obesity and hypertension. Int J Obes 5:1-7.

Bernstein, E. and B. M. Diskant. 1982. Phenylpropanolamine: a potentially hazardous drug. Ann Emerg Med 11:311-15.

Center for Science in the Public Interest. 1984. Diet pills linked with 17 cases of strokes and seizures. News release. Washington, D.C. January 26.

Curatolo, P. W. and D. Robertson. 1983. The health consequences of caffeine. Ann Intern Med 98:641-53.

Elliott, C. F. and J. C. Whyte. 1981. Phenylpropanolamine and hypertension. Med J Aust 1:715.

Health and Human Services, Food and Drug Administration (FDA). 1983. Enforcement action under the new drug provisions of the Federal Food, Drug and Cosmetic Act: certain OTC drug products; advisory opinion. FDA docket no. 83A-0339. Federal Register 48:52513-14. November 18.

———. 1982. Establishment of a monograph for weight control drug products for over-the-counter human use. FDA docket no. 81N-0022. Federal Register 47:8466-84. February 26.

Health, Education and Welfare. 1979. Report of the Hypertension Task Force: scientific survey and recommendations. PHS, HSH, publication 79:1624. Washington, D.C.: U.S. Government Printing Office.

Johnson, D. A., H. S. Etter, and D. M. Reeves. 1983. Stroke and phenylpropanolamine use. Lancet 2:970.

Kannel, W. B. et al. 1967. The relation of adiposity to blood pressure and development of hypertension. Ann Intern Med 67:48-59.

King, J. 1979. Hypertension and cerebral haemorrhage after Trimolets ingestion. Med J Aust 2:258.

Mueller, S. M. 1983. Neurologic complications of phenylpropanolamine use. Neurology 33:650-52.

Mueller, S. M., J. D. Graham, and D. Duggan. 1985. Neurologic signs and symptoms related to over-the-counter diet pills. Indiana Med. In press.

Mueller, S. M., J. Muller, and S. M. Asdell. 1984. Cerebral hemorrhage associated with phenylpropanolamine in combination with caffeine. Stroke 15:119-23.

Mueller, S. M. and E. B. Solow. 1982. Seizures associated with a new combination "pick-me-up" pill. Ann Neurol 11:322.

Rall, T. W. 1980. Central nervous system stimulants: xanthines. In The pharmacological basis of therapeutics, edited by A. G. Goodman, L. S. Goodman, and A. Gilman, 6th ed., 592–607. New York: Macmillan.

Sattin, A. 1971. Increase in the content of adenosine 3'5'-monophosphate in mouse forebrain during seizures and prevention of the increase by methylxanthines. J Neurochem 18:1087-96.

Schlemmer, R. F. et al. 1984. Caffeine potentiates phenylpropanolamine (PPA) lethality but not motor behavior. Fed Proc 43:572.

Smith, R. L. and L. G. Dring. 1970. Patterns of metabolism of beta-phenylisopropylamines in man and other species. In Amphetamines and related compounds: proceedings of the Mario Negri Institute for Pharmacological Research, edited by E. Costa and S. Garattini. New York: Raven Press.

Snoddy, A. M., S. M. Mueller, and W. L. Black. 1985. Inhibition of para-hydroxylation does not alter phenylpropanolamine's effect in the rat. Fed Proc 44:1637.

Zeman, W. and J.R.M. Innes. 1963. Craigie's neuroanatomy of the rat, 45. New York: Academic Press.

ACKNOWLEDGMENT

Dr. Mueller was the recipient of a Young Investigator Award (#HL 26378) from the National Institutes of Health, which supported this research.

15

ASSESSING EPIDEMIOLOGICAL RELATIONSHIPS BETWEEN STROKES AND PHENYLPROPANOLAMINE USE

Charles Winick

INTRODUCTION

The existence of a link between the use of phenylpropanolamine (PPA) and the occurrence of stroke has been suggested in a variety of sources: occasional newspaper articles (Green 1984), a statement by a consumer advocacy organization (U.S. Congress, House 1983a), testimony by four consumers before the Select Committee on Aging of the U.S. House of Representatives (U.S. Congress, House 1983b), and several case reports, usually in the form of letters to the editor (Humberstone 1969; King 1979; Elliott and Whyte 1981; Bernstein and Diskant 1982; Johnson, Etter, and Reeves 1983).

The purpose of this paper is to contribute to the evaluation of this possible connection between phenylpropanolamine consumption and stroke. First, the available information on the characteristics of stroke and of phenylpropanolamine use will be summarized. Next, six case reports of the appearance of stroke-related symptoms following phenylpropanolamine ingestion will be assessed. Finally, the following four comparative studies of phenylpropanolamine use and stroke incidence will be presented:

(1) An analysis of the relationship between phenylpropanolamine use and the occurrence of stroke among members of a large health maintenance organization;

(2) A comparison of the demographic characteristics of users of different kinds of phenylpropanolamine products and of persons who have strokes;

(3) An analysis of the relationships between the trends over time in the volume of sales of phenylpropanolamine products and in incidence of stroke; and

(4) A comparison of the seasonal occurrence of stroke and phenylpropanolamine sales.

SOME CHARACTERISTICS OF STROKE

A stroke is any sudden paralysis, the usual cause of which is a vascular disturbance of the brain. Stroke is third to coronary heart disease and cancer as a cause of death in the United States, accounting for approximately 11% of total mortality.

A diagnosis of stroke is usually made on the basis of a combination of symptoms and results of various tests and other specialized procedures. Stroke is probably misdiagnosed more often than any other neurological disease because its diagnosis depends on a composite picture rather than on any specific deficit. Correct diagnosis of death due to stroke requires an examination of the brain but autopsies are performed in only 11.9% of stroke deaths (Walker, Robins, and Weinfeld 1981). Even when autopsies are performed, the brain is removed in only about one-half of those examinations. If the brain _is_ examined, the findings are seldom available in less than a week and thus may not influence what is recorded on the death certificate. In a Framingham, Massachusetts, longitudinal study of vascular disease begun in 1948 under the auspices of the U.S. Public Health Service, it was estimated that, based on death certificate diagnoses, one-third of actual stroke cases are not detected and one-fourth of recorded stroke cases are incorrectly listed as such (Wolf, Kannel, and Dawber 1978).

Moreover, there is a lack of uniformity in stroke data. The several kinds of stroke have different pathogeneses and do not necessarily share the same epidemiological characteristics. Some data on strokes are derived from special population groups and other data are based on hospitalized cases. In some studies, only first strokes are reported; in others, all strokes may be counted. Some investigations include transient ischemic attacks under the definition of stroke; others do not. It may be difficult to distinguish between a thrombotic and a hermorrhagic stroke, even if the spinal fluid is examined.

Estimates of Stroke Incidence

Kurtzke (1976a, 1976b) has estimated that 69% of first strokes are cerebral infarctions (thrombosis or embolism), 12% cerebral hemorrhages, and 8% subarachnoid hemorrhages (11% were unspecified types of stroke). In the National Survey of Stroke, 82% of initial attacks were identified as thrombotic; subarachnoid hemorrhages, intraparenchymal hemorrhages, and embolic strokes each accounted for about 6% (Weinfeld 1981).

The most complete stroke data have been compiled in the National Survey of Stroke, which sampled the 6,140 short-term general hospitals in the United States for stroke cases from 1971 through 1976 (Weinfeld 1981). Sampled cases included those categorized under the International Classification of Disease as subarachnoid hemorrhage (category 430), cerebral hemorrhage (431), cerebral thrombosis or thrombotic infarction of the brain (433), cerebral embolism or embolic infarction of the brain (434), occlusion or stenosis of precerebral arteries (432), and acute but ill-defined cerebrovascular disease (436) (National Center for Health Statistics 1980). Patients with transient ischemic attacks (category 435) were not included.

Risk Factors for Stroke

The occurrence of stroke is not randomly distributed in the population. The likelihood of stroke increases with age, approximately doubling with every ten years of age between 45 and 85. If the relatively older age distribution of females in the United States is taken into account, the standardized incidence ratio of stroke is 1.21 for men and 0.84 for women, so that a male has a 44% greater likelihood of having a stroke than a female of comparable age (Robins and Baum 1981). Approximately 14.0% of stroke cases (Baum 1981), but 13.4% of the total population, is nonwhite.

Risk factors for stroke should be analyzed in terms of the kinds of stroke, the relationships of risk factors to underlying vascular disease, the onset of clinical disease, and the morbidity/mortality of the stroke. Other risk considerations include demographic and regional factors and dose-response evaluations, including threshold levels, for substances ingested (Kuller 1978). For example, the use of oral contraceptives could have contributed to an increase in strokes in premenopausal women.

The available data do not provide a clear-cut picture of the relationship between obesity and stroke. Only the Framingham prospective study has produced evidence that obesity plays a role independent of increased blood pressure in the occurrence of stroke (Gordon and Kannel 1976). However, increased salt consumption often accompanies a high intake of calories and this could contribute to the development of hypertension in genetically or otherwise susceptible individuals.

In a study attempting to define the relative contribution of elevated blood pressure as a factor leading to stroke, it was estimated that 56% of the strokes in black males and 76% in black females could be attributed to high blood pressure (Heyman et al. 1971). Persons with diabetes, heart disease, and hypertension are six, six, and four times more likely, respectively, to have a stroke as persons in the same age group who do not have these conditions (Westat Research 1983).

In the Framingham study, a number of risk factors that predispose to stroke were identified, including high blood pressure, diabetes, cigarette smoking, left ventricular hypertrophy, and increased serum cholesterol. It was found that 50% of strokes occurred in the 10% of the population in which these risk factors were highest. It is possible that many strokes result from a slight elevation of several risk factors rather than from an exceptionally high level of any single factor.

There is a wide variation in the frequency of stroke in different parts of the world, in different regions within the United States, and even within individual states. Rates of stroke vary not only by gender, age, and race, but also on geographic, ethnic, and perhaps even sociocultural dimensions. For example, the rates of cerebrovascular disease in Japanese men who migrate to California or Hawaii are much lower than those of their counterparts in Japan (Worth et al. 1975). Different population subgroups may have a greater likelihood of experiencing a particular kind of stroke. For instance, women are more liable to suffer subarachnoid hemorrhagic strokes, while infarction strokes are more common among men. The younger the population, the higher is the proportion of hemorrhagic stroke.

SOME DIMENSIONS OF PHENYLPROPANOLAMINE USE

Phenylpropanolamine is found in four types of products: prescription cough, cold, and allergy medications, over-the-counter (OTC) cough, cold, and allergy preparations, OTC appetite suppressants, and "look-alike" combinations (the availability of which has probably been diminished by recent federal and state regulatory actions).

Prescription Drugs

Phenylpropanolamine, which ranks sixth among all generic drugs contained in prescriptions, is included in 2.7% of all prescriptions dispensed in a typical year. The six most popular prescription products containing phenylpropanolamine are widely prescribed for the relief of allergies and cough and cold symptoms. These six products (Dimetapp®, Ornade®, Naldecon®, Tuss Ornade®, Dimetane® Expectorant, and Dimetane® Expectorant DC) accounted for 31.4 million prescriptions in 1980 (National Prescription Audit 1980). These products contain from 5 to 50 mg of phenylpropanolamine per recommended dose, usually taken several times a day. The cough and cold preparations are typically taken for three to five days and the allergy products for several weeks. Approximately one billion doses of prescription products containing phenylpropanolamine are consumed each year in the United States (Consumer expenditure study, annuals 1973-83). It is likely that these products are most often given to children.

OTC Cough, Cold, and Allergy Products

OTC cough, cold, and allergy preparations containing phenylpropanolamine are used by vast numbers of people. In a typical year, 64% of the population consume cold/allergy products, 51% take lozenges, 40% use cough syrup, and 31% take cough drops. Approximately four billion doses of phenylpropanolamine were ingested in these products in the United States in 1984.

Since 1976, phenylpropanolamine has been replacing pseudoephedrine as the most widely used nasal decongestant in OTC products. Some representative products, the amount of phenylpropanolamine per dose they contain, and their recent shares of their respective markets are given below:

Product	Dosage	Market share
Contac® (the major nonaspirin product)	75 mg	28%
Vicks Formula 44D® (the leading proprietary cough drop)	37.5 mg	51%
Sucrets (the major lozenge)	25 mg	70%

These products may be taken one or more times daily for days or weeks while symptoms persist.

Appetite Suppressants

Phenylpropanolamine was first marketed on a large scale as an OTC appetite suppressant in 1974; about one billion doses are currently taken by some ten million consumers in the United States annually. Representative products include

Dietac™ (50 mg of phenylpropanolamine per recommended dose), Appedrine® (25 mg), Dexatrim Extra Strength™ (75 mg), and Prolamine™ (37.5 mg). The smaller-dose products are usually sold in immediate-release forms, while those containing higher doses are available only as sustained-release preparations. Recommended maximum daily dosages vary, but none exceeds 75 mg. Users typically take these products to achieve specific weight loss goals. Package instructions usually specify that the products should not be taken for more than three consecutive months.

Look-Alike Combinations

Combination products, which are simulated controlled substances often resembling amphetamine in appearance and containing various combinations of phenylpropanolamine, caffeine, and ephedrine, became popular in the 1970s. Although these products were declared new drugs by the Food and Drug Administration (FDA) in 1982 and have been prohibited for sale in most states, some versions are still sold by mail order and in retail stores and an unknown number of people continue to use them. These products are called look-alikes because they are deliberately manufactured to resemble controlled substances like amphetamine even though all their ingredients are available on a nonprescription basis. Phenylpropanolamine became an important ingredient in look-alikes only in 1980-82; before that time, it was seldom included (see Morgan, Puder, and Kagan, chapter 9, this volume).

PUBLISHED CASE REPORTS OF STROKE SYMPTOMS FOLLOWING PHENYLPROPANOLAMINE INGESTION

In a recent literature search, six published case reports were found that cited a link between the ingestion of a phenylpropanolamine product and the subsequent occurrence of stroke-related symptoms.

Humberstone (1969), in England, reported the case of a 36-year-old woman with a "longstanding somewhat hysterical personality" who was hospitalized with severe headache symptoms following ingestion of multiple drugs, including phenylpropanolamine. A lumbar puncture confirmed a subarachnoid hemorrhage and there was the possibility of an aneurysm. Treated conservatively, she recovered completely. During the previous six months, she had been taking 30 mg daily of phenelzine, an inhibitor of monoamine oxidase (MAO) that may cause hypertensive crises. A few hours before her headache symptoms appeared, she had taken two tablets of the decongestant Mucron, each containing 30 mg of phenylpropanolamine, phenacetin, ipecacuanha, and vitamin C. Although the patient's blood pressure was not elevated, the author suggested it was likely that "the interaction of phenelzine and phenylpropanolamine resulted in the rupture of a berry aneurysm." Since the early 1970s, prescriptions containing MAO inhibitors in the United States have included detailed warnings regarding possible drug interactions.

King (1979), in Australia, cited the case of a 37-year-old woman who had taken two Trimolets tablets before going to bed; the following morning, her speech was slurred and she had a right hemiparesis. A computerized axial tomography (CAT) scan showed several small hemorrhages in the region of the left internal capsule. Two weeks later, she recovered completely. Trimolets contains 85 mg of phenylpropanolamine in an immediate-release form described as "D-phenylpropanolamine," which could be very different from the (±)-phenylpropanolamine sold in the United States (see Morgan, chapter 11, this volume). No product containing 85 mg of phenylpropanolamine in immediate-release form has ever been available in the United States, where 37.5 mg is the maximum dosage permitted for an immediate-release anorexiant; Trimolets in this dosage form has since been withdrawn from the market in Australia.

Also from Australia, Elliott and Whyte (1981) reported on a 54-year-old diabetic woman who had a left occipital hemorrhage after she had taken one capsule of the appetite suppressant Dietgard™ (containing 75 mg of phenylpropanolamine) that day and the previous day. She subsequently died. The authors noted, however, that "this report does not prove any association between phenylpropanolamine and intra-cerebral hemorrhage." An autopsy demonstrated no evidence of hypertensive change in cerebral vessels.

Bernstein and Diskant (1982) reported on two men in New Mexico who suffered intracerebral hemorrhages culminating in death after they had taken look-alike products. One of the men, 26 years of age, had drunk three to six ounces of whiskey and taken two black look-alikes (each containing 200 mg of caffeine, 25 mg of ephedrine, and 50 mg of phenylpropanolamine). He died 11 hours after he was hospitalized. Extensive subarachnoid and intraventricular hemorrhage was found at autopsy.

The other man, who was 17 years old, had also ingested two black look-alikes and was brought to the emergency department 17 hours later. On the fourth day after admission, he died. At autopsy, a massive intracerebral hemorrhage in the left parieto-occipital area and intraventricular hemorrhage on the left were noted. The authors found these cases to be dramatic examples of the "combination and synergistic effect" of the phenylpropanolamine/caffeine/ephedrine combination. Ephedrine was found in the blood samples of both men; an analysis for phenylpropanolamine was not ordered. Since both men exhibited increased blood pressure, it is possible that they had taken more than the reported dosages of the look-alike substances.

In a case reported from the United States by Johnson, Etter, and Reeves (1983), a 24-year-old man had been taking eight to ten capsules daily of the sustained-release appetite suppressant Dexatrim™ (each containing 50 mg of phenylpropanolamine and 200 mg of caffeine) for three months before an episode of right-sided hemiparesis. A brain scan was consistent with a left middle cerebral artery cardiovascular accident and a CAT scan reflected a lesion in the left front parietal area suggestive of an evolving infarct. Another man, 34 years old, who had been taking three to eight tablets daily of the appetite suppressant Dietac™ (containing 37.5 mg of phenylpropanolamine per tablet) for four months, developed right-sided hemiparesis. Both patients recovered. The authors noted that the "neurological complications [of the patients] seem to be at least temporally related to the use of diet pills."

Mesnard and Ginn (1984), in the United States, reported the case of a 25-year-old man who experienced a severe frontal headache 30 minutes after he had taken approximately five times the recommended dose of "a liquid PPA diet preparation" in an attempt to achieve an altered mental state. He went to an emergency room but left before receiving any treatment. Five days later, he returned with symptoms of headache and a stiff neck, both of which responded to treatment within 36 hours. The patient was normotensive throughout his hospitalization. The authors suggested that the patient's ingestion of phenylpropanolamine had led to a transient hypertensive episode causing a subarachnoid hemorrhage, although this diagnosis was not confirmed.

In assessing adverse drug reactions such as those summarized above, it is often difficult to identify the contribution of a specific substance, in a context of drug interactions, preexisting disease conditions, the possibility of overdose, and the hazards of accepting patient identification of drugs without verification of their presence by analysis of body fluids.

The relative paucity of reports linking stroke to phenylpropanolamine is noteworthy. Although some 50 billion doses of phenylpropanolamine have probably been consumed in the United States alone in the last 15 years, only six reports involving eight patients have been published during this period. Two reports came from Australia, one from England, and three from the United States. The presence of phenylpropanolamine was not verified by analysis of the body fluids in any of the cases. The British case undoubtedly reflected a drug interaction; one of the Australian reports dealt with a high-dosage form of phenylpropanolamine never available in the United States and not currently available anywhere; the other Australian report involved a preexisting chronic disease; and patients in two of the reports from the United States had taken multiple-ingredient products. The look-alikes ingested by the two men in the first U.S. case report have been illegal since 1982. In the second case report from the United States, both patients had been taking much greater than the recommended doses of appetite suppressants for several months. In the third U.S. report, the patient had taken an overdose.

STUDY OF THE RELATIONSHIP BETWEEN STROKE AND PHENYLPROPANOLAMINE USE AMONG MEMBERS OF A HEALTH MAINTENANCE ORGANIZATION

One source of data for the empirical study of phenylpropanolamine/stroke relationships is the health maintenance organization, which maintains medical records on its members, including medications ingested and illnesses treated. The availability of such records makes it possible to compare the relative incidence of stroke among persons who have taken phenylpropanolamine and those who have not. This approach offers a real-life situation representing a natural experiment in which not only the number of cases of stroke among users and nonusers but also the number of days during which users are "at risk" can be determined. A statistical comparison can then be made in order to establish the degree to which phenylpropanolamine use is related to stroke.

Such a study has been conducted using data from the Group Health Cooperative of Puget Sound, a health maintenance organization in the state of Washington whose approximately 300,000 participants receive prescription drugs and medical and hospital care through the Cooperative. In joint studies with the Boston Collaborative Drug Surveillance Program, the Cooperative has examined the relationships between the use of a number of specific drugs and the presence of various symptoms and conditions. Established in 1966, the Boston Collaborative Drug Surveillance Program (1974) has analyzed many drug/illness relationships, including those between reserpine use and breast cancer.

Jick, Aselton, and Hunter (1984) have reported the results of the Cooperative/Program joint study of the relationship between phenylpropanolamine use and cerebral hemorrhage. Four prescription preparations containing phenylpropanolamine are available through the Cooperative, with a recommended daily dosage for adults ranging between 45 and 150 mg. Between 1977 and 1981, 216,189 prescriptions for products containing phenylpropanolamine were filled for Cooperative members under 65 years of age (no data were available on those over 65). Assuming that every person for whom a phenylpropanolamine prescription was filled was at risk of cerebral hemorrhage (including subarachnoid, intracranial, and subdural hemorrhage) for 30 days after the prescription was filled, there was a total of 6,485,670 (30 x 216,189) "at risk" person-days of phenylpropanolamine use (assuming no simultaneous use of more than one phenylpropanolamine product or overlap of 30-day "at risk" periods for any individual).

A comparison was made between the incidence of stroke per "at risk" person-days of phenylpropanolamine use (defined as all 30-day periods after the filling of phenylpropanolamine prescriptions) versus the incidence of stroke per "not at risk" person-days of no phenylpropanolamine use (including "not at risk" days for persons who had had prescriptions filled at some other time). Multiplying the number of Cooperative members under 65 years of age times the number of days they were members during the five-year study period (not all persons were members throughout the entire study) gives the total number of person-days. Subtracting the number of "at risk" person-days leaves 425,850,342 "not at risk" person-days of no phenylpropanolamine use. One person was hospitalized for cerebral hemorrhage during an "at risk" period of phenylpropanolamine use, for an incidence rate of 1/6,485,670 "at risk" person-days. There were 113 individuals admitted to the hospital for cerebral hemorrhage during "not at risk" periods of no phenylpropanolamine use, for an incidence rate of 113/425,850,342 "not at risk" person-days. The 95% upper confidence limit for risk attributable to phenylpropanolamine use in this population is less than one per million "at risk" person-days. The authors concluded that "These data indicate that the risk of cerebral hemorrhage requiring hospital admission and attributable to taking PPA-containing cough and cold remedies, if present at all, is very small. This conclusion was not affected by changing the assumption about the risk period from thirty days to ninety days" (Ibid.) No indication was given in the brief report about the ages of the patients for whom phenylpropanolamine prescriptions had been filled. It is possible that many phenylpropanolamine prescriptions were given to children and this may have contributed to the noncomparability regarding stroke incidence as well.

DEMOGRAPHIC RELATIONSHIPS BETWEEN STROKE AND PHENYLPROPANOLAMINE USE

What relationships exist between the demographic characteristics of persons who have had a stroke and persons who use each of the several types of phenylpropanolamine products? In order to examine this question, the demographic composition of the stroke population can be compared to that of three groups of phenylpropanolamine consumers, those who use (1) appetite suppressants, (2) OTC cough, cold, and allergy preparations, and (3) prescription products. (Because look-alike products are illegal and are not monitored by the syndicated national retail audit services, there is no information available on the characteristics of their users.) Each group compared has been classified according to three demographic variables (tables 15.1 and 15.2): age (20-44, 45-64, and 65 and over), race (white or other), and gender (male or female). Data on characteristics of phenylpropanolamine consumers have been derived from a number of sources (Baum 1982). Each phenylpropanolamine consumer subgroup can be compared separately to the same subgroup in the stroke population in order to ascertain whether or not the two groups are homogeneous. For example, if a particular phenylpropanolamine consumer group is 60% female, then the stroke patient group would be at least statistically similar if it was also 60% female.

It is hypothesized that the two groups being compared are homogeneous, and then an attempt is made to disprove the hypothesis. It would, for instance, be expected that the proportions for age, gender, and race would be the same for both groups being compared if phenylpropanolamine has a prominent effect.

Four generalized hypotheses are tested for each of the comparisons between groups:

(1) The proportion of white and other races is the same for both the stroke and phenylpropanolamine groups.

(2) The proportion of males and females is the same for both groups.

(3) The proportion in each age category is the same for both groups.

(4) All the proportions--age, gender, and race--are the same for both groups.

Two different statistics are used in this section. The dichotomous variables--those divided into two categories,

TABLE 15.1

Stroke patients and phenylpropanolamine consumers classified by race, sex, and age

Category	U.S. population over 20		Stroke patients		Individuals using phenylpropanolamine products					
					Appetite suppressants		Cough/cold and allergy products		Prescription products	
	Number	Percent	Number	Percent	Number	Percent	Number	Percent	Number	Percent
Total	168,421,000	(100.0)	2,692,145	(100.0)	10,000,000	(100.0)	113,600,000	(100.0)	31,400,000	(100.0)
Race										
White	145,899,000	(86.6)	2,314,382	(86.0)	9,700,000	(97.0)	97,696,000	(86.0)	—	—
Other	22,522,000	(13.4)	377,763	(14.0)	300,000	(3.0)	15,904,000	(14.0)	—	—
Sex										
Male	80,234,000	(47.6)	1,315,884	(48.9)	1,000,000	(10.0)	60,208,000	(53.0)	13,502,000	(43.0)
Female	88,187,000	(52.4)	1,376,261	(51.1)	9,000,000	(90.0)	53,392,000	(47.0)	17,898,000	(57.0)
Age (years)										
20–44	95,082,000	(56.5)	287,165	(10.7)	7,959,255	(79.6)	63,161,600	(55.6)	20,724,000	(66.0)
45–64	44,666,000	(26.5)	880,662	(32.7)	2,016,158	(20.2)	35,556,800	(31.3)	5,966,000	(19.0)
65 and over	28,673,000	(17.0)	1,524,318	(56.6)	24,587	(0.2)	14,881,600	(13.1)	4,710,000	(15.0)

—: Data not available.

Source: Compiled by the author. Data derived from Department of Commerce. 1980. Statistical abstracts of the United States. Washington, D.C.: U.S. Government Printing Office; National disease and therapeutic index. 1980. Ambler, PA: IMS America. December; Baum, H. M. 1982. Stroke prevalence: an analysis of data from the 1977 Health Interview study. Public Health Rep 97:24–30; unpublished studies available from various manufacturers.

such as male and female—are tested using a standard difference of proportions test and the results are evaluated using the normal distribution. From the actual data an observed value of z is calculated. This value is compared to a critical value of z that has been chosen at a 1% level of significance (i.e., corresponding to a probability of occurrence of one chance in 100). If the absolute value of the calculated (observed) value of z is greater than the critical value of z, then the hypothesis of equality (or similarity) is rejected and an alternative hypothesis of inequality is accepted (Blalock 1979).

The other statistic used here is the chi-square statistic. This statistic measures the difference between the actual data and what the data would be expected to be if the hypothesis of equality was true. In other words, the value of the chi-square statistic represents the degree to which the original equality hypothesis is violated. If the observed (calculated) value of chi-square is larger than the critical value of chi-square (here again, at a 1% level of significance)--larger than the difference expected by chance—then the hypothesis of equality is rejected and the alternative hypothesis of inequality is accepted (Siegel 1956).

All observed values reported below were calculated on the basis of data summarized in tables 15.1 and 15.2.

Race

The demographic variable of race is divided here into two categories, white and "other" ("other" consists of approximately four-fifths blacks). Since this is a dichotomous variable, it makes no difference whether the proportions of whites or of other races are compared.

The following hypotheses concerning race are being tested:

(1) The proportion of white and other races is the same for the stroke patient group as it is for the phenylpropanolamine appetite suppressant user group.

(2) The proportion of white and other races is the same for the stroke patient group as it is for the OTC phenylpropanolamine cough, cold, and allergy product user group.

(There are no data on the racial composition of prescription phenylpropanolamine users.)

The observed value of z calculated to test the first hypothesis is 714.63 and the critical value of z is 2.576. The hypothesis is rejected because the proportion of white

TABLE 15.2

Comparison of stroke patients and phenylpropanolamine users on three demographic variables

Age (years)	Sex	Race	U.S. population over 20		Stroke patients		Individuals using phenylpropanolamine products: Appetite suppressants		Cough/cold and allergy products		Prescription products	
			Number	Percent	Number	Percent	Number	Percent	Number	Percent	Number	Percent
20–44	Male	White	40,581,000	(24.1)	120,666	(4.5)	772,047	(7.7)	28,789,057	(25.3)	8,911,320	(28.4)
20–44	Male	Other	6,920,000	(4.1)	19,696	(0.7)	23,878	(0.2)	4,686,591	(4.1)		
20–44	Female	White	40,066,000	(23.8)	126,204	(4.7)	6,948,430	(69.5)	25,529,919	(22.5)	11,812,680	(37.6)
20–44	Female	Other	7,515,000	(4.5)	20,599	(0.8)	214,900	(2.1)	4,156,033	(3.7)		
45–64	Male	White	18,879,000	(11.2)	370,054	(13.7)	195,568	(2.0)	16,206,789	(14.3)	2,565,380	(8.2)
45–64	Male	Other	2,381,000	(1.4)	60,402	(2.2)	6,048	†	2,638,315	(2.3)		
45–64	Female	White	20,434,000	(12.1)	387,032	(14.4)	1,760,105	(17.6)	14,372,059	(12.7)	3,400,620	(10.8)
45–64	Female	Other	2,972,000	(1.8)	63,174	(2.3)	54,435	(0.5)	2,339,637	(2.1)		
65 and older	Male	White	10,380,000	(6.2)	640,518	(23.8)	2,385	†	6,783,033	(6.0)	2,025,300	(6.5)
65 and older	Male	Other	1,093,000	(0.6)	104,548	(3.9)	74	†	1,104,215	(1.0)		
65 and older	Female	White	15,559,000	(9.2)	669,908	(24.9)	21,465	(0.2)	6,015,143	(5.3)	2,684,700	(8.6)
65 and older	Female	Other	1,641,000	(1.0)	109,344	(4.1)	663	†	979,209	(0.9)		
		TOTAL	168,421,000	(100.0)	2,692,145	(100.0)	10,000,000	(100.0)	113,600,000	(100.0)	31,400,000	(100.0)

*A breakdown by race of users of phenylpropanolamine prescription products was not available; comparisons by age and sex only are given.

†Less than 0.1%.

Source: Compiled by the author. Data derived from Department of Commerce. 1980. Statistical abstracts of the United States. Washington, D.C.: U.S. Government Printing Office; National disease and therapeutic index. 1980. Ambler, PA: IMS America. December; Baum, H. M. 1982. Stroke prevalence: an analysis of data from the 1977 Health Interview study. Public Health Rep 97:24–30; unpublished studies available from various manufacturers.

stroke patients differs significantly from the proportion of whites using a phenylpropanolamine appetite suppressant.

The observed value of z calculated to test the second hypothesis is 1.50 and the critical value of z is 2.576. The hypothesis of the similarity of the two groups with respect to race is accepted, because the proportion of white stroke patients is the same as the proportion of whites who use phenylpropanolamine in the form of OTC cough, cold, and allergy preparations. It is also the same as the proportion of whites in the general population in the 1980 census, suggesting the possibility that the similarity of the proportions may be coincidental.

Gender

The demographic variable of gender is also divided into two categories, male and female. The following hypotheses concerning gender are being tested:

(1) The proportion of males and females is the same for the stroke patient group as it is for the phenylpropanolamine appetite suppressant user group.

(2) The proportion of males and females is the same for the stroke patient group as it is for the OTC phenylpropanolamine cough, cold, and allergy preparation user group.

(3) The proportion of males and females is the same for the stroke patient group as it is for the prescription phenylpropanolamine user group.

The observed values of z calculated to test these three hypotheses are shown below. The critical value of z for all three tests is 2.576.

User group	Observed value of z
Appetite suppressants	-1,466.05
Cough/cold and allergy products	133.90
Prescription products	-186.74

In all three tests, the absolute value of the observed value of z is greater than the critical value of z. All three hypotheses of similarity are rejected because the proportion of male stroke patients is significantly different from the proportion of males using each of the three types of phenylpropanolamine products. The gender profile of each group of phenylpropanolamine users clearly differs from that of stroke patients.

Age

The demographic variable of age is divided into three categories: 20-44, 45-64, and 65 and older. Since the variable of age has more than two categories, chi-square tests will be used. Degrees of freedom here represent a proportion of the number of cells in the tables. The general hypothesis concerning age being tested is that the age distribution of stroke patients is the same as the age distribution of each of the three phenylpropanolamine consumer groups.

The observed values of chi-square calculated to test the three hypotheses of homogeneity between the stroke patient and phenylpropanolamine user groups are shown below. In all three tests, there are 2 degrees of freedom and the critical value of chi-square is 9.210.

User group	Observed value of chi-square
Appetite suppressants	7,221,261.40
Cough/cold and allergy products	4,505,642.70
Prescription products	3,812,869.68

In all three tests, the observed value of chi-square is greater than the critical value of chi-square. All three hypotheses of homogeneity are rejected because the age distribution of stroke patients differs significantly from that of each group of phenylpropanolamine consumers.

The size of the observed value of chi-square is a direct function of the sample size. In other words, if the size of the sample is multiplied by 100, the resulting observed value of chi-square will be exactly 100 times greater. Since such large numbers are being examined in this attempt to ascertain whether a relationship exists between phenylpropanolamine consumers and stroke patients, it was decided that additional statistical tests should be employed.

The data were therefore further analyzed using two-by-two comparisons of proportions and the results were interpreted using the normal distribution. It is hypothesized that the age distribution of stroke patients is the same as that of each group of phenylpropanolamine users when two-by-two comparisons are made. For example, it is hypothesized that the proportion of stroke patients in the age group 20-44 is the same as the proportion of phenylpropanolamine appetite suppressant consumers in the same age group.

The results of this analysis are presented on the next page.

User group	Age (years) 20-44	45-65	65 and over
Appetite suppressants	2,104.24	1,463.44	1,791.77
Cough/cold and allergy products	-435.53	-49.38	-538.97
Prescription products	-2,508.34	-2,027.49	-1,695.45

The range of the absolute values of the observed z values shown in the table is 49.38 to 2,508.34 and the critical value of z is 2.576. The hypothesis is rejected because the age distribution of stroke patients is significantly different from that of each group of phenylpropanolamine users.

All Demographic Variables Combined

The users of each of the three categories of phenylpropanolamine products can also be compared to stroke patients across all three demographic variables combined.

It is hypothesized that the distribution of age, race, and gender combined is the same for the stroke patients as it is for each group of phenylpropanolamine consumers (age and gender only for the prescription phenylpropanolamine user group). The observed values of chi-square calculated to test these hypotheses (using data summarized in table 15.2), the degrees of freedom, and the critical values of chi-square are given below.

User group	Observed value	Degrees of freedom	Critical value
Appetite suppressant	8,115,252.32	11	24.725
Cough/cold and allergy products	4,546,818.41	11	24.725
Prescription products	3,871,577.04	5	20.517

In all three tests, the observed value of chi-square is greater than the critical value of chi-square. All three hypotheses of homogeneity between the stroke patient population and each of the three phenylpropanolamine user groups are therefore rejected since the distribution of age, race, and gender combined is significantly different for stroke patients compared to that for each group of phenylpropanolamine consumers.

As was done in the previous section on age, z values were calculated for all two-by-two comparisons (table 15.3). It is again hypothesized that the distribution of age, race, and gender combined is the same for the stroke patients as it is for each group of phenylpropanolamine consumers. The absolute values of the observed values of z range between 8.94 and 1,893.96, with a critical value of 2.576 for z. The hypothesis of similarity of demographic characteristics for stroke patients and phenylpropanolamine users is therefore rejected.

TABLE 15.3

Observed values of z for two-by-two comparisons
(across all demographic variables)
of stroke patients and phenylpropanolamine users

<table>
<tr><th>Age (years)</th><th>Sex</th><th>Race</th><th>Appetite suppressants</th><th>Cough/cold and allergy products</th><th>Prescription products</th></tr>
<tr><td>20-44</td><td>Male</td><td>White</td><td>199.32</td><td>782.57</td><td rowspan="2">825.97</td></tr>
<tr><td>20-44</td><td>Male</td><td>Other</td><td>-119.69</td><td>279.41</td></tr>
<tr><td>20-44</td><td>Female</td><td>White</td><td>1,893.96</td><td>695.58</td><td rowspan="2">1,061.48</td></tr>
<tr><td>20-44</td><td>Female</td><td>Other</td><td>138.03</td><td>252.33</td></tr>
<tr><td>45-64</td><td>Male</td><td>White</td><td>-821.35</td><td>23.64</td><td rowspan="2">-435.28</td></tr>
<tr><td>45-64</td><td>Male</td><td>Other</td><td>-434.96</td><td>8.94</td></tr>
<tr><td>45-64</td><td>Female</td><td>White</td><td>123.88</td><td>-84.00</td><td rowspan="2">-292.81</td></tr>
<tr><td>45-64</td><td>Female</td><td>Other</td><td>-287.64</td><td>-32.00</td></tr>
<tr><td>65 and older</td><td>Male</td><td>White</td><td>-1,577.18</td><td>-1,183.44</td><td rowspan="2">-1,223.86</td></tr>
<tr><td>65 and older</td><td>Male</td><td>Other</td><td>-625.17</td><td>-464.41</td></tr>
<tr><td>65 and older</td><td>Female</td><td>White</td><td>-1,583.74</td><td>-1,364.66</td><td rowspan="2">-1,062.40</td></tr>
<tr><td>65 and older</td><td>Female</td><td>Other</td><td>-639.20</td><td>537.06</td></tr>
</table>

*A breakdown by race of users of phenylpropanolamine prescription products was not available; comparisons by age and sex only are given.
<u>Source</u>: Compiled by the author.

Even though the statistical tests evaluated above using the normal distribution are not as sensitive to large numbers as are the chi-square tests, the normal distribution results are still influenced by the size of the groups. In order to further check these test results, a "what if" analysis was performed using the Kolmogorov-Smirnov nonparametric test. The principle of this test is that if two populations are identical, then their cumulative frequency distributions should be similar. The test statistic used is the maximum difference between the two cumulative frequency distributions. If the maximum difference is larger than would be expected by chance, then the distributions are considered to be significantly diffferent.

First, the data from table 15.2 were tested, given all possible rankings within each group; all three phenylpropanolamine user groups were found to be significantly different from the stroke patient group. In the second step, it was assumed that the proportional relationship between group sizes remained constant and the minimum stroke patient sample size necessary for the two groups to be significantly different was calculated. The results of this analysis are presented below.

User group	Minimum sample size	
	Stroke patients	PPA users
Appetite suppressants	9	34
Cough/cold and allergy products	63	2,569
Prescription products	28	327

These data can be interpreted as follows. Given that the group proportions remain the same, a sample of nine stroke patients and 34 phenylpropanolamine appetite suppressant users would be sufficiently large to demonstrate that the two groups are significantly different at a 1% significance level.

Thus, all three "overview" tests yield the same conclusion: the distribution of demographic characteristics for the stroke patients is different, at a statistically significant level, from that for each phenylpropanolamine consumer group.

TRENDS IN THE INCIDENCE OF STROKE AND OF PHENYLPROPANOLAMINE USE

Another approach that may be used in evaluating the relationship between stroke and phenylpropanolamine involves an examination of the comparative trends in the incidence of stroke and of phenylpropanolamine consumption. If there is a powerful correlation between phenylpropanolamine use and stroke, it might be expected that as phenylpropanolamine use increased, there would also be an increase in the occurrence of stroke. Similarly, it has been observed that as alcohol consumption rises, there is a proportionate increase in alcoholism and in conditions like cirrhosis of the liver (Winick 1978). The following section examines the trends in the incidence of stroke and of phenylpropanolamine use and possible connections between them.

Trends in the Incidence of Stroke over Time

Worldwide, stroke has been declining steadily for several decades; although this decline is the most noticeable epidemiological trend in the incidence of stroke, the reasons for the drop are not completely understood. It is possible that aspirin, which has been so widely used in the last half-century, might help to prevent stroke. Another contributing factor may be that, as refrigerators and freezers have become more widely available, the use of salt for curing, pickling, and preserving food has declined, and this could have led to a generalized drop in high blood pressure and thus in stroke. Long-term studies of blood pressure, such as the Framingham study, indicate that the incidence of high blood pressure has decreased (Wolf, Kannel, and Dawber 1978).

The decline in the incidence of stroke has been so dramatic that Ostfeld (1980) concluded a major review of stroke epidemiology by observing that "stroke may be the first of the great current pandemics to yield." The decrease in stroke incidence, which began around 1920, has been noted in all age groups, among both males and females, and blacks and whites. Even in a country like Japan, which has had one of the world's highest stroke rates, the incidence of stroke is now diminishing steadily (Ueda et al. 1981).

Perhaps related to the decrease in the incidence of new cases of stroke is the decline in stroke deaths. Mortality rates from stroke fell at an average annual rate of less than 1% from 1900 to 1950. From 1950 to the early 1970s, stroke mortality dropped at an annual rate of about 1.5%. Since 1976, the mortality rate has been decreasing at an average annual rate of 4% to 5%. The decrease in stroke mortality began long before recent advances in treatment.

Whether the period of observation and data collection is relatively short or long, all available studies concur in the conclusion that stroke incidence is declining. Between 1971 and 1977, there was a drop in the percentage of stroke patients among the members of the largest health maintenance organization in the United States, the Kaiser-Permanente Medical Plan (Friedman 1979). In the Framingham study, the incidence of stroke among women declined over a 24-year period of observation (Wolf, Kannel, and Dawber 1978). In the only national survey of hospital cases, age-adjusted incidence rates of initial strokes declined 15% between 1971 and 1976; the decline was even greater among the elderly (Robins and Baum 1981).

The most complete data on trends in the incidence of stroke have been compiled by the Mayo Clinic in Rochester, Minnesota, a city of 58,000 persons in Olmsted County. The Mayo Clinic is an ideal center for the documentation of trends in the incidence of stroke. It administers a standard, quantifiable clinical examination for all neurological disorders, its neurology department is closely involved in the diagnosis and management of stroke, stroke diagnoses are confirmed by CAT scan or autopsy in 67% of the cases, and the Clinic utilizes an automated record-retrieval system (Garraway, Whisnant, and Drury 1983). Diagnoses made at other medical facilities in and around Olmsted County are also entered into the centralized diagnostic index at the Mayo Clinic. This medical records linkage and indexing system, begun in 1907, permits almost complete identification of all residents in the area who have ever received medical care. No other population anywhere in the world has been studied for so long or so carefully.

The decreased incidence of stroke seen elsewhere has also taken place in the Rochester area. For every 100 initial episodes of stroke per unit of population that occurred in Rochester from 1945 through 1949, only 55 occurred between 1970 and 1974 (Garraway et al. 1979). When the total stroke rate per 100,000 persons for each five-year period from 1945-49 through 1975-79 is compared with that for the immediately preceding period, it is found that that rate declined in every consecutive period, with a range of decrease between 6% and 25% and an average drop of 12%. The two five-year periods with the largest declines compared to the previous period were 1970-74 (25%) and 1975-79 (14%). The 1975-79 rate was 46% of the comparable rate in 1945-49.

In the Rochester area, rates for cerebral infarction have gradually decreased, intracerebral hemorrhage rates have declined less consistently, and subarachnoid hemorrhage rates have shown no clear trend (Ibid.). Since 1945, there has been no change in the age of onset of stroke.

What has caused this decline in stroke incidence in Rochester? It does not appear to be related either to the improved treatment of transient ischemic attacks and carotid stenosis or to decreases in cholesterol levels and cigarette smoking. Nor does it seem to be related to improved treatment of diabetes. Among nonhypertensive individuals in the

Rochester area, diabetics did not have significantly more strokes than did nondiabetics. Improved treatment of hypertension remains as a probably significant contributor to the decline (Whisnant 1984).

However, why did the incidence of stroke begin to decline before the emergence of the new hypertensive agents of the 1960s? The population in the United States is growing older, and age-adjustments to the 1940 population may be artificially reducing stroke rates slightly. Another small drop in rates could have resulted from the increased accuracy in diagnosis in recent years. A third reason for the decline is demographic: there has been a substantial black migration from the rural South to the urban North and the blood pressure of such migrants usually declines (National Center for Health Statistics 1964). A fourth factor may be related to a blood pressure testing program begun by the American Heart Association in the late 1960s. During about the first decade of this program (from its inception to the late 1970s), about 15 million people were screened for high blood pressure, of whom approximately four million were identified as hypertensive (Ostfeld 1980). Many of these persons may have sought help for their condition and thus reduced their likelihood of stroke.

Although these four factors are plausible, the major underlying reasons for the decline in stroke incidence are still not completely clear. In the United States, the 1964 warnings by the Surgeon General against smoking cigarettes and by the American Heart Association against diets high in saturated fat could have contributed to an overall drop in vascular disease (Walker 1977). Recent dietary reductions in salt intake may have further reduced the likelihood of hypertension and thus of stroke. Since 1974, the national High Blood Pressure Education Program has worked to improve the public's awareness of the implications of high blood pressure and has encouraged treatment of hypertension.

The major programs established in the 1960s to facilitate access to hospital care for the disadvantaged and the elderly, such as the Regional Medical Programs and Medicaid, have undoubtedly contributed to the decline in stroke incidence among those segments of the population. Ironically, however, since increased availability of hospital care is often accompanied by improvements in the accuracy and completeness of incidence statistics, it is possible that, if these programs had not been established, the decline in <u>reported</u> stroke incidence would have been even greater (although the decline in <u>actual</u> incidence would have been smaller in the absence of expanded hospital care).

Trends in the Incidence of Phenylpropanolamine Use over Time

Although there are prescription audit services that report on the number of prescriptions filled for various medicinal products, changes in the databases of the several services over the last decade make it impossible to evaluate prescription phenylpropanolamine sales trends over time. However, sales of OTC cough and cold remedies and appetite suppressants are reported each year in trade publications, by syndicated audit services such as the A. C. Nielsen Company, and in reports of individual companies and trade associations.

During the last 15 years, sales of OTC cough, cold, and allergy remedies containing phenylpropanolamine have greatly increased. Such increases are due to a variety of factors, including the emergence of new products and new formats for existing products, marketing initiatives, the reclassification of products from prescription to OTC, price reductions in OTC medications, reports in consumer publications and other media favorable to OTC products, more frequent self-medication, population growth, and colder weather conditions.

The use of phenylpropanolamine as an appetite suppressant was first reported almost two generations ago (Hirsh 1939). A major surge in its popularity has occurred over the last decade. It is sold throughout the United States in drugstores, convenience stores, and supermarkets. By 1981, one in five women on diets had tried an OTC phenylpropanolamine weight loss product.

Even when adjusted for inflation and population growth, the sales of both cough, cold, and allergy preparations and appetite suppressants containing phenylpropanolamine have increased substantially. Many more millions of people used them in the decade from 1974 to 1983 than in the previous ten-year period.

Statistical Examination of Trends in the Incidence of Phenylpropanolamine Use and of Stroke

Data on the sales of phenylpropanolamine-containing cough, cold, and allergy preparations from 1972 through 1982 and of appetite suppressants from 1974 through 1983 can be analyzed by means of a trend line, or linear least squares equation, that is fitted to each set of data. In addition, a trend line can be fitted to the incidence of stroke per 100,000 population from 1945 through 1979, using the Mayo

Clinic reports, the only reliable data available. The Rochester, Minnesota, and Olmsted County areas, from which the Mayo Clinic incidence data were derived, are typical of many other communities in the United States in demography and purchases of OTC phenylpropanolamine cough, cold, and allergy products and appetite suppressants. Every one of the area's convenience stores, supermarkets, and chain and independent drugstores carries both types of products.

If there is a strong relationship between stroke and the use of phenylpropanolamine, the incidence of stroke would be expected to rise as the consumption of phenylpropanolamine increased. Because most reports linking phenylpropanolamine use to elevations in blood pressure suggest that such effects usually occur after the first few ingestions, the large numbers of consumers trying phenylpropanolamine products for the first time make it plausible to be concerned that strokes will increase along with any jump in phenylpropanolamine use.

In the classical statistical approach to time series analyses, the independent variable is time, which is the horizontal axis in figures 15.1-15.4. The dependent variables are retail sales, shown in figures 15.1-15.3, and the incidence of stroke, shown in figure 15.4. Stroke data are shown for the last three decades for which Minnesota data are available (1945-79) to indicate the long-term trend. Phenylpropanolamine retail sales data are shown for approximately the last decade, during which the greatest increase occurred; data for earlier periods are not available. A least squares linear regression line was fitted to each set of sales and stroke data. Each of these straight lines, or trend lines, represents an average of the ups and downs in the actual data (Gujarati 1978).

The slope of each trend line was also calculated in order to statistically determine whether it was significantly different from zero, reflecting a significantly positive or negative trend. Hypothesis 1 is that the slope of each trend line is not significantly different from zero (i.e., there is no positive or negative trend). Alternative hypothesis 2 is that there is a significant positive or negative trend. If the observed (calculated) value of t is greater than the critical value of t at the 1% level of significance, then hypothesis 1 is rejected and alternative hypothesis 2 is accepted.

The actual data and the trend line for the retail sales of phenylpropanolamine cough and cold preparations are shown in figure 15.1. The observed value of t is 10.391, with 9 degrees of freedom, and the critical value of t is 2.82. The hypothesis of a significant positive trend in the sales of these preparations is confirmed.

FIGURE 15.1

Retail sales of
phenylpropanolamine cough/cold preparations,
1972-82

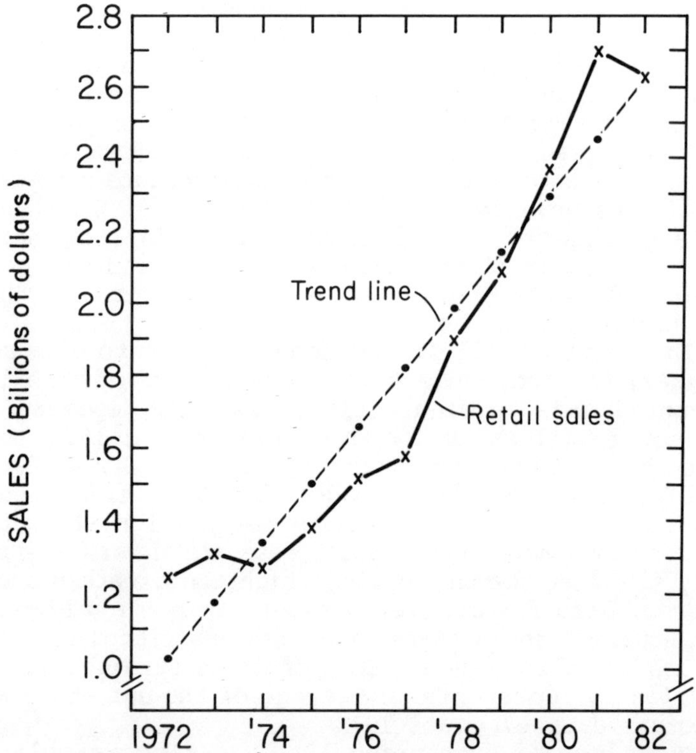

Source: Compiled by the author. Data derived from report on cough/cold product demographics, 1984, by the Marschalk Company, New York City; Consumer expenditure study, annuals. 1973-83. Product Marketing. July.

In figure 15.2, the actual data and the trend line for the retail sales of phenylpropanolamine appetite suppressants are given. The observed value of t is 7.54, with 8 degrees of freedom, and the critical value of t is 2.90. The hypothesis of a significant upward trend in the sales of these preparations is confirmed.

FIGURE 15.2

Retail sales of phenylpropanolamine appetite suppressants, 1974-83

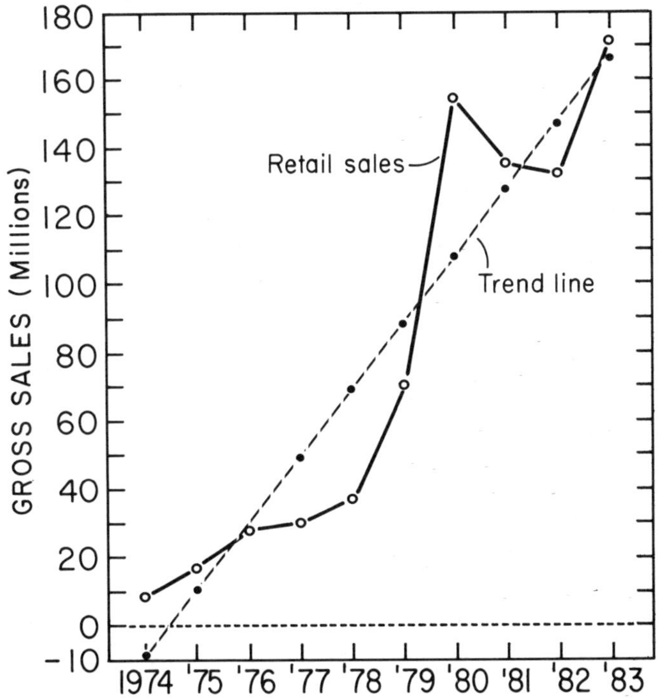

Source: Compiled by the author. Data derived from Dieting aids seasonality indices. 1984. Chicago: A. C. Nielsen; Consumer expenditure study, annuals. 1973-83. Product Marketing. July; Total dieting aids sales trends. 1984. Chicago: A. C. Nielsen; information made available by Thompson Medical Company: New York.

It is possible that the increase in retail sales of phenylpropanolamine products in this period was entirely a result of inflation. When the data are expressed in 1967 dollars, however, the trends remain similar (figure 15.3), indicating that the rate of inflation made only a small contribution to the upward sales trend of these products.

FIGURE 15.3

Retail sales of phenylpropanolamine appetite suppressants adjusted for inflation, 1974-83

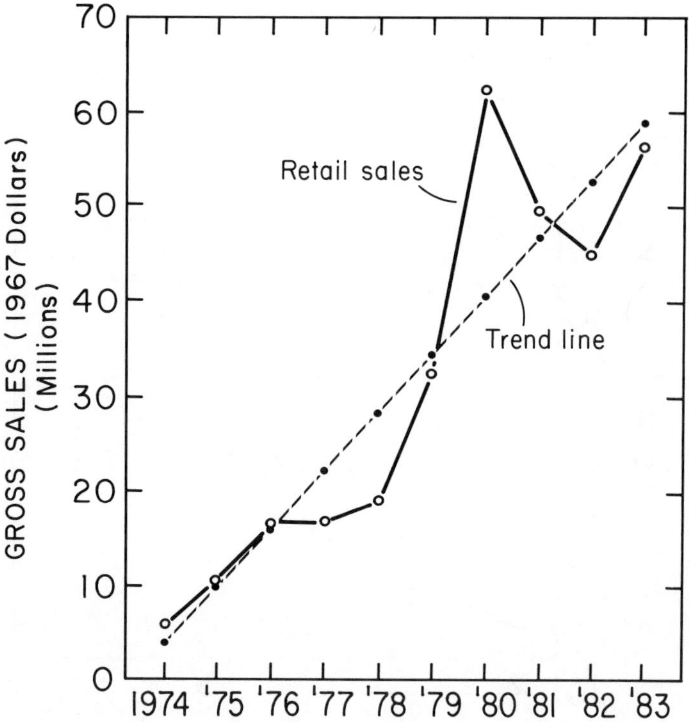

Source: Compiled by the author. Data derived from Dieting aids seasonality indices. 1984. Chicago: A. C. Nielsen; Consumer expenditure study, annuals. 1973-83. Product Marketing. July; Total dieting aids sales trends. 1984. Chicago: A. C. Nielsen; information made available by Thompson Medical Company: New York.

Figure 15.4 shows the actual data and the trend line for the Minnesota figures on stroke incidence between 1945 and 1979 (with each five-year interval indicated by its midpoint). The hypothesis of a significant downward or negative trend in the incidence of stroke is confirmed.

If there were a positive relationship between the increase in the use of phenylpropanolamine and the occurrence of stroke, there ought to have been significant increases in the number of strokes. In fact, however, during the decade in which sales of OTC phenylpropanolamine allergy, cough, and cold products doubled, sales of phenylpropanolamine appetite suppressants increased by 1,500%, and the total number of doses of phenylpropanolamine annually consumed probably tripled, the incidence of stroke dropped by 20%. There is no observed connection between the breadth and amount of phenylpropanolamine use and the incidence of stroke.

FIGURE 15.4

Stroke incidence per 100,000 population, 1945-79

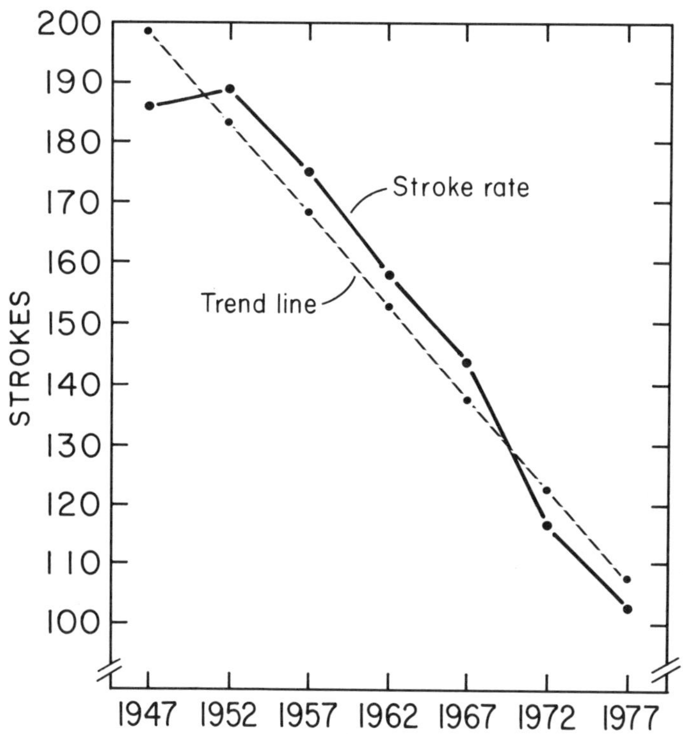

Source: Compiled by the author. Data derived from Baum, H. M. 1982. Stroke prevalence: an analysis of data from the 1977 Health Interview study; Public Health Rep 97:24-30; National Disease and Therapeutic Index. 1980. Ambler, PA: IMS America; Garraway, W. M., J. P. Whisnant, and I. Drury. 1983. The continuing decline in the incidence of stroke. Mayo Clin Proc 58:520-23.

Even though the trends in phenylpropanolamine use and in the incidence of stroke are moving in opposite directions, a statistical test was nonetheless employed in order to determine if the trends were significantly different. Comparison of trends in phenylpropanolamine appetite suppressant sales and stroke incidence yielded an observed value of t of 6.15, with 11 degrees of freedom, and a critical value of t of 3.11. A similar comparison of trends in stroke incidence and sales of phenylpropanolamine cough, cold, and allergy preparations yielded an observed value of t of 6.62, with 12 degrees of freedom, and a critical value of t of 3.06. In both cases, the trends were significantly different. Any contribution of phenylpropanolamine use to stroke did not alter the downward trend in the incidence of stroke.

INVESTIGATION OF SEASONALITY CONSIDERATIONS

Another approach to an evaluation of the relationship between stroke and phenylpropanolamine use is to examine the dimension of seasonality. In this section, the seasonality factors in the occurrence of stroke and in phenylpropanolamine sales are studied in order to determine if there is any connection between the month in which phenylpropanolamine products are bought (and presumably used) and the month in which strokes occur.

A four-city hospital consortium is currently investigating seasonality factors in the occurrence of stroke, as part of the National Stroke Data Bank Project, but is not expected to publish findings for several years. There are a few published reports on seasonality factors in blood pressure changes, cholesterol levels, and stroke (Takakashi et al. 1957; Wylie 1962; Thulin, Bengtsson, and Schersten 1978; Doyle et al. 1965). One report has been published on the month of occurrence of strokes based on data from Bellevue Hospital in New York City (McDowell, Louis, and Monahan 1970). However, the population of Bellevue's catchment area is not representative, and the study was done before the recent expansion of phenylpropanolamine consumption and will therefore not be used here. Instead, it was decided to generate a database from a major New York City medical center for use in this study of seasonality factors.

Data are available on the monthly sales of both prescription and OTC allergy and cough/cold remedies containing phenylpropanolamine. Similar data are available on the sales of OTC phenylpropanolamine appetite suppressants.

New York City is typical of the United States in both the rate and demographic characteristics of stroke and the rate and month of purchase of phenylpropanolamine products. Since most reports linking blood pressure changes to phenylpropanolamine consumption cite incidents that occur a day or two after initial ingestion of the product (Morgan 1985), the sales of phenylpropanolamine products each month can be compared to the incidence each month of new cases of stroke at the medical center.

The month of admission for all patients admitted to this center with a primary diagnosis of stroke from 1972 through 1982 was tabulated (n = 4,281). Patients were included if they had been admitted with a primary diagnosis of cerebral thrombosis, intracerebral hemorrhage, subarachnoid hemorrhage, unspecified cerebral hemorrhage, or acute but ill-defined cerebrovascular disease. Stroke categories for 1980 to 1982 admissions were based on the ninth revision of the International Classification of Disease; the seventh and eighth editions were used to determine stroke categories for admissions in previous years (World Health Organization 1980). The greatest number of admissions occurred in October, followed by March and July. The winter months had lower than average rates of admission. These trends were independent of the overall pattern in the total number of monthly admissions of patients to the hospital. The data on admissions to the medical center for stroke were indexed, with 100 representing the average of the 12 months. The monthly data for stroke admissions to the facility are summarized in figure 15.5.

To facilitate direct comparisons, the monthly data on the retail sales of each of the three kinds of phenylpropanolamine products were also indexed. It was then possible to compare the monthly data on admissions to the medical center for stroke with the monthly data on sales of the three types of phenylpropanolamine products.

The hypothesis being investigated is that admissions to the hospital for stroke are related to phenylpropanolamine consumption, as represented by sales of phenylpropanolamine products. A simple linear correlation is employed. The correlation coefficient (r) is used to measure the degree of association between sales of phenylpropanolamine products and hospital admissions of stroke patients. The correlation coefficient ranges from -1 to +1. A perfect negative correlation is indicated by a correlation coefficient of -1, a value of 0 indicates there is no correlation, and a value of +1 represents perfect positive correlation. If the absolute value of the observed value of t is greater than the critical value of t (at a 1% level of significance), then the hypothesis that the correlation coefficient is zero is rejected.

FIGURE 15.5

Average monthly admissions
to a New York City medical center for stroke

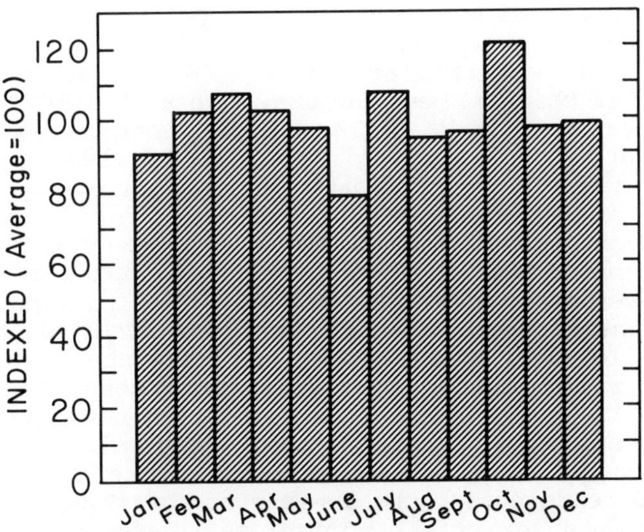

Source: Compiled by the author.

Figure 15.6 shows the monthly variation in sales of prescription phenylpropanolamine products compared with stroke admissions to the medical center. The observed value of t is -0.25, with 10 degrees of freedom, and the critical value of t is 2.76; r is -0.08. Therefore, there is no statistically significant correlation between stroke admissions to this center and sales of prescription phenylpropanolamine products by month.

The monthly variations in sales of phenylpropanolamine cough, cold, and allergy preparations are also summarized in figure 15.6. A comparison of these sales data with admissions to the medical center for stroke yields an observed value of t of -0.20, with 4 degrees of freedom, and a critical value of t of 3.75; r is -0.10. There is no statistically significant correlation between month of phenylpropanolamine purchase and of admission for stroke.

FIGURE 15.6

Average monthly sales of
phenylpropanolamine prescription and cough/cold products
compared to monthly New York City medical center
admissions for stroke

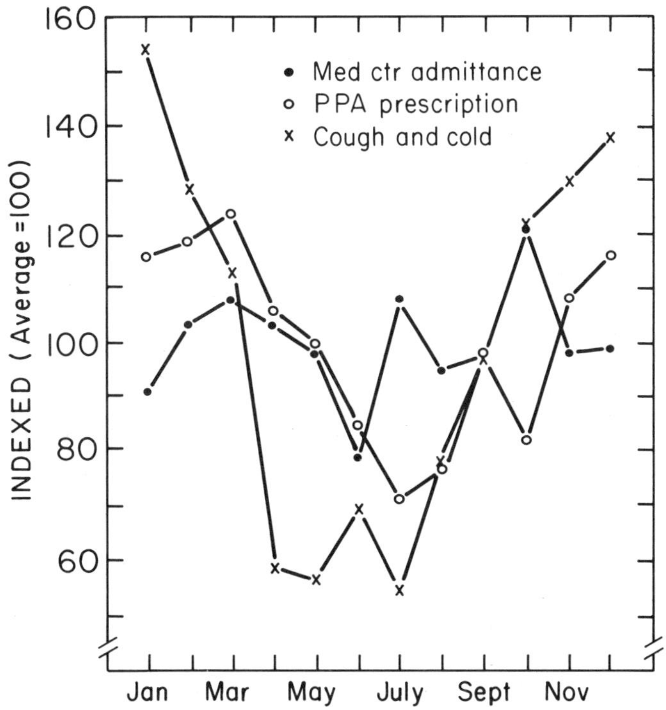

Source: Compiled by the author. Data derived from National Prescription Audit. 1982. Ambler, PA: IMS America; National Prescription Audit. 1983. Ambler, PA: IMS America.

Bimonthly variations in the sales of phenylpropanolamine appetite suppressants and in admissions to the medical center for stroke are indicated in figure 15.7. The observed value of t is -0.20, with 4 degrees of freedom, and the critical value of t is 3.75; r is 0.05. No statistically significant correlation is found between appetite suppressant sales and admissions for stroke, by month.

In all these comparisons, no significant correlation was found betwen sales (and thus ingestion) of any phenylpropanolamine product and admission to the medical center for stroke.

FIGURE 15.7

Average monthly sales of phenylpropanolamine appetite suppressants compared to monthly New York City medical center admissions for stroke

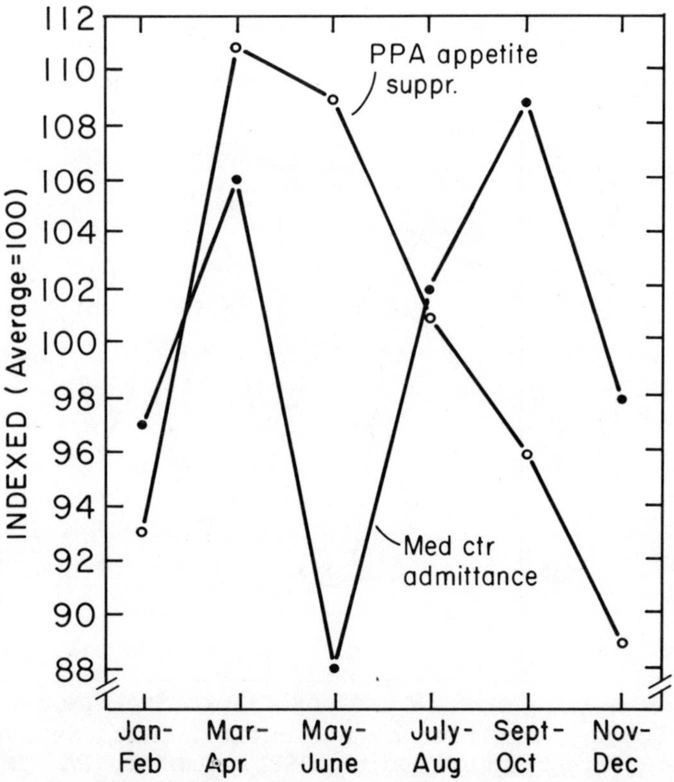

<u>Source</u>: Compiled by the author. Data derived from <u>Dieting aids seasonality indices</u>. 1984. Chicago: A. C. Nielsen Company; <u>Seasonality or growth trends by category: health and beauty aids</u>. 1982. New York: Selling Areas--Marketing, Inc.; Consumer expenditure study, annuals. 1973-83. <u>Product Marketing</u>. July; information made available by Thompson Medical Company: New York.

DISCUSSION

In this article, the published case reports linking stroke to phenylpropanolamine ingestion and the only systematic empirical study (in Washington state) of the occurrence of stroke following use compared to nonuse of prescription phenylpropanolamine products have been examined. Neither the published case reports nor the Washington study provides any solid evidence to confirm a link between phenylpropanolamine consumption and the subsequent occurrence of a stroke.

On the basis of three statistical studies, it has been similarly concluded that taking phenylpropanolamine in the form of appetite suppressants or OTC or prescription cough, cold, and allergy products is not related to the occurrence of stroke. Demographic characteristics of phenylpropanolamine users and stroke victims differ. As phenylpropanolamine use has increased in the last few decades, stroke incidence has decreased. The month in which phenylpropanolamine is sold (and presumably ingested) is unrelated to the month of occurrence of stroke. All these differences are statistically significant at very high levels of significance.

However, these studies showing no correlation between some characteristics of phenylpropanolamine users and stroke victims are not conclusive and must, like the case reports, be interpreted with caution and open-mindedness. I feel that it was appropriate to examine these available statistics but multiple interpretations are possible. They most likely indicate that, at the present state of our knowledge, there appear to be no generalizable or predictable relationships between phenylpropanolamine use and strokes in the general population. However, since it is likely that any contribution of phenylpropanolamine to stroke is small and necessarily interactive with other variables, an effect could be present and not detectable by these examinations. The number of case reports is small and they are, in themselves, not convincing. A prospective study or a retrospective case control study (if data collection on phenylpropanolamine use was improved) could yield a more probative answer but it is not likely that such a study will be done. It is my opinion that the case incriminating phenylpropanolamine is not strong enough to require that such a costly study be done.

REFERENCES

Baum, H. M. 1982. Stroke prevalence: an analysis of data from the 1977 Health Interview study. Public Health Rep 97:24-30.

———. 1981. An examination of the demographics of stroke victims using prevalence and mortality data. Public Health (London) 95:1-14.

Bernstein, E. and B. M. Diskant. 1982. Phenylpropanolamine: a potentially hazardous drug. Ann Emerg Med 11:311-15.

Blalock, H. M. 1979. Social statistics. New York: McGraw-Hill.

Boston Collaborative Drug Surveillance Program. 1974. Reserpine and breast cancer. Lancet 2:669-71.

Consumer expenditure study, annuals. 1973-83. Product Marketing. July.

Department of Commerce. 1980. Statistical abstracts of the United States. Washington, D.C.: U.S. Government Printing Office.

Dieting aids seasonality indices. 1984. Chicago: A. C. Nielsen.

Doyle, J. T. et al. 1965. Seasonal variations in serum cholesterol concentration. J Chronic Dis 18:657-64.

Elliott, C. F. and J. C. Whyte. 1981. Phenylpropanolamine and hypertension. Med J Aust 1:715.

Friedman, G. 1979. Declines in hospitalizations for coronary heart disease and stroke: the Kaiser-Permanente experience in Northern California. In Proceedings of the conference on the decline in coronary heart disease mortality, edited by R. J. Havlik and M. Feinleib. Bethesda, MD: National Institutes of Health.

Garraway, W. M., J. P. Whisnant, and I. Drury. 1983. The continuing decline in the incidence of stroke. Mayo Clin Proc 58:520-23.

Garraway, W. M. et al. 1979. The declining incidence of stroke. N Eng J Med 300:449-52.

Gordon, T. and W. B. Kannel. 1976. Obesity and cardiovascular diseases: the Framingham study. Clin Endocrinol Metab 5:367-75.

Green, F. 1984. Dieter's dilemma: who is right about appetite pills' effects? Hattiesburg (Mississippi) American, July 5, Sec. D, 1.

Gujarati, D. C. 1978. Basic econometrics. New York: McGraw-Hill.

Heyman, A. et al. 1971. Cerebral vascular disease in the biracial population of Evans County. Stroke 2:509-18.

Hirsh, L. S. 1939. Controlling appetite in obesity. J of Medicine (Cincinnati) 20:84-86.

Humberstone, P. M. 1969. Hypertension from cold remedies. Letter. Br Med J 1:846.

Jick, H., P. Aselton, and J. R. Hunter. 1984. Phenylpropanolamine and cerebral haemorrhage. Letter. Lancet 1:1017.

Johnson, D. A., H. S. Etter, and D. M. Reeves. 1983. Stroke and phenylpropanolamine use. Lancet 2:970.

King, J. 1979. Hypertension and cerebral haemorrhage after Trimolets ingestion. Med J Aust 2:258.

Kuller, L. H. 1978. Epidemiology of stroke. In Advances in neurology, neurological epidemiology: principles and clinical applications, edited by B. S. Schoenberg, 281-312. New York: Raven Press.

Kurtzke, J. F. 1976a. Epidemiology of cerebrovascular disease. In Cerebrovascular survey report, edited by the Joint Council Subcommittee on Cerebrovascular Disease, 213-27. Bethesda, MD: National Institutes of Health.

———. 1976b. An introduction to the epidemiology of cerebrovascular disease. In Cerebrovascular diseases, 10th Princeton conference, edited by P. Scheinberg, 139-53. New York: Raven Press.

McDowell, F. H., S. Louis, and K. Monahan. 1970. Seasonal variation of non-embolic cerebral infarction. J Chronic Dis 23:29-32.

Mesnard, B. and D. R. Ginn. 1984. Excessive phenylpropanolamine ingestion followed by cerebral hemorrhage. South Med J 77:939.

Morgan, J. P. 1985. Phenylpropanolamine: an analysis of reported adverse reactions and overdosages. Fort Lee, NJ: Jack K. Burgess.

National Center for Health Statistics. 1964. Blood pressure of adults by race and area, United States, 1960-62. Series 11, no. 5. Hyattsville, MD: National Center for Health Statistics.

National disease and therapeutic index. 1980. Ambler, PA: IMS America. December.

National prescription audit. 1983. Ambler, PA: IMS America.

———. 1982. Ambler, PA: IMS America.

———. 1980. Ambler, PA: IMS America.

Ostfeld, A. M. 1980. A review of stroke epidemiology. Epidemiologic Reviews 2:136-52.

Robins, M. and H. M. Baum. 1981. Incidence. In The national survey of stroke, edited by F. D. Weinfeld. Stroke (Suppl 1) 12:45-57.

Seasonality or growth trends by category: health and beauty aids. 1982. New York: Selling Areas-Marketing Inc.

Siegel, S. 1956. Nonparametric statistics. New York: McGraw-Hill.

Takakashi, E. et al. 1957. The geographic distribution of cerebral hemorrhage and hypertension in Japan. Hum Biol 29:139.

Thulin, T., B. Bengtsson, and B. Schersten. 1978. Assessment of casual blood pressure variations. Postgrad Med J 54:10-15.

Total dieting aids sales trends. 1984. Chicago: A. C. Nielsen.

Ueda, T. et al. 1981. Decreasing trend in incidence and mortality from stroke in Hisayama residents, Japan. Stroke 12:154-60.

U.S. Congress, House. 1983a. Statement to the Subcommittee on Health and Long-Term Care, the Select Committee on Aging, by B. B. Young. Given before the 97th Congress, 2nd session, July 21.

———.1983b. Select Committee on Aging, Subcommittee on Health and Long-Term Care. 97th Congress, 2nd session. Record of hearing, July 21.

Walker, W. J. 1977. Changing United States life style and declining vascular mortality: cause or coincidence. N Eng J of Med 297:163-65.

Weinfeld, F. D., ed. 1981. The national survey of stroke. Stroke (Suppl 1) 12:2.

Westat Research. 1983. National survey of stroke. Rockville, MD: National Institutes of Health.

Whisnant, J. P. 1984. The decline of stroke. Stroke 15:160-67.

Winick, C. 1978. The alcohol offender. In Psychology of crime and criminal justice, edited by H. Toch, 347-72. New York: Holt, Rinehart and Winston.

Wolf, P. A., W. B. Kannel, and T. R. Dawber. 1978. Prospective investigations: the Framingham study and the epidemiology of stroke, in Advances in neurology, neurological epidemiology: principles and clinical applications, edited by B. S. Schoenberg, 107-20. New York: Raven Press.

Wolf, P. A. et al. 1977. Epidemiology of stroke. In Stroke: advances in neurology, edited by R. A. Thompson and J. R. Green, 5-19. New York: Raven Press.

World Health Organization. 1980. International classification of diseases: clinical modification, 9th revision, 2nd edition. Geneva: World Health Organization.

Worth, R. M. et al. 1975. Epidemiologic studies of coronary heart disease and stroke in Japanese men living in Japan, Hawaii and California: mortality. Am J of Epidemiol 102:481-90.

Wylie, C. 1962. Cerebrovascular accident deaths in the United States and England and Wales. J Chronic Dis 15:85-90.

16

A REVIEW OF REPORTED ADVERSE CARDIOVASCULAR REACTIONS TO PHENYLPROPANOLAMINE

Marcus M. Reidenberg

Phenylpropanolamine (PPA) is a primarily indirectly acting sympathomimetic amine. Its effects are dose-related and reported cases of cardiovascular toxicity following its use can be interpreted as resulting from its sympathomimetic effects.

CASE REPORTS

A number of cases of adverse cardiovascular events following phenylpropanolamine ingestion have been reported. In nearly all these cases, blood pressure increased and symptoms occurred so that the patient sought medical care. Some of these patients had taken overdoses of phenylpropanolamine in either cough/cold or diet aid products (Salmon 1965; Ostern and Dodson 1965; Mueller 1983; Pentel and Mikell 1982; Duffy 1981; Weesner, Denison, and Roberts 1982; Bernstein and Diskant 1982; Duvernoy 1969; Misage 1970). Other case reports failed to specify the exact dose taken (Peterson and Vasquez 1973; Shapiro 1969; Livingston 1966; Clark and Simon 1983). Thus, a portion of the reported cases of adverse cardiovascular reactions to phenylpropanolamine occurred in people who had taken large or unknown doses. That large doses of a sympathomimetic amine can produce hypertension, cardiac tachyarrhythmias, headaches, encephalopathy, and even acute renal tubular or myocardial necrosis should not be surprising in view of the known pharmacologic effects of such a drug.

There have been reports, however, of hypertensive episodes occurring in patients who did not take obviously excessive doses of phenylpropanolamine. These include:

- A 58-year-old diabetic woman with a cerebral hemorrhage who took one Dietgard™ capsule (containing 75 mg phenylpropanolamine) the day before and another the day of her stroke (Elliott and White 1979);
- A 29-year-old woman who took one Trimolets tablet (85 mg phenylpropanolamine) (King 1979);
- A 37-year-old woman who took two Trimolets and had a stroke (King 1979);
- A 23-year-old man who took two Contac 500 capsules, each containing 50 mg phenylpropanolamine (Teh 1979).
- An 18-year-old woman who took two Comtrex™ tablets (Bernstein and Diskant 1982);
- A 13-year-old girl who took two Dex-A-Diet II® capsules (75 mg phenylpropanolamine, 200 mg caffeine in each) (Howrie and Wolfson 1983);
- A 24-year-old woman who experienced chest pain, hypertension, and inferior and lateral electrocardiographic ST-segment depression after taking a single capsule of phenylpropanolamine (50 mg), chlorpheniramine (4 mg), and belladonna alkaloids (0.2 mg) (Pentel, Mikell, and Zavorall 1982);
- A 41-year-old woman who took two Trimolets (McEwen 1983);
- A 32-year-old woman who took one Trimolets (McEwen 1983);
- A 28-year-old woman who took one Trimolets (McEwen 1983);
- A 38-year-old woman who took one Trimolets (McEwen 1983);
- A 19-year-old woman who took two Trimolets (McEwen 1983);
- A 22-year-old woman who took two Trimtabs™, each containing 50 mg phenylpropanolamine (McEwen 1983);
- A 34-year-old woman who took two Trimolets (McEwen 1983);
- A 49-year-old woman who took one Trimolets (McEwen 1983).

While it seems likely that in these cases the hypertension and associated adverse events following drug ingestion were due to the drug, case reports alone cannot be used as proof of a cause-and-effect relationship. To better understand these case reports, the results of some clinical trials must be reviewed.

CLINICAL TRIALS

Horowitz et al. (1979) gave six normotensive medical students (four male and two female, ages 22 to 24), one Trimolets or a placebo in a double-blind crossover study. All subjects given Trimolets experienced a rise in blood pressure. Horowitz and other co-investigators (1980) then carried out a more extensive study. Thirty-seven subjects ingested one Trimolets capsule and 35 took a placebo in a randomized, double-blind, parallel group, single-dose study. The mean diastolic blood pressure increased from 70 to 96 mm Hg in the Trimolets-treated group ($p < .001$) with peak supine diastolic pressure exceeding 100 mm Hg in 12 of the Trimolets-treated subjects and one of the controls ($p < .001$). Six of the 37 Trimolets-treated subjects showed an increase in diastolic pressure of more than 20 mg Hg, while others of this group had virtually no rise in blood pressure at all.

An identical protocol was used to study the blood pressure response to Contac 500 containing 50 mg phenylpropanolamine in 34 subjects while 35 took matching placebo (Ibid.). The mean diastolic blood pressure increased from 78 to 83 mm Hg in the Contac-treated group ($p < .05$); four of these subjects but none of the placebo-treated patients developed peak diastolic pressures above 100 mm Hg. Thus, in this study, an acute increase in blood pressure was found to occur after ingestion of each of these phenylpropanolamine-containing drug products. The effect was observed after a single dose, was apparently dose-dependent, and peaked one and one-half to three hours after ingestion. There was also marked individual variability in the hypertensive response.

Saltzman, Dolan, and Doyne (1983) conducted a randomized crossover study in which 14 normotensive males ages 20 to 40 received 25 mg of phenylpropanolamine three times daily or 75 mg in a controlled-release preparation once daily for four days. The crossover was separated by a ten-day washout period and no placebo period was used. No increase in blood pressure was detected; however, the results of blood pressure measurements following the first dose were not reported. What was reported is that there was no progressive increase in blood pressure with duration of therapy nor any correlation at steady state between blood pressure and serum concentration of phenylpropanolamine.

In another study of the blood pressure response to phenylpropanolamine (Mitchell 1968), 32 healthy subjects took 50 mg of sustained-release phenylpropanolamine twice daily. Blood pressure was measured daily from the second to the sixth day of treatment and no effect on blood pressure was found. As in the previous study, however, blood pressure measurements following the first dose were not reported.

The discrepancy between, on the one hand, the findings of Saltzman, Dolan, and Doyne and of Mitchell and, on the other, of Horowitz et al.'s two studies requires comment. Horowitz et al. observed that 85 mg in an immediate-release preparation (Trimolets) (1980, 1979) produced more hypertension than 50 mg in a sustained-release preparation (Contac 500) (1980). In the studies by Saltzman, Dolan, and Doyne (1983) and by Mitchell (1968), lower doses were given either as such or through sustained-release preparations so that the initial peak concentrations were lower than in the Horowitz et al. studies of Trimolets. Thus, on the basis of dose alone, 85 mg of immediate-release phenylpropanolamine caused substantial hypertension (diastolic pressure > 100 mm Hg) in one-third, 50 mg in a sustained-release form caused this in a little more than one-tenth (Horowitz et al. 1980), and 25 mg caused it in too few to be detectable (Saltzman, Dolan, and Doyne 1983) in small groups of healthy, young subjects.

Any hypertensive response to phenylpropanolamine should also be considered in the context of the moment-to-moment fluctuations in blood pressure seen in individuals who have their blood pressure measured repeatedly. These fluctuations in blood pressure have been studied extensively by Pickering et al. (1982) and Harshfield et al. (1984). They measured blood pressure every 15 minutes for 24 hours with an automated device while normal and hypertensive subjects went about their ordinary activities. They found that, in normal subjects, the daily range between the highest and lowest diastolic blood pressure measurements in any one individual averaged 46 ± 11 mm Hg. The maximum systolic pressure achieved by a normotensive subject averaged 90 mm Hg higher than the lowest systolic pressure measured in that subject during the 24-hour period. These examples should indicate to those not familiar with the subject how much moment-to-moment variation in blood pressure normally exists. It should be considered, therefore, whether the blood pressure response to specific doses of phenylpropanolamine raises an individual's blood pressure above the levels that occur in response to exercise, anxiety, or fear.

Another difference between the studies of blood pressure response to phenylpropanolamine discussed above is the time when the observations began. In the Horowitz et al. studies (1979; 1980), blood pressure was measured immediately after the first dose and evidence of a blood pressure response was found. In the Saltzman, Dolan, and Doyne (1983) and the Mitchell (1968) studies, on the other hand, blood pressure measurements following the first dose were not reported and no increase in blood pressure was detected in the later measurements which were taken. If tachyphylaxis to this indirectly acting sympathomimetic amine occurs in humans (tachyphylaxis is characteristic of indirectly acting sympathomimetic amines), then, all things being equal, a greater hypertensive response might be expected after the first dose than after subsequent doses. In this context, it is of interest to note that in nearly all the reported cases of hypertensive episodes in which patients took doses of phenylpropanolamine that were not excessive, the hypertensive episode occurred after the initial dose of the phenylpropanolamine-containing product. This supports the hypothesis that tachyphylaxis to the hypertensive effects of phenylpropanolamine occurs in man. The therapeutic implications of this hypothesis are clear for initiating therapy with this drug as well as for interpreting the results of clinical trials.

Phenylpropanolamine Interactions with Other Medications

Cuthbert, Greenberg, and Morley (1969) did a study which confirmed the dose-dependent hypertensive effects of phenylpropanolamine and also demonstrated a predictable drug interaction enhancing the hypertensive effect. Three subjects took either 50 or 100 mg of phenylpropanolamine or placebo. A dose-dependent increase in blood pressure was observed. When a monoamine oxidase (MAO) inhibitor was given before the phenylpropanolamine, a profound enhancement of the hypertensive response occurred. This was to be expected since it is well-known that MAO inhibition enhances the response to indirectly acting sympathomimetic drugs.

Hypertensive reactions have been reported in patients taking MAO inhibitors and phenylpropanolamine (Tonks and Lloyd 1965; Mason and Buckle 1969; Smookler and Bermudez 1982). Recently Goldin et al. (1982) studied the variation in platelet MAO in 309 individuals. They found a range of enzyme activity of one to 25 nmoles of product formed/10^9 platelets/hour, with eight of the 309 subjects having values below 2.3. Thus, some people who are not taking drugs have naturally low levels of MAO and may thus be sensitive to the hypertensive effects of phenylpropanolamine. A difference in innate MAO activity may be one of the reasons some people have a greater blood pressure response than others to a dose of phenylpropanolamine.

Oguchi et al. (1982) observed that several compounds in the phenethylamine class are MAO inhibitors and slow tyramine metabolism. Tyramine is an indirectly acting sympathomimetic amine that occurs naturally in some foods and causes hypertension in people taking MAO inhibitors who eat these foods. Thus, these phenethylamine compounds might enhance the hypertensive response to tyramine by MAO inhibition. Although phenylpropanolamine was not evaluated in this study, it is similar in structure to compounds that were evaluated and were found to inhibit MAO. In this context, one case was reported in which the combination of phenylpropanolamine and a cheese meal containing substantial amounts of tyramine was considered to be the cause of a hypertensive episode (Gibson and Warrell 1972). In addition to mature cheese, some red wines and pickled herring contain large amounts of tyramine and might act in conjunction with phenylpropanolamine to cause an adverse cardiovascular event at doses that, if taken alone, would be too low to be harmful.

Thus, in addition to genetically determined MAO activity, dietary factors and drugs acting on the sympathetic nervous system can also modify sensitivity to the blood pressure raising effects of phenylpropanolamine. Two published reports suggest the possibility that the factors that can cause hypertension from oral contraceptive use can also increase sensitivity to the hypertensive effects of phenylpropanolamine. In one report, two women currently taking oral contraceptives experienced hypertensive episodes following phenylpropanolamine ingestion (McEwen 1983). In the other report, a woman who had stopped using oral contraceptives the previous month suffered a hypertensive episode after taking phenylpropanolamine (Frewin, Leonello, and Frewin 1978). This raises the possibility that the factors that can cause hypertension from oral contraceptive use can also increase sensitivity to the hypertensive effects of phenylpropanolamine.

The phenothiazines can cause arrhythmias and sudden death. A 27-year-old patient who exhibited electrocardiogram (ECG) abnormalities while on chloropromazine (900 mg/day) was switched to thioridazine (100 mg/day). A month after this, she took a Contac - C and died suddenly two hours later. Although it is not certain that the drugs played a role in this death, the suspicion is very strong. In retrospect, this patient's ECG abnormalities during chloropromazine could have suggested a predisposition to adverse cardiac effects from these drugs.

A patient on methyldopa and oxprenolol had a hypertensive episode when he took two tablets of Triogesic (phenylpropanolamine, 12.5 mg, and acetaminophen, 500 mg) three times daily for two days. It is presumed that beta-blockade permitted the vasoconstrictor effects of the catecholamine released by the phenylpropanolamine to occur while the vasodilator effects were blocked, leading to marked hypertension (McLaren 1976). This same hypertensive effect of catecholamines can be seen in patients with pheochromocytoma given beta-blockers without concurrent alpha-adrenergic blockade.

Other conditions that impair the balance and control of the sympathetic nervous system can increase susceptibility to the hypertensive effects of phenylpropanolamine. Autonomic dysfunction has been reported to be one such condition (Pentel and Mikell 1982). Drugs that block the reuptake of norepinephrine into sympathetic nerve endings can also enhance the blood pressure raising effect of phenylpropanolamine (Misage and McDonald 1970; Rumack et al. 1974). These include the antihypertensive drugs bethanidine, guanethidine, and debrisoquine and the tricyclic antidepressants.

A case report of phenylpropanolamine/indomethacin interaction raises the suspicion that another whole class of drugs may increase sensitivity to the hypertensive effects of phenylpropanolamine. A 27-year-old woman had a marked hypertensive episode when she took 25 mg of indomethacin after taking one Trimolets capsule daily for several months. The Trimolets capsule alone did not raise her blood pressure and the indomethacin alone raised it only slightly. The authors concluded that the indomethacin blocked prostaglandin synthesis, thereby reducing the prostaglandin-controlled negative feedback of catecholamine release at sympathetic nerve endings and also reducing the amount of vasodilator prostaglandins available to counteract the vasoconstrictor effects of the catecholamines released by the phenylpropanolamine (Lee, Beilin, and Vandongen 1980, 1979). If the proposed mechanism is correct, then any drug that inhibits cyclooxygenase, even aspirin, could sensitize a person to a hypertensive response to phenylpropanolamine. Furthermore, cyclooxygenase can be inhibited by chemicals in the environment as well as by drugs. For example, phenylhydrazine, a common industrial product which is also a postulated metabolite of the common yellow food color tartrazine, is a potent inhibitor of platelet cyclooxygenase (Leipzig et al. 1984). It could also be noted that phenylpropanolamine is very frequently combined with aspirin in widely used cough/cold preparations.

CONCLUSION

It is possible to speculate about other innate or environmental factors that might enhance the hypertensive effects of phenylpropanolamine, but several facts seem clear from this review of case reports and the pharmacology underlying them:

1. There appears to be a steep dose-response curve for the blood pressure raising effects of phenylpropanolamine. Single doses of 85 mg raised blood pressure substantially in one-third of the subjects, 50 mg in one-tenth, and 25 mg in none of the subjects in the clinical studies summarized in this review. This blood pressure elevation should be evaluated in the light of the normal moment-to-moment variation in an individual's blood pressure.
2. Many factors can increase the degree of blood pressure elevation per unit dose of phenylpropanolamine. These include MAO inhibition and impairment of the sympathetic neurone catecholamine reuptake mechanism by antihypertensive or tricyclic antidepressant drugs. Other contributing factors might be hyperthyroidism, autonomic dysfunction, cyclooxygenase inhibitors, beta blockers, and ingestion of large amounts of tyramine. Moreover, all of the drug interactions probably have their own dose-response relationships and susceptibility factors.
3. Tachyphylaxis to the blood pressure raising effects of phenylpropanolamine is likely to occur and this may explain why nearly all cases of adverse reactions are reports of events occurring after the first dose of this drug.

REFERENCES

Bernstein, E. and B. M. Diskant. 1982. Phenylpropanolamine: a potentially hazardous drug. Ann Emerg Med 11:311-15.

Clark, J. D. and W. A. Simon. 1983. Cardiac arrhythmias after phenylpropanolamine ingestion. Drug Intell Clin Pharm 17:737-38.

Cuthbert, M. F., M. P. Greenberg, and S. W. Morley. 1969. Cough and cold remedies: a potential danger to patients on monoamine oxidase inhibitors. Br Med J 1:404-6.

Duffy, W. B. et al. 1981. Acute renal failure due to phenylpropanolamine. South Med J 74:1548.

Duvernoy, W. 1969. Positive phentolamine test in hypertension induced by a nasal decongestant. N Engl J Med 280:877.

Elliott, C. F. and J. C. Whyte. 1981. Phenylpropanolamine and hypertension. Med J Aust 1:715.

Frewin, D. B., P. P. Leonello, and M. E. Frewin. 1978. Hypertension after ingestion of Trimolets. Med J Aust 2:497-98.

Gibson, G. J. and D. A. Warrell. 1972. Hypertensive crises and phenylpropanolamine. Lancet 2:492-93.

Goldin, L. R. et al. 1982. Segregation and linkage studies of plasma dopamine-beta-hydroxylase (DBH), erythrocyte catechol-o-methyltransferase (COMT), and platelet monoamine oxidase (MAO): possible linkage between ABO locus and a gene controlling DBH activity. Am J Hum Genet 34:250-62.

Harshfield, G. A. et al. 1984. Ambulatory blood pressure monitoring: recorders, applications, and analyses. In Ambulatory blood pressure monitoring, edited by M. A. Weber and J.I.M. Drayer, 1-7. Darmstadt: Steinkopff.

Horowitz, J. D. et al. 1980. Hypertensive responses induced by phenylpropanolamine in anorectic and decongestant preparations. Lancet 1:60-61.

Horowitz, J. D. et al. 1979. Hypertension and postural hypotension induced by phenylpropanolamine (Trimolets). Med J Aust 1:175-76.

Howrie, D. L. and J. H. Wolfson. 1983. Phenylpropanolamine-induced hypertensive seizures. J Pediatr 102:143-45.

King, J. 1979. Hypertension and cerebral haemorrhage after Trimolets ingestion. Med J Aust 2:258.

Lee, K. Y., L. J. Beilin, and R. Vandongen. 1980. Severe hypertension after ingestion of an appetite suppressant (phenylpropanolamine) with indomethacin. Letter. Aust NZ J Med 10:122.

———. 1979. Severe hypertension after ingestion of an appetite suppressant (phenylpropanolamine) with indomethacin. Lancet 1:1110-11.

Leipzig, R. M. et al. 1984. Inhibition of human platelet aggregation by phenylhydrazine and acetylphenylhydrazine. Clinical Research 32:243A.

Livingston, P. H. 1966. Transient hypertension and phenylpropanolamine. Letter. JAMA 196:1159.

Mason, A.M.S. and R. M. Buckle. 1969. "Cold cures" and monoamine oxidase inhibitors. Br Med J 1:845-46.

McEwen, J. 1983. Phenylpropanolamine-associated hypertension after the use of "over-the-counter" appetite suppressant products. Med J Aust 2:71-73.

McLaren, E. H. 1976. Severe hypertension produced by interaction of phenylpropanolamine with methyldopa and oxprenolol. Br Med J 2:283-84.

Misage, J. R. and R. H. McDonald. 1970. Antagonism of hypotensive action of bethanidine by "common cold" remedy. Br Med J 4:347.

Mitchell, C. A. 1968. Possible cardiovascular effect of phenylpropanolamine and belladonna alkaloids. Current Therapeutic Research 10:47-53.

Mueller, S. M. 1983. Neurologic complications of phenylpropanolamine use. Neurology 33:650-52.

Oguchi, K. et al. 1982. Binding and deamination of various substrates by types A and B monoamine oxidase in bovine brain mitochondria. Biochem Pharmacol 31:1515-20.

Ostern, S. and W. H. Dodson. 1965. Hypertension following Ornade ingestion. Letter. JAMA 194:472.

Pentel, P. and F. Mikell. 1982. Reaction to phenylpropanolamine/chlorpheniramine/belladonna compound in a woman with unrecognized autonomic dysfunction. Lancet 2:274.

Pentel, P. R., F. L. Mikell, and J. H. Zavoral. 1982. Myocardial injury after phenylpropanolamine ingestion. Br Heart J 47:51-54.

Peterson, R. B. and L. A. Vasquez. 1973. Phenylpropanolamine-induced arrhythmias. JAMA 223:324-25.

Pickering, T. G. et al. 1982. Blood pressure during normal daily activities, sleep, and exercise. JAMA 242:992-96.

Rumack, B. H. et al. 1974. Ornade and anticholinergic toxicity: hypertension, hallucinations, and arrhythmias. Clin Toxicol 7:573-81.

Salmon, P. R. 1965. Hypertensive crisis with Eskornade. Letter. Br Med J 1:193.

Saltzman, M. B., M. M. Dolan, and N. Doyne. 1983. Comparison of effects of two dosage regimens of phenylpropanolamine on blood pressure and plasma levels in normal subjects under steady state conditions. Drug Intell Clin Pharm 17:746-50.

Shapiro, S. R. 1969. Hypertension due to anorectic agent. N Engl J Med 280:1363.

Smookler, S. and A. J. Bermudez. 1982. Hypertensive crisis resulting from an MAO inhibitor and an over-the-counter appetite suppressant. Ann Emerg Med 11:482-84.

Teh, A.Y.F. 1979. Phenylpropanolamine and hypertension. Med J Aust 2:425.

Tonks, C. M. and A. T. Lloyd. 1965. Hazards with monoamine-oxidase inhibitors. Letter. Br Med J 1:589.

Weesner, K. M., M. Denison, and R. J. Roberts. 1982. Cardiac arrhythmias in an adolescent following ingestion of an over-the-counter stimulant. Clin Pediatr 21:700-701.

ACKNOWLEDGMENT

I wish to thank Drs. John P. Morgan and Robert L. Marlin for their help in assembling the referenced list of publications about phenylpropanolamine.

B. DOES PHENYLPROPANOLAMINE CAUSE CENTRAL NERVOUS SYSTEM STIMULATION AND BEHAVIORAL TOXICITY?

17

DOES PHENYLPROPANOLAMINE CAUSE PSYCHIATRIC DISORDERS?

C. Raymond Lake, Sheryl W. Alagna, Rosemarie S. Quirk, Kathleen M. Moriarty, and Audrey A. Reid

INTRODUCTION

A Case Study

The authors first became interested in the drug phenylpropanolamine (PPA) in 1982 when Dr. Lake was called to consult on a case involving a 21-year-old male recently hospitalized for acute mania (Lake et al. 1983). The patient's symptoms warranted the diagnosis of mania by DSM-III* criteria: decreased need for sleep without concurrent fatigue; euphoria with grandiose delusions; increased activities including excessive phone calling, business dealings, and spending; racing thoughts; pressured speech; and increased irritability. The patient's work and social life were sufficiently impaired that he required hospitalization. Following treatment with a neuroleptic (haloperidol) and then lithium, his condition was resolved and he was discharged for outpatient follow-up approximately two months after admission.

The patient's drug and alcohol history revealed an average of two marihuana cigarettes and two to three beers per day during the months preceding admission without ingestion of any other drugs for over six months. The patient had never had a manic or hypomanic episode, but two years earlier had been briefly treated on an outpatient basis without medication for depression. His family's psychiatric history, however, was remarkable. Two of his brothers, both older, had been previously hospitalized for mania. Both had

---

*DSM-III refers to the 3rd edition of the Diagnostic and Statistical Manual of Mental Disorders (American Psychiatric Association 1980).

been diagnosed as having major affective disorder, bipolar, and both were currently taking lithium prophylactically. The patient's father and two of his older brothers (including one with bipolar disorder) also had had psychiatric contact for alcohol abuse.

On the evening before the manic episode began, the patient had taken four "black beauty" capsules which he had been told contained "weak speed." Within about 30 minutes, he began to experience mild to moderate signs of central nervous system (CNS) stimulation, including hyperalertness, increased talkativeness, tachycardia, and sweating. These effects subsided five hours after ingestion, and he slept through the night and woke at the usual time for work the next morning. Over the next three days, manic symptoms developed and on the fourth day the patient was hospitalized. A broad urine drug analysis performed at the time of admission, including tests for tetrahydrocannabinol (THC), amphetamine, cocaine, barbiturates, morphine derivatives, phencyclidine hydrochloride (PCP), and lysergic acid diethylamide (LSD), was negative for all drugs screened.

Amphetamine Look-Alikes

These black beauty capsules probably contained no amphetamine, but rather some combination of phenylpropanolamine, caffeine, and ephedrine. This assumption is based on information from such sources as the medical literature (Lake et al. 1983), the Drug Enforcement Administration (DEA) (Franzosa 1983), laboratory analyses of street drugs (Morgan and Kagan 1978), and various experts in the field (Morgan 1983). Although it is difficult to obtain a precise figure on the amount of "street speed" which consists of drugs other than amphetamine, one study found that only 17% of drugs sold as street speed actually included amphetamine, with the majority of the remaining 83% comprised of combinations of phenylpropanolamine, ephedrine, and caffeine (Saxena and Kingston 1981). These combinations are representative of "look-alike" drugs, defined as "tablets, capsules or other substances containing noncontrolled, 'over-the-counter' (OTC) ingredients, which closely resemble well-known, highly abused controlled drug products" (Haislip 1983).

The proliferation of amphetamine look-alike drugs is a direct result of the passage and enforcement of the Federal Controlled Substances Act of 1970 (Patrick 1977). This legislation was prompted by the large amount of legitimately produced amphetamine that was being diverted to illegal markets (Morgan and Kagan 1978). At the time of the legislation, less than 50% of manufactured amphetamine could be accounted for by examining the legal retail market and other legitimate sales (McGlothlin 1973). The legislation imposed severe limitations on prescribers and stringent security, inventory, and export/import controls and production quotas on manufacturers of amphetamine. By 1972, enforcement had cut amphetamine production by 88%; legitimate production fell from a peak of 12 billion units in 1971 to less than two million in 1981 (Morgan 1981). Thus, large legitimate and illicit markets were left without a product until the look-alikes were manufactured and marketed.

Although the look-alikes are manufactured and sold legally, often through mail-order houses, large quantities are subsequently sold deceptively as amphetamine on the street. Not surprisingly, the biggest market for this distribution consists of young people between junior high and college age (Humphrey 1983). The use of stimulants among high school students is increasing, according to the 1982 High School Senior Drug Use Survey. In 1982, 36% of the high school seniors sampled reported using some type of stimulant, compared to only 26% in 1980. These percentages almost surely reflect use of look-alikes as well. In response to a specific question added in 1982 to estimate look-alike use, 15% of the seniors said they had tried a look-alike (Johnston, Bachman, and O'Malley 1982).

One of the dangers of look-alikes is that they lead naive drug users (which young people usually are) to believe that they have a greater capacity for drugs than they actually do, possibly resulting in serious complications when the user ingests the real thing. The growing problem of look-alike abuse has been recognized since the early 1980s, and laws aimed at limiting sales have been passed in 41 states with even more stringent legislation advocated in recent U.S. Senate hearings devoted to the look-alike drug phenomenon (Humphrey 1983). The 1982 classification by the U.S. Food and Drug Administration (FDA) of the triple combination of phenylpropanolamine, caffeine, and ephedrine as a new drug requiring extensive testing before being approved for use (Health and Human Services 1982) essentially prohibits look-alike manufacturers from continuing to market this combination legally. A similar ruling for phenylpropanolamine/caffeine combinations was made in December 1983 (Short 1984). In response, manufacturers have simply eliminated one of the drugs in their products and increased the concentrations of the others. In fact, by adapting its methods to circumvent restrictions while technically "playing by the rules," the look-alike industry has survived attempts by the FDA, DEA, and U.S. Post Office to regulate it. For instance, legislation banning counterfeiting has prompted look-alike manufacturers to redesign their products so as not to meet the definition of counterfeit drugs (Humphrey 1983).

Even though phenylpropanolamine combined with other products has now replaced amphetamine in some legitimate markets as well as on the street, it did not become well-known until more than 50 years after it was synthesized in 1910. The earliest use of phenylpropanolamine was as a substitute for ephedrine (Jarvik 1977). Its anorexiant properties were recognized as early as the 1930s, but phenylpropanolamine was marketed almost exclusively as a nasal decongestant until 1970 when, after passage of the Controlled Substances Act, which imposed tight controls on amphetamine, its use in OTC diet aids expanded rapidly. By late 1983, there were more than 139 preparations marketed in the United States that contained phenylpropanolamine alone or in various combinations (primarily with antihistamines or caffeine) (figure 17.1). Most of these are anorexiants or nasal decongestants. Sixty-one of these require a prescription, while the rest are available over-the-counter (Physicians' desk reference 1984; Physicians' desk reference for nonprescription drugs 1983). Worldwide, several billion legitimate doses of phenylpropanolamine are consumed annually (Waggonner 1983). It is estimated that patients in general medical outpatient clinic populations receive prescription products containing phenylpropanolamine in one out of every four visits (Jick 1984).

The reasons phenylpropanolamine has replaced amphetamine can be traced to parallels between the two drugs (Blum 1981). Their chemical structures differ only by a beta-carbon hydroxyl group (figure 17.2). Both have been widely used legitimately for weight loss and for the relief of cold symptoms and illicitly for CNS stimulation. They produce similar effects, including vasoconstriction in nasal passages, anorexia, increased blood pressure and heart rate, greater alertness, and elevated mood potentially extending to psychosis. Further, both initially had reputations for safety. As observed by Ellinwood, "historical analysis shows that major CNS stimulant abuse epidemics are preceded by the introduction of large segments of the population to a drug's effects for medical and recreational purposes" (Ellinwood 1974).

FIGURE 17.1

Phenylpropanolamine products available in the United States, 1983

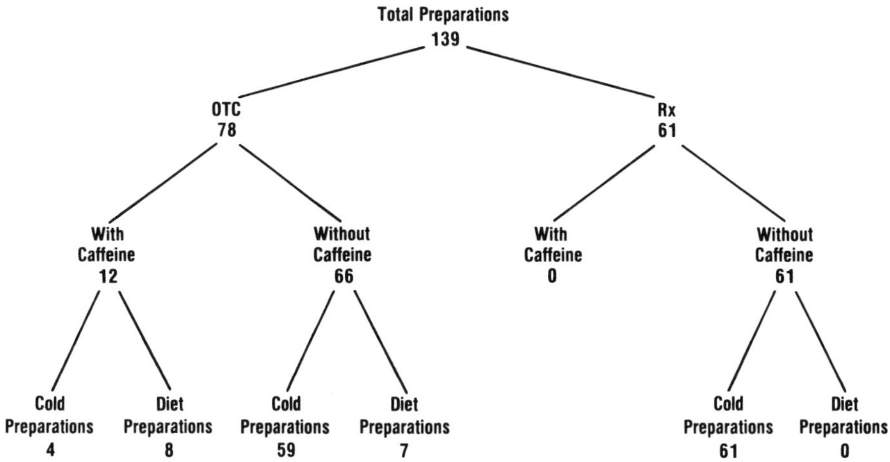

Source: Compiled by the authors. Data derived from Physicians' desk reference. 1984. Oradell, NJ: Medical Economics; Physicians' desk reference for nonprescription drugs. 1983. Oradell, NJ: Medical Economics.

FIGURE 17.2

Corresponding structures of endogenous neurotransmitters and sympathomimetic phenethylamines

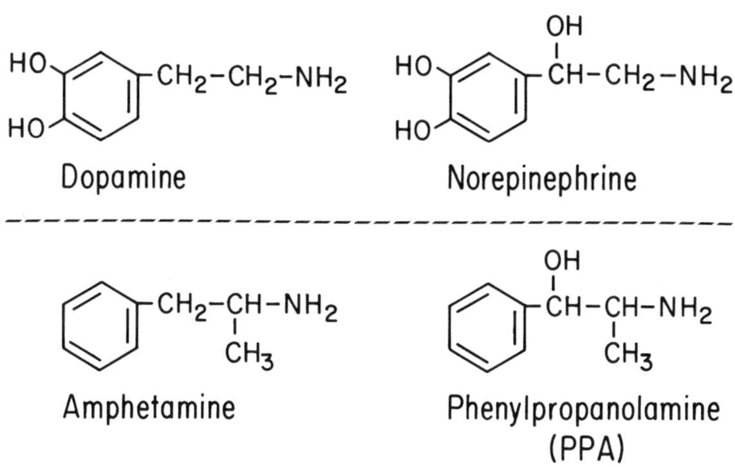

Source: Compiled by the authors.

Norephedrine Isomers

However, even the most potent isomer of phenylpropanolamine, (+)-norpseudoephedrine, which is contained in European products, stimulates motor activity in rats only 10% as much as amphetamine. The form of phenylpropanolamine sold in the United States, a racemic mixture of (+)- and (-)-norephedrine, is reported to cause only minimal stimulation (Fairchild and Alles 1967). (+)-Norpseudoephedrine is also contained in the leaves of the khat plant (Catha edulis), which have been chewed for centuries by peoples of Africa and the Arabian peninsula to produce euphoria and to increase alertness and CNS stimulation (Zelger and Carlini 1980; Luqman and Danowski 1976). The active ingredients in khat leaves are (+)-norpseudoephedrine (cathine) and the more potent (-)-alpha-aminopropiophenone (cathinone), which contains a beta-ketone instead of a beta-hydroxyl group (Alles, Fairchild, and Jensen 1961). Many speculate that cathinone is the more important psychoactive ingredient. A case of manic-like psychosis due to khat-chewing was reported in 1982 (Giannini and Castellani 1982). However, since only (±)-norephedrine (which is not contained in khat) is used in the United States, this case does not indicate that phenylpropanolamine in U.S. diet aids causes psychosis. Similarly, adverse reactions following ingestion of European phenylpropanolamine products cannot be considered evidence that phenylpropanolamine-containing products sold in the United States are dangerous.

Safety Studies of Phenylpropanolamine

The status of phenylpropanolamine as an OTC drug is based on unpublished and published research indicating its safety in prescribed dosages. One published study of 70 patients who had accidentally or purposefully overdosed with phenylpropanolamine or a phenylpropanolamine/caffeine combination found that no serious long-range consequences ensued (Ekins and Spoerke 1983). Sixteen of these patients were advised to see a physician, but only two were hospitalized. Although this study is quoted to support the safety of phenylpropanolamine, it has a significant shortcoming in that 54 patients were evaluated by telephone only. In another study of phenylpropanolamine's safety, it was shown that baboons do not chronically self-administer phenylpropanolamine as they do amphetamine and cocaine (Griffiths, Brady, and Snell 1978). Also, one study of phenylpropanolamine in mice found it to have minimal CNS-stimulating effects (Fairchild and Alles 1967).

However, the fact that many safety studies remain unpublished, were poorly controlled, administered phenylpropanolamine in doses of only 25 or 50 mg (whereas 75 mg is the daily dose approved by the FDA), observed side effects only acutely, used too few subjects, or were funded by one of the drug companies which produce phenylpropanolamine undercuts their significance. Furthermore, the potential health hazards of phenylpropanolamine are suggested by the increasing frequency of reports of adverse side effects (figure 17.3) and phenylpropanolamine-related emergency room visits.

FIGURE 17.3

Frequency of published reports of psychiatric side effects associated with phenylpropanolamine use, 1966-84

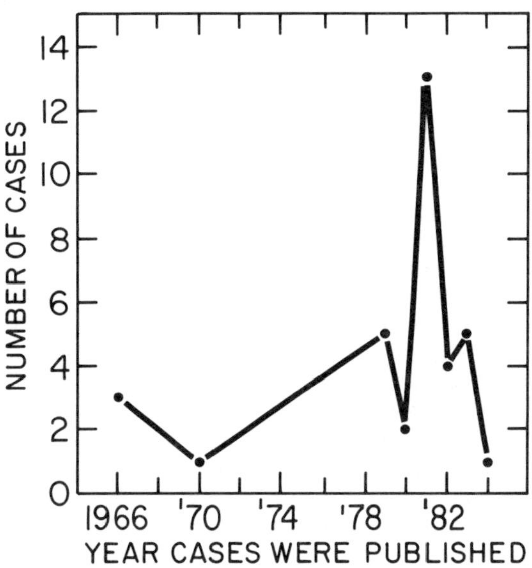

Source: Compiled by the authors. Data derived from articles listed in table 17.1.

From 1975 through 1980, the occurrence of dangerous side effects following ingestion of phenylpropanolamine products reported to the National Clearinghouse of Poison Control Centers (NCPCC) increased from 0.1% to 0.9% of the total cases reported (Phenylpropanolamine for weight control products 1981). Between 1978 and 1980, the percentage of phenylpropanolamine-related emergency room visits reported to the Drug Abuse Warning Network (DAWN) doubled, from 0.3% to 0.6% of the total reported visits (Bernstein and Diskant 1982). The actual number of phenylpropanolamine-related emergency room visits is probably much higher since there may often be a failure to recognize phenylpropanolamine as a contributor to or cause of the problem. The adverse effects recorded include hypertensive episodes (in several cases leading to death by cerebrovascular accident) (Ibid.), arrhythmias (Pentel, Mikell, and Zavoral 1982), renal failure, and psychoses (Lake et al. 1983).

CASE REPORTS OF PSYCHIATRIC DISORDERS RELATED TO PHENYLPROPANOLAMINE (ALONE OR IN COMBINATION)

This paper reviews 34 cases of phenylpropanolamine-related psychiatric side effects that have been reported in 13 articles in the U.S. or European literature since 1960 (table 17.1*).

Kane and Green (1966)

The first article appeared in 1966, when Kane and Green reported in the American Journal of Psychiatry three cases of acute psychosis associated with the ingestion of nasal decongestants containing phenylpropanolamine and other drugs (Kane and Green 1966). The first case was a 68-year-old woman who had been prescribed Ornade®, a nasal decongestant which contains phenylpropanolamine (50 mg) and chlorpheniramine maleate (8 mg). She had taken Ornade® for three weeks (having also taken syringoserpine, chloroquin, iron, and aspirin during the four months prior to hospitalization) before abnormal emotional symptoms prompted her to discontinue all medication. Two days later, a doctor again prescribed Ornade® and, after taking the drug for five days, she experienced a psychotic episode characterized by persecutory delusions, auditory and visual hallucinations, confusion, and disorientation. She was hospitalized, the Ornade® was discontinued, and she was given chlorpromazine (150 mg) intramuscularly daily for two weeks, after which she was discharged in a normal condition.

*Table 17.1 lists reports of psychiatric side effects by authors' names and in reverse chronological order.

Case 2 involved a 35-year-old man with no history of psychiatric problems who was given a common OTC antihistaminic/decongestant combination drug containing phenylpropanolamine for his perennial allergic rhinitis (hay fever). The other drugs contained in this preparation were not discussed, nor was the trade name of this drug given. He developed symptoms of a classical paranoid schizophrenic episode, with disordered thinking, delusions of reference, and feelings of grandiosity, inordinate influence, and persecution. He was hospitalized and treated with 1,650 mg of chlorpromazine daily along with phenylpropanolamine for rhinitis. After about two months, he was discharged on 300 mg of chlorpromazine per day, presumably with the diagnosis of paranoid schizophrenia. He discontinued all medication several months after discharge and was doing well until about a year later when he again developed allergic respiratory symptoms. He bought an OTC nasal decongestant which probably contained phenylpropanolamine and, after consuming two bottles within one week, had a second episode of paranoid schizophrenia requiring hospitalization. The relationship of hay fever pill ingestion to both episodes was noted and his nasal congestion was treated only with nose drops which did not contain phenylpropanolamine. He was discharged on 600 mg of chlorpromazine per day and was said to be doing well 12 weeks later.

Case 3 was a 36-year-old woman hospitalized in 1963 for acute undifferentiated schizophrenia without any mention of OTC drug ingestion. After treatment with chlorpromazine, she recovered and was discharged. Seven months later, she was prescribed Ornade® for sinusitis. She took one capsule each morning for two days without experiencing side effects but, after adding a second capsule on the third day, she developed schizophrenic symptoms with paranoid features including fears that her husband was going to kill her or the children and that her medication was poison. She also experienced auditory hallucinations and demonstrated impaired thought and speech, all with an intact sensorium. She again responded well to chlorpromazine (800 mg daily), was discharged on 500 mg daily, and was asymptomatic on 300 mg daily five months later.

Wharton (1970)

In 1970, in the British Journal of Psychiatry Wharton described a case of paranoid psychosis associated with nasal decongestants (Wharton 1970). A 37-year-old married man with no psychiatric history took 30 tablets of Anahist®

TABLE 17.1

Summary of published reports of psychiatric side effects associated with phenylpropanolamine use, 1966-84

Author, date (country)	Case # age/ sex	Drug (source)	Contents of drug (dose)	OCD	Symptoms	Diagnosis	Patient history	Family history
Cornelius, Soloff, and Reynolds 1984 (U.S.)	1 28/F	Triaminicol®, 12 oz (OTC)	PPA (900 mg), pheniramine maleate (450 mg), pyrilamine maleate (450 mg), dextromethorphan (1,080 mg)	-	paranoid ideation, homicidal actions, grand mal seizure	"transient psychotic experience" (H)	borderline personality, multiple suicide attempts	-
Lake et al. 1983 (U.S.)	1 21/M	4 black beauties (street)	caffeine, ephedrine, PPA	+	grandiose delusions, pressured speech	bipolar disorder, manic, with psychotic features (H)	previously suicidal, mild depression	+
Mueller 1983 (U.S.)	1 29/M	at least 2 black beauties (street)	PPA	+	bizarre behavior, PPA in urine	disturbances of thought processes (NH)	ni	ni
	2 25/F	white pill (street)	PPA	ni	auditory and visual hallucinations, PPA in urine	acute psychosis (ni)	chronic undifferentiated schizophrenia	ni
	3 13/M	ni	PPA	ni	attempted suicide, PPA in urine	disturbances of thought processes (NH)	ni	ni
	4 17/F	several black beauties (street)	PPA	ni	alleged sexual assault with no evidence, PPA in urine	disturbances of thought processes (NH)	ni	ni

Tornatore and Gilderman 1982 (U.S.)	1 24/F	anorexiant agents (OTC; Rx)	PPA; amphetamine	+	loose associations, paranoid delusions, autistic thinking	schizophrenia, drug-induced mental disorder (H)	-	-
Dougherty 1982 (U.S.)	1 24/F	alcohol, 12-20 pseudo-speed capsules (street)	PPA, caffeine, ephedrine (?)	+	increased anxiety, decreased job performance, agitation, auditory hallucinations	psychotic episode (H)	ni	ni
	2 14/M	20 pseudo-speed capsules (street)	PPA, caffeine, ephedrine (?)	+	failing grades, absenteeism, tardiness at school	psychological dependence (ni)	ni	ni
	3 17/M	marihuana, 3-6 pseudo-speed capsules, methamphetamine (street)	PPA, caffeine, ephedrine (?); methamphetamine	+	ni	drug abuse (ni)	anti-social personality	ni
Dietz 1981 (U.S.)	1 20/F	anorexiant agent (OTC)	PPA (75 mg)	ni	moderate anxiety, severe agitation, mild dizziness	severe agitation (NH)	ni	ni
	2 27/F	anorexiant agent (OTC)	PPA (75 mg), caffeine (200 mg)	ni	severe anxiety, moderate agitation, mild hallucinations, severe dizziness	acute psychotic episode (NH)	ni	ni

OCD = Other Concurrent Drugs | + = positive | (H) = hospitalized | (?) = speculation by cited author
ni = not indicated (no data in article) | - = negative | (NH) = not hospitalized

TABLE 17.1. (continued)

Author, date (country)	Case # age/ sex	Drug (source)	Contents of drug (dose)	OCD	Symptoms	Diagnosis	Patient history	Family history
Dietz 1981 (U.S.) (cont.)	3 17/F	anorexiant agent (OTC)	PPA (50 mg)	ni	moderate agitation, severe dizziness	moderate agitation (NH)	ni	ni
	4 22/F	anorexiant agent (OTC)	PPA (75 mg)	ni	mild agitation, moderate dizziness	mild agitation (NH)	ni	ni
	5 45/F	anorexiant agent (OTC)	PPA (50 mg), caffeine (200 mg)	ni	mild agitation, severe hallucinations	acute psychotic episode (H)	ni	ni
	6 22/F	anorexiant agent (OTC)	PPA (75 mg), caffeine (200 mg)	ni	severe anxiety, severe agitation	severe agitation (NH)	ni	ni
	7 24/F	anorexiant agent (OTC)	PPA (75 mg)	ni	moderate anxiety, mild agitation, severe dizziness	moderate anxiety (NH)	previous hospitalization	ni
Achor and Extein 1981 (U.S.)	1 32/F	Dexatrim Extra-strength™ (OTC)	PPA (75 mg), caffeine (200 mg)	ni	uncontrollable behavior, delusional thinking	bipolar disorder, mixed, with psychotic features (H)	postpartum dysphoric moods	ni
	2 51/F	Control® (OTC)	PPA (75 mg)	+	violent behavior, pressured speech, irritable mood	bipolar disorder, manic, without psychotic features (H)	irritability and impulsivity	ni

	3 19/M	Dexatrim™ (OTC)	PPA (50 mg), caffeine (200 mg)	ni	hypertalkativeness, hyperactivity, irritability	bipolar disorder, manic, with psychotic features (H)	possible depressive episode	+
Rieger 1981 (West Germany)	1 34/F	Amorphan (Rx)	(+)-norpseudoephedrine, other contents*	ni	paranoid delusions, sleep disturbance, bizarre delusions, ideas of reference, euphoria	emotionally disturbed with paranoid depressive thoughts (H)	-	-
	2 41/F	Recatol (OTC)	(+)-norpseudoephedrine, vitamins B_1, B_6, C	ni	auditory hallucinations, ideas of reference, bizarre delusions, paranoid delusions	possible schizophrenia (H)	probable anorexia nervosa during puberty	ni
	3 22/M	Amorphan (Rx)	(+)-norpseudoephedrine, other contents*	ni	paranoid delusions, euphoria, decreased sleep	paranoid hallucinatory psychoses (H)	drug and ethanol dependence for 15 years	ni
Renfordt and Wirtz 1980 (West Germany)	1 36/F	Boxogetten (OTC)	(+)-norpseudoephedrine, guaiacol glycerol ether, bisacodyl	ni	depression, mania, apathy, paranoid delusions, suicide attempt, auditory hallucinations	paranoid hallucinatory psychoses (H)	analgesics abuse	+
		Recatol (OTC)	(+)-norpseudoephedrine, vitamins B_1, B_6, C					

*Other contents of Amorphan include extract and leaf of Betulae, oil of juniper, Aloe, Cort. Frangulae, root of Gantianae, root of Calami.

OCD = Other Concurrent Drugs   + = positive   (H) = hospitalized
ni = not indicated (no data in article)   - = negative   (NH) = not hospitalized

TABLE 17.1. (continued)

Author, date (country)	Case # age/ sex	Drug (source)	Contents of drug (dose)	OCD	Symptoms	Diagnosis	Patient history	Family history
Schaffer and Pauli 1980 (U.S.)	1 23/F	Dexatrim™ (OTC) Permathene® (OTC)	PPA (50 mg), caffeine (200 mg) PPA (75 mg), caffeine (140 mg)	–	disorganized thoughts, paranoid delusions, decreased sleep, poor judgment and insight, some combativeness, hyperactivity	acute psychotic episode (H)	–	–
Norvenius, Widerlov, and Lonnerholm 1979 (Sweden)	1 3/M	Rinexin (Rx)	PPA	ni	confusion	psychotic episode (NH)	ni	ni
	2 8/M	Rinexin (Rx)	PPA	ni	confusion	psychotic episode (NH)	ni	ni
	3 4/F	Lunerin® (ni)	PPA (50 mg), brompheniramine (12 mg)	ni	visual hallucinations, grand mal seizure	psychotic episode (H)	ni	ni
	4 25/F	Monhydrin® (ni)	PPA (100 mg)	ni	increased excitation, decreased concentration, sleep disturbances, paranoia	psychotic episode (H)	ni	ni
	5 17/M	Rimonar (ni) Rinexin (Rx)	PPA, brompheniramine PPA	ni	motor excitation, aggressive behavior, elevated mood, hallucinations, confusion	acute mania-like psychosis (H)	ni	ni

Wharton 1970 (England)	1 37/M	Anahist (ni)	PPA (12.5 mg), thorsylamine HCl (6.25 mg), phenyltoxolamine citrate (6.25 mg), phenacetin (97.2 mg), caffeine, aspirin, vitamin C	ni	increased physical activity, paranoid delusions	acute paranoid episode (H)	-	ni
Kane and Green 1966 (U.S.)	1 68/F	Ornade (Rx)	PPA (50 mg), chlorphenir-amine (8 mg), isopropamide (2.5 mg)	+	running thoughts, persecutory delusions, hallucinations, confusion	psychotic episode with paranoid ideation (H)	-	ni
	2 35/M	combined antihistamine and PPA (OTC)	PPA, an unknown antihistamine	-	grandiose and paranoid delusions, ideas of reference	paranoid schizophrenia (H)	acute undifferentiated schizophrenia	-
	3 36/F	Ornade (Rx)	PPA (50 mg), chlorphenir-amine (8 mg), isopropamide (2.5 mg)	+	auditory hallucinations, gross thinking disorder, neologisms, clang associations	acute schizophrenia (H)	ni	ni

OCD = Other Concurrent Drugs + = positive (H) = hospitalized
ni = not indicated (no data in article) - = negative (NH) = not hospitalized

Source: Compiled by the authors.

(phenylpropanolamine, 12.5 mg; thorsylamine hydrochloride, 6.25 mg; phenyltoxolamine citrate, 6.25 mg; phenacetin, 97.2 mg; and caffeine, aspirin, and ascorbic acid in unspecified amounts) over eight days (a total of 375 mg of phenylpropanolamine), after which he was forcibly hospitalized with paranoid psychotic delusions. He showed increased physical activity and garrulousness, and developed ideas of reference and fears that his food was being poisoned and that there was a plot in his office to overthrow the government. He recovered rapidly on 300 mg of chlorpromazine given daily for three days (with, presumably, the simultaneous withdrawal of the Anahist®). Upon discharge, his position at work was tenuous and a second episode occurred some eight weeks later in which he "complained, in irrational terms, that he was being tested and investigated" at his job. Anahist® was not associated with this relapse, which was less severe than the first episode, and he improved quickly. When followed up three months later, the patient still had his job.

Norvenius, Widerlov, and Lonnerholm (1979)

Norvenius, Widerlov, and Lonnerholm (1979), of the pediatric clinic at Ostra Sjukhuset in Gothenburg, Sweden, published a letter in _Lancet_ summarizing the Swedish Adverse Drug Reaction Committee's experience with phenylpropanolamine-containing products during that year. Sixty-one cases of adverse effects were noted, 48 of which occurred in children 15 years old or younger. Five involved psychotic episodes. Two boys, ages three and eight, exhibited confusion and did not recognize their parents several hours after ingesting an unnoted amount of phenylpropanolamine; their symptoms abated a few hours later. A four-year-old experienced "visual hallucinosis" and a grand mal seizure after taking 50 mg of phenylpropanolamine in combination with 12 mg of brompheniramine, an antihistamine also capable of inducing adverse effects. A 25-year-old woman developed manic-like symptoms of increasing excitement, decreased ability to concentrate, a vaguely described sleep disturbance, and "vivid paranoid misconceptions" during treatment for allergies with phenylpropanolamine alone. It was not explicitly stated whether the phenylpropanolamine had been taken in prescribed amounts. The fifth case was a patient hospitalized three times within several months for acute manic-like psychoses with excessive motor excitement, aggressive behavior, and elevated mood. Each episode was linked to consumption of "large quantities" of phenylpropanolamine alone or in combination with brompheniramine.

Schaffer and Pauli (1980)

The first published case of a psychotic episode following ingestion of OTC diet aids containing phenylpropanolamine appeared in 1980 in the <u>American Journal of Psychiatry</u> (Schaffer and Pauli 1980). The patient was a 23-year-old woman who did not use alcohol or drugs to a significant degree and who had no personal or family history of psychiatric treatment. Desiring to lose weight, she took two diet pills a day for two days and then "copious amounts" for three days (estimated at a daily intake of three to five Dexatrim® capsules containing 50 mg phenylpropanolamine and 200 mg caffeine and three to five capsules of Permathene®, containing 75 mg phenylpropanolamine and 140 mg caffeine). She began to sleep less, developed paranoid ideations, and exhibited impulsivity. Upon hospitalization she was agitated, disoriented, disorganized in her thinking, and hyperactive to the extent that physical restraint was needed. After three days without any medication, she recovered fully.

Renfordt and Wirtz (1980)

Two articles that appeared in the West German publication <u>Der Nervenarzt</u> in 1980 and 1981 reported psychotic episodes in four individuals following ingestion of diet aids containing (+)-norpseudoephedrine (Renfordt and Wirtz 1980; Rieger 1981). The first describes a 36-year-old woman who, in an effort to lose weight, became psychologically dependent on diet aids containing (+)-norpseudoephedrine (Renfordt and Wirtz 1980). She increased her intake from the prescribed amount to four to six pills a day in order to maintain the stimulant effects and subsequently developed symptoms characterized at various times as depressive, paranoid, and manic. Her condition required several psychiatric hospitalizations, and she was treated with haloperidol on at least one admission but concealed her abuse of diet aids from several of her doctors. Elimination of the diet aids coincided with resolution of her psychiatric symptoms.

Rieger (1981)

The second West German article (Rieger 1981) discusses three cases of schizophrenic-like syndromes associated with appetite suppressants containing (+)-norpseudoephedrine. In one case, a 34-year-old woman with no personal or family history of psychiatric illness tried to lose weight with a diet preparation prescribed by her doctor that contained a number of ingredients, including (+)-norpseudoephedrine. At first, the drug improved her mood and enabled her to get more work done. However, she developed paranoid delusions and required hospitalization. Her symptoms were resolved once the diet aids were discontinued and she was given a neuroleptic.

The second case was a 41-year-old woman with a questionable earlier diagnosis of anorexia nervosa. She had taken a diet drug containing (+)-norpseudoephedrine primarily on weekends and during vacations for about ten years. When under the influence of the drug, she felt euphoric, was not hungry, and needed less sleep. However, during the reported episode she developed auditory hallucinations, agitation, and inability to concentrate to a degree necessitating hospitalization. Treatment was similar to that described in the first Rieger-reported case above and resulted in complete remission.

The third patient was a 22-year-old male multiple drug and alcohol abuser who took (+)-norpseudoephedrine pills solely for their stimulating effects. He regularly increased his dose as he developed tolerance and eventually experienced a paranoid psychosis. Similar to the above cases, his symptoms were resolved during hospitalization after withdrawal of the diet drugs.

Achor and Extein (1981)

In the American Journal of Psychiatry, Achor and Extein (1981) published a "Letter to the Editor" which described three cases of adverse reactions related to phenylpropanolamine use. One case involved a 32-year-old woman three months postpartum with a past history of mild postpartum dysphoric mood. Two weeks after she began taking Dexatrim® Extra-Strength® (containing 75 mg phenylpropanolamine and 200 mg caffeine), she required hospitalization because of "uncontrolled behavior" and delusional thinking. She was diagnosed as having bipolar disorder, mixed, with psychotic features.

The second case was a 51-year-old postmenopausal woman, with a past history of episodic irritability and impulsivity. Two weeks before she was hospitalized for violent behavior, pressured speech, and irritability, she had begun taking Control® (75 mg phenylpropanolamine) along with her three cups of coffee or tea per day. Her diagnosis was bipolar disorder, manic, without psychotic features. These two patients had personal histories of psychiatric illness but whether they had family histories of psychiatric illness was not indicated.

The third patient was a 19-year-old man with a positive family history of bipolar disorder and the suggestion of a personal history of a minor depressive episode. He had taken two Dexatrim® (50 mg phenylpropanolamine and 200 mg caffeine) capsules daily for three months prior to becoming hypertalkative, hyperactive, and irritable. He was hospitalized and diagnosed as having bipolar disorder, manic type, with psychotic features. It is not indicated whether any of these three patients abused alcohol or other drugs.

Dietz (1981)

Dietz (1981) published a report of emergency room visits associated with phenylpropanolamine use based on a review of emergency room records over a six-month period. Seven cases were found, all female, ages 17 to 45. Symptoms reportedly developed within one to two hours after ingesting a single pill. No indications were given as to personal or family psychiatric history or drug or alcohol abuse for six of the seven patients. Common side effects in all patients were agitation and anxiety, symptoms of which included hyperventilation, tachypnea, tremor, tachycardia, and dizziness. Five of the seven patients were judged to have moderate to severe anxiety and/or agitation. One had severe hallucinations requiring hospitalization, while a second had "mild" hallucinations along with severe anxiety. All side effects subsided within two to four hours for the six patients who did not require hospitalization. One of these had been hospitalized with moderate anxiety and severe dizziness about a year earlier after having taken 75 mg of phenylpropanolamine. At that time, presumably the history of phenylpropanolamine ingestion had not been elicited or considered important since the patient had undergone a thorough neurological workup including a computerized axial tomography (CAT) scan and lumbar puncture. Five of these patients had consumed 75 mg of phenylpropanolamine, and in two of these five cases the phenylpropanolamine was combined with 200 mg of caffeine (one was the patient who developed mild hallucinations). The patient who experienced severe hallucinations had taken 50 mg of phenylpropanolamine in combination with 200 mg of caffeine. The remaining patient had ingested 50 mg of phenylpropanolamine only.

Dougherty (1982)

Dougherty (1982) reported three cases of excessive "pseudospeed" capsule use. His first case was a 24-year-old woman who took 12 to 20 capsules per day in order to work two jobs averaging 50 to 60 hours per week. She also used alcohol in unspecified amounts. She hospitalized herself because of increasing anxiety, marked agitation, decreased job performance, and, finally, auditory hallucinations.

The second case was a 14-year-old boy, a chronic drug abuser who, after two years of abuse, needed 20 capsules per day to get the same high that a few had given him initially. He was referred to the adolescent drug treatment unit because of failing grades, absenteeism, and continual tardiness at school. He also used some alcohol and smoked "a few joints per week."

Dougherty's third case was a 17-year-old male, a multiple drug abuser who had used about an ounce of marihuana per week, drunk two to four six-packs of beer per day, and snorted two grams of methamphetamine HCl per week over a three-month period. Family and personal psychiatric histories of these three patients were not given; neither was treatment nor clinical course. These cases were complicated by simultaneous use of multiple drugs and/or alcohol abuse. No laboratory identification of the specific drugs ingested was conducted, so that conclusions about the role of phenylpropanolamine are tentative.

Tornatore and Gilderman (1982)

Also published in 1982 was the case of a 24-year-old obese woman brought to a psychiatric clinic because of bizarre behavior, including the belief that her parents were part of a devil cult that was poisoning her food (Tornatore and Gilderman 1982). She was diagnosed as schizophrenic, hospitalized for four days, and given haloperidol, 30 mg per day. She had no family or personal history of mental illness but had reputedly taken amphetamine and phenylpropanolamine-containing diet aids for approximately a year before admission. Upon discovery of this information, her diagnosis was changed to "drug-induced organic mental disorder" and her medication discontinued. She recovered during hospitalization and remained well eight months after she was released.

Mueller (1983)

In a 1983 issue of Neurology, Mueller reported 11 cases involving neurologic and/or psychiatric complications following phenylpropanolamine use. In four of these patients, the psychiatric side effects were primary. One was a 29-year-old male who, after taking at least two black beauty capsules and smoking two joints, began acting in a bizarre manner, which included taking off his clothes at an airport. A second case involved a 25-year-old female who overdosed on an unknown number of "white pills" and developed an acute psychosis with auditory and visual hallucinations. She had previously been diagnosed as having chronic undifferentiated schizophrenia. A third case was a 13-year-old boy who, after taking some phenylpropanolamine-containing drugs, attempted suicide by hanging. The fourth was a 17-year-old female who, after taking several black beauties, alleged a sexual assault in the absence of any evidence of such an event. All of these patients had complete urine drug screens capable of identifying 130 drugs, including amphetamine, phenylpropanolamine, caffeine, and ephedrine. In each case, the drug screens showed only phenylpropanolamine. Details of the drug-screening method, treatment, and family and personal psychiatric histories (with the exception of one patient who had been previously diagnosed as having chronic undifferentiated schizophrenia) were not given.

Lake et al. (1983)

One additional case report of psychiatric complications following phenylpropanolamine use was published in 1983 by Lake et al. in the American Journal of Psychiatry. This case is described in detail in the beginning of this paper.

Cornelius, Soloff, and Reynolds (1984)

The case described by Cornelius, Soloff, and Reynolds (1984) is the only instance of phenylpropanolamine-related psychiatric side effects reported in 1984. The patient was a 28-year-old woman with a personal history but no family history of psychiatric illness. The case is unique in that it is the first in which phenylpropanolamine ingestion was related to violent, almost homicidal, behavior. It is also the first time a phenylpropanolamine challenge was administered in the hospital to reproduce the admitting symptoms. This patient had abused various substances, attempted suicide many times, and been previously diagnosed as a borderline personality. During the two years preceding admission, she had abused Triaminicol®, an OTC cough syrup containing phenylpropanolamine, pheniramine maleate, pyrilamine maleate, and dextromethorphan. The day before admission she had consumed approximately 12 ounces of this syrup (which amounts to about 900 mg phenylpropanolamine, 450 mg pheniramine, 450 mg pyrilamine, and 1,080 mg dextromethorphan), after which she began to feel that her mother was "sadistically sabotaging her life." She attempted to kill her mother by stabbing her repeatedly, resulting in severe but not lethal injury. At the time of the hospitalization, she was confused, tearful, mute, and fearful. On the third day she had a 50-second grand mal seizure; her electroencephalogram (EEG) was abnormal the next day but normalized within a week. A challenge test with 50 mg phenylpropanolamine caused focal temporal lobe seizure activity and behavioral changes including expressions of fear, apprehension, confusion, and isolation. Symptoms cleared within six hours and her EEG was normal the next day.

SUMMARY

The most striking finding in these 34 cases is the severity of the phenylpropanolamine-linked psychiatric disturbances, as reflected by diagnoses and hospitalizations. Acute psychoses occurred in 20 cases: ten of the 24 cases cited in the United States and all ten cited in the European literature. Twenty patients required hospitalization for periods varying from days to months: 12 in the United States (in three other cases insufficient data were given) and eight in Europe. Several patients demonstrated two or more symptom complexes. Five had manic symptoms and prominent paranoid delusions, plus other symptoms of schizophrenia. Five had predominantly manic symptoms, five predominantly schizophrenic symptoms, and, in an additional five, the disorder was not clearly affective or schizophrenic. In several cases, information was inadequate to make a diagnosis.

Where the psychosis was recognized as drug-related, the hospital stay tended to be shorter; however, despite knowledge of the drug-relatedness of the symptoms, at least nine of those hospitalized were discharged on antischizophrenic drugs or lithium. In another 11 cases, no discharge medication data were given.

The severity of these side effects makes it important to determine whether phenylpropanolamine had a causative role in their development. To evaluate this, we sought to assess whether the severity of the effects had been influenced by (1) the type of phenylpropanolamine ingested (($\pm$)-norephedrine versus (+)-norpseudoephedrine); (2) the combination of phenylpropanolamine with other drugs; (3) the amount of phenylpropanolamine that had been used; (4) the family and personal psychiatric history; and (5) any other factors that may have potentially predisposed the patient to adverse reactions. This assessment was hampered by the considerable amounts of missing data. Often dosages were unknown or not indicated or the length of time over which an individual had ingested phenylpropanolamine-containing products was not specified. Family and personal psychiatric histories were not consistently provided.

DISCUSSION

1. An important factor to consider when examining these phenylpropanolamine-related case reports is which isomer was used. Even though animal data indicate that the isomer used in European drugs containing phenylpropanolamine ((+)-norpseudoephedrine) is a more potent CNS stimulant than the U.S. form (($\pm$)-norephedrine), the reactions described appear to have been similar. Common to cases from both the United States and Europe were mania, paranoid ideations, and psychotic reactions, which suggests that the isomer of phenylpropanolamine sold in Europe cannot be regarded as the only potentially dangerous form. The percentage of European patients requiring hospitalization (80%) was somewhat higher than that in the United States (57% of the 21 cases for whom information was available). From the limited data, the European (+)-norpseudoephedrine preparations do appear to have been more chronically abused for their CNS stimulant properties: five of the ten European patients chronically abused phenylpropanolamine preparations, compared to only five of the 24 U.S. patients.

2. Another factor to be considered is whether other drugs were ingested simultaneously with phenylpropanolamine since it appears that combination products produce greater side effects. Individuals who took U.S. phenylpropanolamine combination products were much more likely to require hospitalization than those who took phenylpropanolamine alone. This relationship was observed even in cases in which recommended dosages were ingested. The most common additional drug consumed with phenylpropanolamine was caffeine: seven of the nine U.S. patients who consumed this combination and for whom hospitalization information was available required

hospitalization; two of these seven may have also taken ephedrine. Nevertheless, seven U.S. cases apparently took phenylpropanolamine alone and four of these took the suggested dosage; all required medical attention but none required hospitalization.

An example of a drug containing a potentially toxic drug combination is Ornade®, which was named specifically in two of the cases reviewed. Like many other OTC cold preparations, Ornade® contains isopropamide (an anticholinergic) and phenylpropanolamine (a sympathomimetic), which act synergistically by different mechanisms to increase the heart rate and to inhibit the beneficial physiologic reflex bradycardia in the presence of acute hypertension.

Other drugs that may produce adverse side effects when taken with phenylpropanolamine include the tricyclic antidepressants, the monoamine oxidase (MAO) inhibitors, and levodopa (Cuthbert et al. 1969; Mason and Buckle 1969). (These reports were not discussed in this paper since only physical side effects, primarily hypertension, occurred with use of these combinations.) Since depression, colds, allergies, weight reduction plans, and caffeine consumption are so prevalent today, it would not be uncommon for an individual to take several of these products at the same time.

Chronic abuse of substances other than phenylpropanolamine may contribute to the development and severity of side effects. History of drug and alcohol abuse was positive for five patients, negative for six, and unreported in the rest, making speculation on the involvement of concurrent substance abuse impossible.

3. A less critical factor appears to be the amount of phenylpropanolamine ingested. Of the cases in the United States in which the amount of phenylpropanolamine taken was recorded, 12 patients took recommended dosages and ten took overdoses; in two cases the dosage taken could not be determined. Eight patients experienced psychotic reactions after taking only recommended amounts of phenylpropanolamine. About the same number of individuals who had ingested recommended doses were hospitalized as those who had taken overdoses.

4. The most consistent characteristic shared by many of these patients is a positive past psychiatric history (13 out of 18, with 16 undetermined). One potential explanation is that phenylpropanolamine products exacerbated trait-related symptoms in patients with positive histories and caused state-related symptoms (acute drug-induced organic brain syndromes) in patients with no psychiatric history. Although this explanation is merely speculative, the reports indicate that patients with past histories of major or minor

affective disorders are at special risk for developing phenylpropanolamine-related psychiatric symptoms. This includes patients with past episodes of mild depression, dysphoric personality disorder, postpartum depression, or mania, hypomania, or cyclothymic personality disorder. Other susceptible individuals may be those who have histories of substance abuse, antisocial or borderline personality disorders, or schizophrenia.

The experience of these cases indicates the need to obtain in-depth personal and family histories. This need is further illustrated by the fact that, in three cases, the association of phenylpropanolamine intake with a past psychiatric hospitalization was not noted initially, either because the physician failed to elicit the history or the patient denied any such drug ingestion (case 2 of Kane and Green 1966; Renfordt and Wirtz 1980; case 7 of Dietz 1981). Routine drug screens also are warranted. When phenylpropanolamine ingestion is documented, it should be considered a possible cause of symptoms and in some cases drug treatment should be withheld to allow symptoms to clear.

5. Groups other than those with past psychiatric problems may also be susceptible to ill effects. Children under five years of age comprise a large percentage of emergency room and poison control center cases involving phenylpropanolamine-containing products. In the United States between 1975 and 1980, the frequency of phenylpropanolamine-related cases in this age group reported to the NCPCC increased sevenfold from 0.1% to 0.7% of all drug cases reported (Phenylpropanolamine for weight control products 1981). Children of this age comprised 56% of cases of phenylpropanolamine overdose reported to a poison control center over a five-month period in 1981 (Ekins and Spoerke 1983). In Sweden in 1979, 67% of reports to the Swedish Adverse Drug Reaction Committee of phenylpropanolamine-related psychiatric disturbances involved children 15 years old or younger (Norvenius, Widerlov, and Lonnerholm 1979). Presumably most of these cases were due to accidental ingestion of phenylpropanolamine-containing cold remedies or the popular diet aids which are readily available over-the-counter and often casually stored in the home.

Since women may be most susceptible to major affective disorders during the postpartum period (Brockington et al. 1981), expectant and postpartum mothers should be advised against taking any sympathomimetic drugs, including phenylpropanolamine. At least two women whose cases are reviewed here began taking diet aids to lose weight gained during pregnancy (case 1 of Achor and Extein 1981; case 1 of Rieger 1981).

Individuals who are sensitive to or who consume large quantities of caffeine may also be at greater risk for adverse psychiatric reactions upon taking phenylpropanolamine-containing drugs. Caffeine and phenylpropanolamine are both sympathomimetic drugs with different but synergistic mechanisms of action. Although in one case consuming five grams of caffeine was not fatal (Syed 1976) and consumption of this amount daily (25 to 50 cups of coffee) is not unheard of, several reports of psychiatric side effects from coffee alone have been published (Mikkelsen 1978; McManamy and Schube 1936; Greden et al. 1978; Orendorff 1914; De Frietas and Schwartz 1979; Herridge and á Brook 1968). Given these data, the FDA's December 1983 decision to require a new drug application for preparations containing phenylpropanolamine/caffeine combinations was probably a wise one, but can hardly be expected to be effective since U.S. residents consume over a billion kilograms of coffee annually (Syed 1976).

REFERENCES

Achor, M. B. and I. Extein. 1981. Diet aids, mania, and affective illness. Am J Psychiatry 138:392.

Alles, G. A., D. Fairchild, and M. Jensen. 1961. Chemical pharmacology of Catha edulis. J Med Pharm Chem 3:323-52.

American Psychiatric Association. 1980. Diagnostic and statistical manual of mental disorders, 3rd ed. Washington, D.C.: American Psychiatric Association.

Bernstein, E. and B. M. Diskant. 1982. Phenylpropanolamine: a potentially hazardous drug. Ann Emerg Med 11:311-15.

Blum, A. 1981. Phenylpropanolamine: an over-the-counter amphetamine? JAMA 245:1346-47.

Brockington, I. F. et al. 1981. Puerperal psychosis. Arch Gen Psychiatry 38:829-33.

Cornelius, J. R., P. H. Soloff, and C. F. Reynolds III. 1984. Paranoia, homicidal behavior, and seizures associated with phenylpropanolamine. Am J Psychiatry 141:120-21.

Cuthbert, M. F., M. P. Greenberg, and S. W. Morley. 1969. Cough and cold remedies: a potential danger to patients on monoamine oxidase inhibitors. Br Med J 1:404-6.

De Freitas, B. and G. Schwartz. 1979. Effects of caffeine in chronic psychiatric patients. Am J Psychiatry 136: 1337-38.

Dietz, A. J. 1981. Amphetamine-like reactions to phenylpropanolamine. JAMA 245:601-2.

Dougherty, R. J. 1982. Pseudo-speed: look-alikes or peashooters. NY State J Med 82:74-75.

Ekins, B. R. and D. G. Spoerke. 1983. An estimation of the toxicity of nonprescription diet aids from seventy exposure cases. Vet Hum Toxicol 25:81-85.

Ellinwood, E. H. 1974. The epidemiology of stimulant abuse. In Drug use: epidemiological and sociological approaches, edited by E. Josephson and E. E. Carroll, 303-29. Washington, D.C.: Hemisphere.

Fairchild, M. D. and G. A. Alles. 1967. The central locomotor stimulatory activity and acute toxicity of the ephedrine and norephedrine isomers in mice. J Pharmacol Exp Ther 158:135-39.

Franzosa, E. 1983. Telephone conversation with author (Lake).

Giannini, A. J. and S. Castellani. 1982. A manic-like psychosis due to khat (Catha edulis Forsk.). J Toxicol Clin Toxicol 19:455-59.

Greden, J. F. et al. 1978. Anxiety and depression associated with caffeinism among psychiatric inpatients. Am J Psychiatry 135:963-66.

Griffiths, R. R., J. V. Brady, and J. D. Snell. 1978. Relationship between anorectic and reinforcing properties of appetite suppressant drugs: implications for assessment of abuse liability. Biol Psychiatry 13: 283-90.

Haislip, G. 1983. Drug Enforcement Administration statement to U.S. Congress, Senate Subcommittee on Alcoholism and Drug Abuse, Committee on Labor and Human Resources. July 14.

Health and Human Services, Food and Drug Administration (FDA). 1982. New drug status of OTC combination drug products containing caffeine, phenylpropanolamine, and ephedrine. FDA docket no. 82N-0266. Federal Register 47:35344-46.

Herridge, C. F. and M. F. ā Brook. 1968. Ephedrine psychosis. Br Med J 2:160.

Humphrey, G. 1983. Hearings on look-alike drugs: opening remarks to U.S. Congress, Senate Subcommittee on Alcoholism and Drug Abuse, Committee on Labor and Human Resources. July 14.

Jarvik, M. E. 1979. Psychopharmacology in the practice of medicine. New York: Appleton-Century-Crofts.

Jick, H. 1984. Telephone conversation with author (Lake). May.

Johnston, L. D., J. G. Bachman, and P. M. O'Malley. 1982. Student drug use, attitudes, and beliefs: national trends, 1975-1982. National Institute on Drug Abuse research report. Washington, D.C.: U.S. Government Printing Office.

Kane, F. J., Jr. and B. Q. Green. 1966. Psychotic episodes associated with the use of common proprietary decongestants. Am J Psychiatry 123:484-87.

Lake, C. R. et al. 1983. Psychomotor stimulant induced mania in a patient with a strong family history: a review of the literature and report of a case. J Clin Psychopharmacol 3:97-100.

Luqman, W. and T. S. Danowski. 1976. The use of khat (Catha edulis) in Yemen: social and medical observations. Ann Intern Med 85:246-49.

Mason, A.M.S. and R. M. Buckle. 1969. "Cold" cures and monoamine oxidase inhibitors. Letter. Br Med J 1:845.

McGlothlin, W. H. 1973. Amphetamines, barbiturates, and hallucinogens: an analysis of use, distribution and control. U.S. Department of Justice, Bureau of Narcotics and Dangerous Drugs, contract no. J-70-33. Washington, D.C.: Drug Enforcement Administration.

McManamy, M. C. and P. G. Schube. 1936. Caffeine intoxication. Report of a case the symptoms of which amounted to a psychosis. N Engl J Med 215:616-20.

Mikkelson, E. J. 1978. Caffeine and schizophrenia. J Clin Psychiatry 3:732-36.

Morgan, J. P. 1983. Telephone conversation with author (Lake).

———. 1981. Amphetamine. In Substance abuse: clinical problems and perspectives, edited by J. H. Lowinson and P. Ruiz, 167-84. Baltimore: Williams and Wilkins.

Morgan, J. P. and D. Kagan. 1978. Street amphetamine quality and the Controlled Substances Act of 1970. J Psychedelic Drugs 10:303-17.

Mueller, S. M. 1983. Neurologic complications of phenylpropanolamine use. Neurology 33:650-52.

Norvenius, G., E. Widerlov, and G. Lonnerholm. 1979. Phenylpropanolamine and mental disturbances. Lancet 2:1367-68.

Orendorff, O. 1914. Letter to the editor. JAMA 62:1828-29.

Patrick, L. 1977. Amphetamine and cocaine: biological mechanisms. In Psychopharmacology: from theory to practice, edited by J. D. Barchas et al., 331-40. New York: Oxford University Press.

Pentel, P. R., F. L. Mikell, and J. H. Zavoral. 1982. Myocardial injury after phenylpropanolamine ingestion. Br Heart J 47:51-54.

Phenylpropanolamine for weight control products. 1981. National Clearinghouse of Poison Control Centers Bulletin 25:16-19.

Physicians' desk reference, 38th ed. 1984. Oradell, NJ: Medical Economics.

Physicians' desk reference for nonprescription drugs, 4th ed. 1983. Oradell, NJ: Medical Economics.

Renfordt, E. and W. Wirtz. 1980. Mißbrauch von d-norpseudoephedrine appetitzuglern. Der Nervenarzt 51:691-93.

Rieger, G. 1981. Paranoid halluzinatorische psychosen nach linnahme von d-norpseudoephedrinhaltigen appetitzuglern. Der Nervenarzt 52:423-25.

Saxena, K. and R. Kingston. 1981. Morbidity of street speed--an update. Vet Hum Toxicol 23:10-12.

Schaffer, C. B. and M. W. Pauli. 1980. Psychotic reaction caused by proprietary oral diet agents. Am J Psychiatry 137:1256-57.

Short, J. 1984. Telephone conversation with author (Lake).

Syed, I. B. 1976. The effects of caffeine. Journal of the American Pharmaceutical Association 16:568-72.

Tornatore, F. L. and A. M. Gilderman. 1982. Substance-induced organic mental disorders. Am Pharm NS22:503-6.

Waggoner, W. C. 1983. Phenylpropanolamine overdosage. Lancet 2:1503.

Wharton, B. K. 1970. Nasal decongestants and paranoid psychosis. Br J Psychiatry 117:439-40.

Zelger, J. L. and E. A. Carlini. 1980. Anorexigenic effects of two amines obtained from Catha edulis Forsk. (khat) in rats. Pharmacol Biochem Behav 12:701-5.

ACKNOWLEDGMENTS

The authors wish to thank Eleanor Gamble for compiling table 17.1, and Robert Whitcher, Rafael Villalobos, Peter Lorenzetti, and Sakeenah Sadrud-din for their help in researching this paper.

18

REPORTED AMPHETAMINE-LIKE REACTIONS TO PHENYLPROPANOLAMINE

Albert J. Dietz, Edward O. Magarian, and David S. Freeman

INTRODUCTION

Phenylpropanolamine (PPA) has been available for the last 40 to 50 years as a component in a number of over-the-counter (OTC), as well as prescription, pharmaceutical preparations. The first use of phenylpropanolamine was as a vasoconstrictor and decongestant to counteract the symptoms of nasal congestion associated with upper respiratory tract infections. Approximately ten years ago, the drug began to be promoted as an OTC appetite suppressant, used alone and in combination with caffeine. Because of the widespread publicizing and promotion of these products in the media recently, many individuals who are concerned with weight reduction have begun to ingest this compound. We became interested in phenylpropanolamine after seeing a number of emergency room patients who had ingested diet aids containing phenylpropanolamine. Many of their reactions were similar to those seen with amphetamine, and this led us to examine the chemical similarity between phenylpropanolamine and amphetamine.

PERTINENT ADRENERGIC PHARMACOLOGY

Therapeutic agents that act by stimulating the dopaminergic and adrenergic systems, whether peripherally or centrally, do so by a variety of mechanisms, including direct receptor activation and various indirect actions, such as the release of endogenous catecholamines from intraneuronal storage vesicles, the inhibition of monoamine reuptake, and the blocking of a major metabolic pathway catalyzed by monoamine oxidase (MAO). One factor that determines the mechanisms of the pharmacological actions of these agents is molecular structure. The functional groups present in a drug can have profound effects on its physicochemical properties, which can significantly modify both receptor activity (efficacy and affinity) and distribution to the biophase (figure 18.1).

FIGURE 18.1

Sites of potential structural variance of sympathomimetic phenethylamines

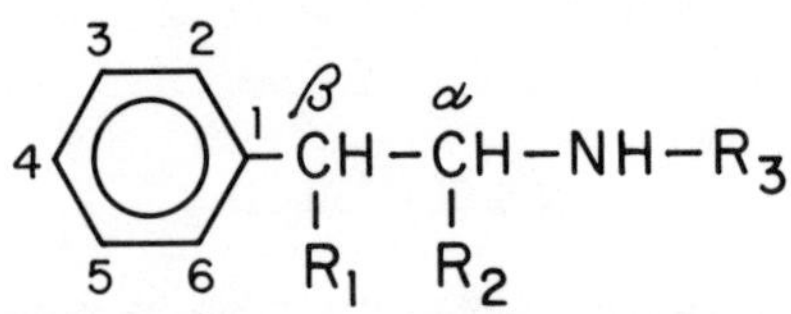

Source: Compiled by the author.

Aromatic Ring Substitution

The catechol nucleus (3,4-dihydroxy phenyl) is required for optimal direct alpha- and beta-receptor activation, but it diminishes central nervous system (CNS) bioavailability of peripherally administered agents. Noncatecholamine derivatives can exhibit alpha and beta effects, mainly by indirect mechanisms (Weiner 1980). Since these noncatecholamines often have higher lipophilic properties and are metabolized more slowly, they are more available to the central nervous system and have been widely employed for their CNS effects.

Alpha-Carbon Substitution

Alpha-methyl substitution yields such isopropyl products as amphetamine, methamphetamine, and other congeners. The biochemical effects of amphetamine include stimulation of the release of catecholamines from neuronal sites and inhibition of their reuptake (Leibowitz 1978; Offermeier and duPreez 1978; Biel 1970; Duhault et al. 1978). The anorexiant effect of amphetamine, which is believed to occur in the rostral and middle hypothalamus, appears to be related to the presence of freshly synthesized, readily available catecholamines (Leibowitz 1978; Sulser et al. 1968; Weissman, Koe, and Tenen 1966). Evidence from several studies strongly supports the hypothesis that amphetamine and most other anorexiants elicit their effects by interacting with dopaminergic and/or beta-adrenergic systems that may be involved in the regulation of feeding (Baez 1974; Goldman, Lehr, and Friedman 1971; Hansen and Whishaw 1973; Heffner, Zigmond, and Stricker 1977; Leibowitz 1978, 1971, 1970a, 1970b; Sanghvi et al. 1975). An interesting finding is that these dopaminergic and beta-adrenergic mechanisms that appear to inhibit feeding are located laterally to another hypothalamic region (the paraventricular nucleus) containing alpha-adrenergic receptors that, when stimulated, produce a vigorous feeding response (Booth 1968; Grossman 1964, 1962; Leibowitz 1978, 1975, 1974, 1973).

The presence of an alpha-methyl group creates an asymmetric center that leads to stereochemical variance of effects. For example, the CNS-stimulating effects of the *dextro* isomers of amphetamine (dextroamphetamine) and methamphetamine are ten to 20 times greater than those of the *levo* isomers (Daniels and Jorgenson 1982). This difference in CNS effect probably occurs because dextroamphetamine has a relative inhibitory potency for blocking ^{3}H-norepinephrine reuptake of 1.5 (relative to norepinephrine), whereas the *levo* isomer has a much lower relative potency of 0.07 (Burgen and Iversen 1965). Methyl substitution also protects these products from oxidation by MAO. Indeed, amphetamine has been shown to inhibit MAO competitively, a fact that has been offered as one explanation of its indirect effects (Clarke 1980). It is interesting to note that amphetamine's ability to inhibit MAO is stereochemically dependent, with dextroamphetamine being several times more potent than levoamphetamine.

Beta-Carbon Substitution

An OH group in the beta-position generally produces diminished CNS effects, including anorexia, often accomplished by a concomitant increase in peripheral alpha and beta effects. Phenylpropanolamine (norephedrine) and ephedrine are less effective than amphetamine as CNS stimulants, but ephedrine is considerably more potent in increasing blood pressure and heart rate (Weiner 1980). The decreased CNS effects may be due in large part to a poorer ability to penetrate the blood/brain barrier. Hydroxyl substitution increases polarity and dramatically reduces lipid solubility. For example, the chloroform/water partition coefficients for dextroamphetamine, ephedrine, and phenylpropanolamine are 146, 0.015, and 0.001, respectively (Vree, Muskens, and van Rossum 1969).

Beta-hydroxyl-substituted products are considered to be indirect agonists (Daniels and Jorgenson 1982; Silverman et al. 1980; Weiner 1980) that, similar to amphetamine, act by enhancing the release of stored catecholamines and/or by inhibiting catecholamine reuptake (Burgen and Iversen 1965). Studies to determine the mechanisms of phenylpropanolamine are not so extensive as those for amphetamine. However, some studies have demonstrated that phenylpropanolamine has significant effects, albeit weaker than amphetamine, on both adrenergic and dopaminergic systems (Biel 1970; Levitt, Cumiskey, and Shargel 1974). Burgen and Iversen (1965) determined the relative inhibitory effects of amphetamine and phenylpropanolamine on norepinephrine reuptake receptors in the isolated rat heart and found phenylpropanolamine to be approximately one-fourth as active as amphetamine. Levitt, Cumiskey, and Shargel (1974) showed that phenylpropanolamine and its analogs may not only block the reuptake of norepinephrine but may also stimulate the release of this neurohormone.

Sinsheimer, Dring, and Williams (1973) investigated the metabolism of phenylpropanolamine, which appears as a minor metabolite of amphetamine and methamphetamine (Caldwell, Dring, and Williams 1972a, 1972b). Volunteers receiving the (^{14}C) labeled drug excreted about 96% of the (^{14}C) during the first day, which was mainly due to unchanged phenylpropanolamine (80% of the dose). Identified minor metabolites were hippuric acid and 4-hydroxyphenylpropanolamine.

Phenylpropanolamine, like ephedrine, contains two asymmetric carbon centers and therefore exists in two diastereomeric pairs. The <u>erythro</u> (see chapter 1, this volume) isomers in a racemic mixture are employed therapeutically.

Thus, phenylpropanolamine produces biochemical effects in adrenergic and dopaminergic systems in a qualitatively similar, but quantitatively different, manner to those produced by amphetamine. This fact, coupled with a decreased CNS bioavailability of phenylpropanolamine due to its diminished lipophilic nature (see above), may explain why these therapeutic agents may produce similar CNS effects but not on an equipotent basis.

CASE REPORTS

The preceding pharmacological review will, we think, facilitate interpretation of the following seven case reports. All seven patients were white females between the ages of 17 and 45 who, after having ingested products containing phenylpropanolamine, reported for treatment to the emergency room of a metropolitan hospital during a six-month period in 1980. Their symptoms varied (table 18.1) but were of sufficient concern to the individuals that they sought emergency medical attention.

Case 1. J.S., 20 years of age, had taken a tablet containing 75 mg of phenylpropanolamine hydrochloride at 9 a.m. The patient stated that one and one-half hours later she became dizzy, had a floating sensation, developed a pounding headache, throbbed all over her body, felt nauseated, and developed numbness in her face. She became very restless and nervous and found it difficult to breathe deeply. Her vision became distorted, with objects appearing to be bent and waving. She denied any other drug use or abuse then or in the past. A physical examination revealed her blood pressure was 120/64 mm Hg, her pulse rate, 110 beats/min, and her respiration rate, 28 breaths/min. Except for the mental aberrations, there were no signs of physical or neurological abnormalities. The patient remained under observation in a darkened room for several hours. Her symptoms gradually abated and she was discharged.

Case 2. D.F., 27 years old, had taken a tablet containing 75 mg of phenylpropanolamine plus 200 mg caffeine at 10 a.m. While driving two hours later, she became dizzy, her heart beat rapidly, and she became faint and short of breath. She pulled off the road, where the highway patrol came to her assistance, and she was brought by ambulance to the emergency room. She complained of feeling severely dizzy, seeing flashing lights, being frightened and nervous, and having difficulty breathing. A physical examination found her blood pressure to be 132/90 mm Hg, her pulse rate, 120 beats/min, and her respiration rate, 34 breaths/min; otherwise her physical examination was normal. The patient remained under observation in a darkened room and, when well, was discharged in the care of her husband.

Case 3. J.K., 17 years of age, was brought into the emergency room after having collapsed in school. In gym class she had become very jittery, felt faint, and developed numbness in her arms, legs, and face. She had stayed in the class despite these symptoms but had become so dizzy that she "passed out." The patient stated that she had taken a diet pill containing 50 mg phenylpropanolamine before leaving for school in the morning. In the emergency room her blood pressure was 126/78 mm Hg, her pulse rate was 98 beats/min, and her respiration rate was 26 breaths/min. Physical examination, blood sugar, and complete blood count (CBC) were all within normal limits. After several hours of observation, she was discharged in the care of her parents.

TABLE 18.1

Summary of emergency room cases involving phenylpropanolamine alone or in combination, January–June 1980

Case no.	Age	Dose (mg) PPA/caffeine	Symptoms: Anxiety	Symptoms: Agitation	Symptoms: Hallucinations	Symptoms: Dizziness	Blood pressure*	Pulse rate†	Respiration rate§
1	20	75/—	moderate	severe	—	mild	120/64	110	28
2	27	75/200	severe	moderate	mild	severe	132/90	120	34
3	17	50/—	—	moderate	—	severe	126/78	98	26
4	22	75/—	—	mild	—	moderate	124/70	110	24
5	45	50/200	—	mild	severe	—	136/84	95	20
6	22	75/200	severe	severe	—	—	140/78	108	26
7	24	75/—	moderate	mild	—	severe	104/70	102	28

*mm Hg †beats/minute §breaths/minute

Source: Adapted from Dietz, A. J. 1981. Amphetamine-like reactions to phenylpropanolamine. JAMA 245:602. Reprinted with permission.

Case 4. R.B., 22 years old, was visiting her parents when she had suddenly developed chest pain, dizziness, ringing in her ears, and epigastric pain. She also had difficulty breathing and complained of numbness and tingling around the mouth. Two hours before her symptoms began, she had taken a diet preparation containing 75 mg phenylpropanolamine. Her blood pressure was 124/70 mm Hg, her pulse rate was 110 beats/min, and her respiration rate was 24 breaths/min. Her physical examination was entirely normal. The patient was observed for several hours and, when her symptoms improved, she was discharged in the care of her parents.

Case 5. M.S., 45 years of age, came to the emergency room complaining that "I don't feel right." According to her husband, she had quite suddenly become confused and nervous, stating that she heard voices. She appeared delusional upon examination and claimed to be on a "secret mission" she could not tell us about. The only medication she stated she had taken that day was a diet pill containing 50 mg phenylpropanolamine plus 200 mg caffeine. When she was examined, her blood pressure was 136/84 mm Hg, her pulse rate was 95 beats/min, and her respiration rate was 20 breaths/min. She was admitted to the hospital for 72 hours and was given a computerized axial tomography (CAT) scan, electroencephalogram (EEG), chest x-ray, electrocardiogram (ECG), a neurological examination, and a psychiatric evaluation, all of which were normal when she was discharged. In subsequent visits she remained normal.

Case 6. M.S., who was 22 years old, came to the emergency room because of difficulty in breathing, which had started approximately one hour after she had ingested a diet pill containing 75 mg phenylpropanolamine and 200 mg caffeine. She stated that her mouth and throat were very dry and that her hands and feet tingled, and she appeared nervous and jittery. A physical examination revealed her blood pressure to be 140/78 mm Hg, her pulse rate 108 beats/min, and her respiration rate 26 breaths/min; both a chest x-ray and ECG were normal. She was observed for several hours, then discharged in the care of her husband with a follow-up appointment in the clinic.

Case 7. D.D., 24 years of age, was admitted to the emergency room complaining of dizziness, faintness, and numbness on the right side of her body. She reported having taken a diet pill containing 75 mg phenylpropanolamine two hours before coming to the emergency room. A physical examination, including a neurological evaluation, was normal, and her blood pressure was 104/70 mm Hg, pulse rate, 102 beats/min, and respiration rate, 28 breaths/min. A similar experience had occurred a year previously following ingestion of a similar diet pill. She had been cautioned about taking diet pills, but in her professional life she was a model and maintained her body weight below the normal range. This second episode elicited stronger warnings about future use of diet aids. When her symptoms improved, she was discharged.

In none of these seven subjects were confirmatory urine or blood tests mentioned.

DISCUSSION

Other writers in this volume (Louis and Horowitz; Krakoff; Mueller; Reidenberg) and in the literature (Frewin, Leonello, and Frewin 1978; Horowitz et al. 1979; Lee, Bielin, and Vandongen 1979; Livingston 1966; Ostern and Dodson 1965) have described the effects of phenylpropanolamine on the vascular system; we will confine our remarks to a comparison of the CNS effects of amphetamine and phenylpropanolamine.

First, amphetamine is one of the most potent sympathomimetic amines with respect to stimulation of the central nervous system. As mentioned previously, the d-isomer (dextroamphetamine) is many times more potent than the l-isomer. The psychic effects of amphetamine include wakefulness, alertness, a decreased sense of fatigue, elevation of mood, elation, and euphoria. There is also an increase in motor and speech activity and in physical and mental task performance. Amphetamine also stimulates the respiratory center and increases the rate and depth of respiration.

Overdosage or prolonged use of amphetamine is frequently followed by mental depression and fatigue. Many individuals taking amphetamine experience headache, palpitations, dizziness, vasomotor disturbance, agitation, confusion, dysphoria, apprehension, delirium, or fatigue. High doses can produce behavioral effects and may precipitate overt psychotic behavior.

Although tolerance develops to some of the CNS effects of amphetamine, namely, the euphorigenic, anorexiant, and hyperthermic actions, it does not develop to certain of the more toxic effects and a toxic psychosis may occur after weeks or months of continued use. If those who develop a psychosis resume use of amphetamine, they will have a lowered threshold during subsequent episodes (Innes and Nickerson 1975).

Phenylpropanolamine, though less centrally active than amphetamine, has nevertheless been cited in case reports as having caused nausea, tremors, dizziness, palpitations, seizures, anxiety, agitation, hallucinations, and psychotic reactions (Lee, Beilin, and Vandongen 1979; Norvenius, Widerlov, and Lonnerholm 1979). Paranoid psychosis has been reported after the use of nasal decongestants (Wharton 1970), and paranoia, homicidal behavior, and psychomotor seizures have been associated with phenylpropanolamine in a more recent case report (Cornelius, Soloff, and Reynolds 1984).

New acceptance has been given to the action of amphetamine as an MAO inhibitor. This action appears to depend on the substrate used in the assay (Clarke 1980; Daniels and Jorgenson 1982). Concurrent use of MAO inhibitors with indirectly acting sympathomimetic amines (including phenylpropanolamine) may lead to increased effects; this is especially important because there has been a growing clinical use of MAO inhibitors for their antidepressant activity. For example, there can be marked CNS stimulation and increased blood pressure after ingesting these drugs in combination (Smookler and Bermudez 1982).

In a three-phase, multisite study, Silverman et al. (1980) examined the effects of phenylpropanolamine when administered in low doses of 25 mg, either alone or in combination with 100 mg caffeine. The subjects were healthy males, ranging in age from 17 to 42. Since the researchers found that phenylpropanolamine produced no significant increase in systolic or diastolic blood pressure, they concluded that phenylpropanolamine is safe to use as an OTC anorexiant. One difficulty with such a study, however, is that healthy male subjects may be reluctant to report side effects spontaneously. Another difficulty with limiting the subject population to healthy males is that it precludes an examination of the effects of sex differences on drug metabolism and pharmacologic action. In addition, responses to medication among the elderly, which are different than the reactions of young people, cannot be considered in such a study.

An additional factor which may limit the applicability of the study is that the effects of only small amounts of phenylpropanolamine were examined. Some consumers of phenylpropanolamine in both legitimate and "look-alike" forms exceed recommended doses.

We conclude that because of the similarity of phenylpropanolamine to amphetamine and because of its CNS activity (at least in larger doses), it use should be carefully monitored to prevent abuse.

REFERENCES

Baez, L. A. 1974. Role of catecholamines in the anorectic effects of amphetamine in rats. Psychopharmacologia 35:91-98.

Biel, J. H. 1970. Structure-activity relationships of amphetamine and derivatives. In Amphetamines and related compounds, edited by E. Costa and S. Garattini, 3-19. New York: Raven Press.

Booth, D. A. 1968. Mechanism of action of norepinephrine in eliciting an eating response on injection into the rat hypothalamus. J Pharmacol Exp Ther 160:336-48.

Burgen, A.S.V. and L. L. Iverson. 1965. The inhibition of noradrenaline uptake by sympathomimetic amines in the rat isolated heart. Br J Pharmacol 25:34-49.

Caldwell, J., L. G. Dring, and R. T. Williams. 1972a. Metabolism of (^{14}C)methamphetamine in man, the guinea pig and the rat. Biochem J 129:11-22.

———. 1972b. Norephedrines as metabolites of (^{14}C)amphetamine in urine in man. Biochem J 129:23-24.

Clarke, D. E. 1980. Amphetamine and monoamine oxidase inhibition: an old idea gains new acceptance. TIPS 1:312.

Cornelius, J. R., P. H. Soloff, and C. F. Reynolds III. 1984. Paranoia, homicidal behavior, and seizures associated with phenylpropanolamine. Am J Psychiatry 141:120-21.

Daniels, T. C. and E. C. Jorgenson. 1982. In Textbook of organic medicinal and pharmaceutical chemistry, 8th ed., edited by R. F. Doerge, 386-87. Philadelphia: J. B. Lippincott.

Dietz, A. J. 1981. Amphetamine-like reactions to phenylpropanolamine. JAMA 245:601-2.

Duhault, J. et al. 1978. Brain serotonergic system and anorectic drugs. In Central mechanisms of anorectic drugs, edited by S. Garattini and R. Samanin, 205-15. New York: Raven Press.

Frewin, D. G., P. P. Leonello, and M. E. Frewin. 1978. Hypertension after ingestion of Trimolets. Med J Aust 2:497-98.

Goldman, H. W., D. Lehr, and E. Friedman. 1971. Antagonistic effects of alpha- and beta-adrenergic coded hypothalamic neurones on consummatory behaviour. Nature 231:453-55.

Grossman, S. P. 1964. Behavioral effects of direct chemical stimulation of central nervous system structures. Int J Neuropharmacol 3:45-58.

———. 1962. Direct adrenergic and cholinergic stimulation of hypothalamic mechanisms. Am J Physiol 202:872-82.

Hansen, M. G. and I. Q. Whishaw. 1973. The effects of 6-hydroxydopamine, dopamine, and dl-norepinephrine on food intake and water consumption, self-stimulation, temperature and electroencephalographic activity in the rat. Psychopharmacologia 29:33-44.

Heffner, T. G., M. J. Zigmond, and E. M. Stricker. 1977. Effects of dopaminergic agonists and antagonists on feeding in intact and 6-hydroxydopamine-treated rats. J Pharmacol Exp Ther 201:386-99.

Horowitz, J. D. et al. 1979. Hypertension and postural hypotension induced by phenylpropanolamine (Trimolets). Med J Aust 1:175-76.

Innes, I. R. and M. Nickerson. 1975. Norepinephrine, epinephrine, and the sympathomimetic amines. In The pharmacological basis of therapeutics, 5th ed., edited by L. S. Goodman and A. Gilman. New York: Macmillan.

Lee, K. Y., L. J. Beilin, and R. Vandongen. 1979. Severe hypertension after ingestion of an appetite suppressant (phenylpropanolamine) with indomethacin. Lancet 1:1110-11.

Leibowitz, S. F. 1978. Identification of catecholamine receptor mechanisms in the perifornical lateral hypothalamus and their role in mediating amphetamine and L-DOPA anorexia. In Central mechanisms of anorectic drugs, edited by S. Garattini and R. Samanin, 39-82. New York: Raven Press.

———. 1975. Ingestion in the satiated rat: role of alpha and beta receptors in mediating effects of hypothalamic adrenergic stimulation. Physiol Behav 14:743-54.

———. 1974. Paraventricular nucleus: a primary site mediating adrenergic feeding-elicitation. Paper presented at symposium, 45th annual meeting of the Eastern Psychological Association.

———. 1973. Brain norepinephrine and ingestive behaviour. In Frontiers in catecholamine research, edited by E. Usdin and S. H. Snyder, 711-13. Oxford: Pergamon Press.

———. 1971. Hypothalamic norepinephrine as an alpha- and beta-adrenergic neurotransmitter active in the regulation of hunger. Proceedings of the 79th annual convention of the American Psychological Association, 741-42.

———. 1970a. Hypothalamic beta-adrenergic "satiety" system antagonizes an alpha-adrenergic "hunger" system in the rat. Nature 226:963-64.

———. 1970b. Reciprocal hunger-relating circuits involving alpha- and beta-adrenergic receptors located, respectively, in the ventromedial and lateral hypothalamus. Proc Nat Acad Sci USA 67:1063-70.

Levitt, M., W. R. Cumiskey, and L. Shargel. 1974. Studies on the physiologic disposition and activity of phenylpropanolamines in the mouse. Drug Metab Dispos 2:187-93.

Livingston, P. H. 1966. Transient hypertension and phenylpropanolamine. Letter. JAMA 196:1159.

Norvenius, G., E. Widerlov, and G. Lonnerholm. 1979. Phenylpropanolamine and mental disturbance. Lancet 2:1367-68.

Offermeier, J. and H. G. DuPreez. 1978. Effects of anorectics on uptake and release of monoamines in synaptosomes. In Central mechanisms of anorectic drugs, edited by S. Garattini and R. Samanin, 217-31. New York: Raven Press.

Ostern, S. and W. H. Dodson. 1965. Hypertension following Ornade ingestion. Letter. JAMA 194:472.

Sanghvi, I. et al. 1975. Anorexigenic effects of d-amphetamine and L-DOPA in the rat. Pharmacol Biochem Behav 3:81-86.

Silverman, H. I. et al. 1980. Lack of side effects from orally administered phenylpropanolamine and phenylpropanolamine with caffeine: a controlled three-phase study. Current Therapeutic Research 28:185-194.

Sinsheimer, J. E., L. G. Dring, and R. T. Williams. 1973. Species differences in the metabolism of norephedrine in man, rabbit and rat. Biochem J 136:763-71.

Smookler, S. and A. J. Bermudez. 1982. Hypertensive crisis resulting from an MAO inhibitor and an over-the-counter appetite suppressant. Ann Emerg Med 11:482-84.

Sulser, F. et al. 1968. The relative role of storage and synthesis of brain norepinephrine in the psychomotor stimulation evoked by amphetamine or by desipramine and tetrabenazine. Psychopharmacologia 12:322-32.

Vree, T. B., A. T. Muskens, and J. M. van Rossum. 1969. Some physicochemical properties of amphetamine and related drugs. J Pharm Pharmacol 21:774-75.

Weiner, N. 1980. Norepinephrine, epinephrine, and the sympathomimetic amines. In The pharmacological basis of therapeutics, 6th ed., edited by A. G. Gilman, L. S. Goodman, and A. Gilman, 141-44. New York: Macmillan.

Weissman, A., B. K. Koe, and S. S. Tenen. 1966. Antiamphetamine effects following inhibition of tyrosine hydroxylase. J Pharmacol Exp Ther 151:339-52.

Wharton, B. K. 1970. Nasal decongestants and paranoid psychosis. Br J Psychiatry 117:439-40.

19

QUANTITATIVE ASSESSMENT OF MOOD AND BEHAVIORAL REINFORCING EFFECT OF PHENYLPROPANOLAMINE

George E. Bigelow

INTRODUCTION

As discussed elsewhere in this volume, phenylpropanolamine (PPA) is a widely employed phenylethylamine, structurally related to amphetamine. Although phenylpropanolamine has been on the market as an over-the-counter product for over 40 years, it is only recently that the question has arisen as to whether it might produce some degree of amphetamine-like mood and behavioral effects--effects which might lead to its abuse.

This concern exists for two major reasons: first, phenylpropanolamine's structural similarity to amphetamine, a known drug of abuse; and second, the inclusion of phenylpropanolamine in the so-called amphetamine "look-alike" products which have been advertised and marketed in ways which would promote their use as central nervous system (CNS) stimulants.

The purpose of the present paper is to review the available experimental data concerning whether phenylpropanolamine produces an amphetamine-like profile of mood and behavioral effects. Specifically, does phenylpropanolamine produce behavior-reinforcing, euphoria-producing, performance-enhancing, or mood-elevating effects which might lead to or sustain its self-administration or use/abuse as a CNS stimulant?

Discussion will be limited to controlled laboratory experiments. Such experiments have been conducted both with animals and with humans. In each case the general procedures that have been developed and used to assess the relative abuse liabilities of the various phenylethylamines will first be considered; then what has been learned concerning phenylpropanolamine using these procedures will be reviewed.

METHODS FOR TESTING ABUSE LIABILITY OF COMPOUNDS IN ANIMAL SUBJECTS

Among the most effective preclinical procedures for assessing drug abuse liability is the animal drug self-administration methodology. Typically in these studies, animals are fitted with indwelling venous catheters for drug administration and operant behavioral procedures are used to place operation of the drug infusion apparatus under the subjects' control. An extensive literature has documented the validity of this animal drug self-administration model for assessing abuse liability and for classifying drugs with respect to their behavior-reinforcing efficacy (Griffiths, Bigelow, and Henningfield 1980). In general, the drugs that sustain self-administration by animals are the same drugs which are self-administered and abused by humans.

Johns Hopkins Medical School Studies

At least two laboratories have examined the effectiveness of phenylpropanolamine in functioning as a reinforcer and in sustaining drug self-administration in animal subjects. At Johns Hopkins Medical School, a drug substitution procedure was used in which primates were trained to self-administer a standard dose of cocaine. Test doses of various CNS stimulant/anorexiant drugs were then substituted for the cocaine to assess the drugs' effectiveness in sustaining continued drug self-administration behavior (Griffiths, Brady, and Snell 1978). Investigators compared the effects of cocaine and of eight phenylethylamines in terms of which dosage levels would sustain drug self-administration and which would suppress food intake (table 19.1).

The reinforcing dose referred to in table 19.1 is the lowest dose which sustained drug self-administration above saline control levels, and the anorexiant dose is the lowest dose which suppressed food intake 50% below saline control levels. The anorexiant/reinforcing ratio is obtained by dividing the anorexiant dose by the reinforcing dose. This ratio represents the number of multiples of the reinforcing dose required to achieve a 50% reduction in food intake; the higher the ratio, the greater the presumed likelihood that the drug will be abused. The relative ratio expresses the same anorexiant/reinforcing ratio relationship, but the relative ratio for (+)-amphetamine has been arbitrarily assigned the value of 1 and all other ratios are expressed as multiples of that value. The reinforcing dose of drugs which were not found to sustain drug self-administration is assumed to be infinite.

TABLE 19.1

Reinforcing efficacies, anorexiant doses, and anorexiant/reinforcing ratios of phenylethylamines and cocaine

Drug	Reinforcing dose (mg/kg)	Anorexiant dose (mg/kg)	Ratio	Relative ratio
Cocaine	0.03	16.0	533.3	14.81
Diethylpropion	0.5	22.0	44.0	1.22
(+)-Amphetamine	0.05	1.8	36.0	1.00
Phenmetrazine	0.5	7.4	14.8	0.41
Chlorphentermine	2.5	20.3	8.1	0.23
Phentermine	0.5	3.7	7.4	0.21
Clortermine	3.0	21.0	7.0	0.19
Fenfluramine	infinite	7.0	0	0
Phenylpropanloamine	infinite	48.1	0	0

Source: Adapted from Griffiths, R. R., J. V. Brady, and J. D. Snell. 1978. Relationship between anorectic and reinforcing properties of appetite suppressant drugs: implications for assessment of abuse liability. Biol Psychiatry 13:285. Reprinted with permission.

There are several points to be noted in these data. First, many of the phenylethylamines—especially those with significant CNS stimulant effects and known abuse liability, such as (+)-amphetamine, phenmetrazine, and diethylpropion—function as reinforcers which sustain drug self-administration by these animal subjects. Second, cocaine, a CNS stimulant compound of high abuse liability which is not used clinically as an anorexiant, has a much higher anorexiant/reinforcing ratio than any of the phenylethylamine anorexiants. Third, the phenylethylamine anorexiants themselves are widely distributed along the anorexiant/reinforcing ratio continuum, suggesting a considerable variability among these compounds with respect to the likelihood that clinical use might involve exposing individuals to reinforcing dose levels of the drug. Fourth, two of the tested phenylethylamines (fenfluramine and phenylpropanolamine) failed to function as reinforcers and did not sustain drug self-administration behavior at any of the doses tested. Fifth, because neither fenfluramine nor phenylpropanolamine function as reinforcers at any dose tested and because they are effective in suppressing food intake, they would appear to be effective anorexiant agents with minimal risk of drug abuse.

University of Chicago Studies

Independent animal experimental studies at the University of Chicago have also indicated that the profile of effects of phenylpropanolamine is distinct from that of amphetamine (Johanson 1984). Investigators used a substitution drug self-administration procedure similar to that of the Johns Hopkins laboratories and corroborated that phenylpropanolamine fails to sustain drug self-administration behavior. In addition, using a drug discrimination procedure in which subjects were trained to make a specific response when administered amphetamine, they tested a range of doses of various CNS stimulant and anorexiant compounds to assess their stimulus similarity to amphetamine. They concluded that phenylpropanolamine did not produce an amphetamine-like profile of subjective effects in the animals tested.

METHODS FOR TESTING ABUSE LIABILITY OF COMPOUNDS IN HUMAN SUBJECTS

Historically, the primary clinical experimental procedures for assessing the potential abuse liability of test compounds have been those developed by the U.S. Public Health Service's Addiction Research Center, which is now an intramural laboratory of the National Institute on Drug Abuse. The core of those procedures is to determine the profile of acute subjective, behavioral, and physiological effects of a range of doses of a test compound in comparison to a standard reference compound of known high abuse liability. The standard reference drug used to measure stimulant/anorexiant compounds has typically been (+)-amphetamine.

The assumption has been that drugs having a profile of effects similar to that of (+)-amphetamine, and especially those having dose-effect functions parallel to those of (+)-amphetamine, will have a potential for abuse similar to that of amphetamine. In general, experimental results have supported the validity of this assumption.

Addiction Research Center Evaluations

The Addiction Research Center methodology has been applied to the clinical evaluation of a number of sympathomimetics and anorexiants. Martin et al. (1971) studied (+)-amphetamine, (+)-methamphetamine (-)-ephedrine, phenmetrazine, and methylphenidate and concluded that all of these compounds had similar effects on blood pressure, respiration, and subjective effects measures. Since then, a number of phenylethylamine anorexiants have been studied using this procedure. Jasinski, Nutt, and Griffith (1974) used both oral and parenteral routes of administration to compare diethylpropion and (+)-amphetamine. They found that the two drugs generally had similar effects, with parallel dose-effect functions. They also observed, however, that diethylpropion was less potent when administered parenterally than orally and concluded that this relatively low parenteral efficacy might result in a lower abuse liability for diethylpropion than for (+)-amphetamine.

Subsequent clinical research from the Addiction Research Center has identified several phenylethylamine anorexiants which appear to have considerably lower abuse liability than (+)-amphetamine, as indicated by their profiles of acute effects being distinctively different from that of (+)-amphetamine. Griffith, Nutt, and Jasinski (1975) compared fenfluramine with (+)-amphetamine and concluded that the two had qualitatively dissimilar profiles of effects, with fenfluramine's being characterized by dysphoria and sedation. A similar conclusion was reached concerning chlorphentermine compared to (+)-amphetamine (Jasinski et al. 1975). Neither fenfluramine nor chlorphentermine produced dose-effect functions parallel to those of (+)-amphetamine.

Unfortunately, the Addiction Research Center has not used its standardized assessment procedures to evaluate phenylpropanolamine. The relevance of the above-described Addiction Research Center evaluations to a consideration of phenylpropanolamine is twofold: first, they demonstrate that the phenylethylamine anorexiants are a pharmacodynamically diverse group of compounds which may or may not produce amphetamine-like profiles of effects; and second, they demonstrate the utility of certain specific experimental measures in differentiating among phenylethylamines with differing profiles of effects.

Addiction Research Center Inventory Evaluations

Some of the experimental measures developed by the Addiction Research Center, most notably the Addiction Research Center Inventory (ARCI) subjective effects scales, has been adapted and utilized by other laboratories to assess phenylpropanolamine.

The ARCI consists of a group of true/false questions about subjective experiences; a number of specific scoring scales have been empirically derived as characterizing the effects produced by various drugs or drug classes (Haertzen 1974). The profiles of drug effects produced on these scales have proven to be among the most sensitive and discriminating indices for identifying drugs which produce amphetamine-like subjective effects and possess amphetamine-like abuse liability. A commonly used version of the ARCI, which provides scores on five scales, has been described by Martin et al. (1971). The Morphine-Benzedrine Group (MBG) scale is characterized as a "euphoria" scale; elevations on this score are generally associated with increased abuse liability. The Pentobarbital-Chlorpromazine-Alcohol Group (PCAG) scale is characterized as a "sedation" scale. The Lysergic Acid Diethylamide (LSD) scale is characterized as a "dysphoria" scale sensitive to unpleasant and unusual drug effects such as those produced by LSD. The Amphetamine (A) scale and the Benzedrine Group (BG) scale are both sensitive to amphetamine-like effects.

Thompson Medical Company, a marketer of phenylpropanolamine, has sponsored recent studies at several different laboratories to assess the effects on the ARCI of clinical dose levels of phenylpropanolamine. These studies used a parallel groups, double-blind design in which normal volunteers were randomly assigned to one of three drug treatment conditions: (1) 25 mg phenylpropanolamine administered three times, at four-hour intervals; (2) 75 mg sustained-release phenylpropanolamine; or (3) placebo. Subjects participated in a single 12-hour session, with ARCI measures collected prior to drug administration and repeatedly during the 12 hours. The laboratory at Johns Hopkins is one of three which have conducted this study; each laboratory enrolled approximately 50 subjects into each of the three study conditions. Analyses of the data from the three sites have found no statistically significant differences in mood effects attributable to the different drug assignment conditions on any of the five scales of the ARCI (Funderburk 1984).

The laboratory at Johns Hopkins has also conducted a crossover study comparing placebo and 75 mg sustained-release phenylpropanolamine. The general procedure was the same as that used in the parallel groups studies described above, but the 59 subjects each participated in two 12-hour sessions, with counterbalanced order of exposure to the two drug conditions. This crossover design is a more sensitive test than the parallel groups design. Also included in this study were visual analog scale measures of subjective drug liking, overall magnitude of drug effect, and "good" and "bad" drug effects. No significant drug treatment effects were found on any of the visual analog scales. Drug treatment did significantly affect two of the ARCI scales: both the PCAG (sedation) score and the LSD (dysphoria) score were significantly reduced in subjects receiving 75 mg sustained-release phenylpropanolamine. None of the scores on ARCI scales reflecting amphetamine-like abuse liability were elevated (Liebson et al. 1984). These data are interpreted as not only indicating a modest mood-elevating effect of phenylpropanolamine--possibly an anti-fatigue or anti-boredom effect during these long and unstimulating experimental sessions--but also as suggesting that phenylpropanolamine lacks significant amphetamine-like subjective effects of the type associated with CNS stimulant abuse liability.

However, it should be noted that these applications of the ARCI subjective effects evaluation to studies of phenylpropanolamine have occurred in contexts quite different from those in which the ARCI was developed and validated. The original Addiction Research Center procedures involved using experienced drug abusers as subjects and administering a range of doses which, at its maximum, exceeded by several multiples typical therapeutic dose levels. Such studies leave unanswered the question whether the ARCI can be considered a valid assessment instrument when applied to normal, nondrug abuser populations who receive only therapeutic level drug dosages. Available data suggest that it is. Most relevant to this issue is a study by Johanson and Uhlenhuth (1982), who used the ARCI in a comparison of placebo and therapeutic dose levels of (+)-amphetamine (5 mg) and fenfluramine (20 mg) in normal volunteers. They found that the MBG, A, and BG scores on the ARCI (i.e., the three scales sensitive to amphetamine-like abuse liability) were all significantly elevated by the 5 mg (+)-amphetamine treatment but not by the fenfluramine or placebo treatments.

Thus, it does appear that the ARCI is an adequately drug-sensitive instrument even when applied to normal populations receiving modest dose levels.

CLINICAL DRUG SELF-ADMINISTRATION STUDIES

One way to assess whether a test compound produces a profile of effects likely to lead to its self-administration and abuse is to test directly whether it will sustain drug self-administration by human subjects. Two research groups have been using this approach in assessment of the phenylethylamines, including phenylpropanolamine.

Johns Hopkins Studies

My colleagues and I have been working with a population of overweight women who participate in clinical studies of phenylethylamines while part of a weight control treatment program. In the first of these studies (Bigelow et al. 1980), participants were randomly assigned to one of three treatment conditions ((+)-amphetamine, 5 mg; fenfluramine, 20 mg; or placebo) in a procedure which allowed subjects a degree of control over the number of capsules taken each day. Sensitivity of the procedure to pharmacological reinforcement effects was illustrated by the fact that patients' self-administration of (+)-amphetamine was sustained above placebo levels, while their self-administration of fenfluramine (an equi-efficacious anorexiant, but one producing some dysphoric effects) was suppressed below placebo levels.

In subsequent studies we used a within-subject, choice procedure in which patients were initially exposed for one week to each of two different medications and were subsequently permitted to choose which of the two medications they preferred to receive next. Using this choice procedure (Bigelow et al. 1982), we reported that (+)-amphetamine was preferred over fenfluramine and that diethylpropion was preferred over chlorphentermine. In a later publication (Bigelow et al. 1985), we presented data from a series of three separate experiments, each of which used this choice procedure and compared placebo to one of the phenylethylamine anorexiants, either diethylpropion, chlorphentermine, or phenylpropanolamine. Figure 19.1 shows the mean percentage of choice occasions that each active drug was chosen in preference to placebo. Patients' self-administration of diethylpropion was sustained at a level significantly above placebo, self-administration of chlorphentermine was suppressed significantly below placebo, and self-administration of phenylpropanolamine did not differ from placebo. These data illustrate the sensitivity of this clinical drug choice procedure to the reinforcing efficacies of these three phenylethylamines and are compatible with other data concerning the relative reinforcing efficacies and abuse liabilities of these compounds.

FIGURE 19.1

Choice comparisons of three phenethylamines and placebo

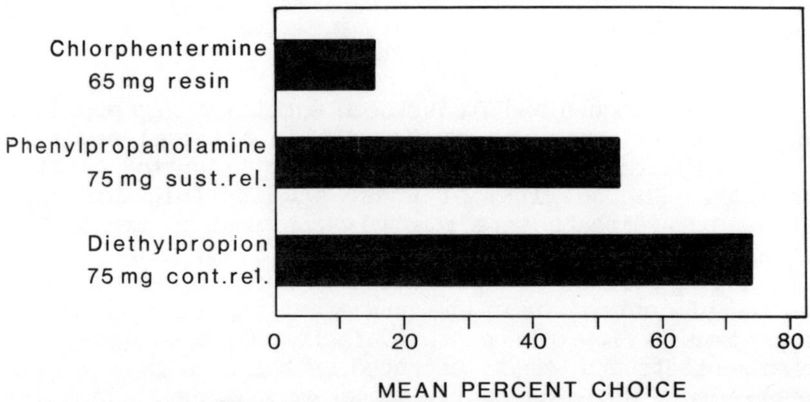

Source: Bigelow, G. E. et al. 1985. Progress report from the Division of Behavioral Biology, the Johns Hopkins University School of Medicine. In Problems of drug dependence, 1984, edited by L. S. Harris, National Institute on Drug Abuse research monograph series. Washington, D.C.: U.S. Government Printing Office.

Additional data concerning the above-mentioned choice comparison of placebo and 75 mg sustained-release phenylpropanolamine are included in another report (Bigelow et al. 1984). The lack of differentiation between the two with respect to self-administration preference was accompanied by equivalent subjective ratings of drug-liking for phenylpropanolamine and for placebo. Interestingly, despite the similarity between phenylpropanolamine and placebo on these behavioral and subjective indices of abuse liability, other data indicated that phenylpropanolamine was an effective anorexiant and that it did produce significant mood-enhancing effects. Specifically, weight loss was significantly greater during phenylpropanolamine treatment, and subjective measures on the Profile of Mood States showed reduced scores on Total Mood Disturbance, Fatigue-Inertia, and Depression-Dejection scales and increased scores on the Vigor-Activity scale following one week of phenylpropanolamine treatment; no significant mood effects were seen after only a single day of phenylpropanolamine treatment, however. The failure of phenylpropanolamine to maintain self-administration above placebo levels is especially noteworthy since in this experiment it also produced significantly greater weight loss and mood enhancement.

Johanson and her colleagues have used a similar choice procedure to evaluate the reinforcing efficacies and subjective effects of various drugs in human volunteers. Their studies are conducted in a purely experimental setting using normal volunteers (typically, college students) who report to the laboratory three times per week to ingest a color-coded drug dose. Following two exposures to each of the two alternatives, subjects are permitted for the next five sessions to choose which drug they prefer to receive. Johanson and Uhlenhuth (1980) compared (+)-amphetamine (5 mg) to placebo and found that (+)-amphetamine was selected on an average of 81% of occasions; they also found (+)-amphetamine to produce significant elevations on the Vigor, Elation, Friendliness, Arousal, and Positive Mood scores of the Profile of Mood States. The sensitivity of this clinical drug choice procedure to the reinforcing effects of amphetamine has been replicated several times (Johanson and Uhlenhuth 1982; Johanson, Kilgore, and Uhlenhuth 1983).

Chait, Uhlenhuth, and Johanson (1984) have reported application of this same drug choice procedure to an evaluation of phenylpropanolamine relative to placebo and have found that, in this context, preference for phenylpropanolamine does not differ from that for placebo.

CONCLUSION

The research reviewed above can be summarized as follows:

1. Phenylpropanolamine is not self-administered by animals in preclinical testing designed to assess drug abuse potential.
2. Phenylpropanolamine does not produce a profile of acute subjective effects similar to amphetamine in clinical testing designed to assess drug abuse potential.

3. Phenylpropanolamine is not chosen and self-administered in preference to placebo in clinical drug self-administration trials.

4. Phenylpropanolamine does produce modest mood-elevating or mood-enhancing effects which are detected under some clinical testing conditions.

Thus, overall these data would indicate that phenylpropanolamine is a compound of low abuse liability which does not produce an amphetamine-like profile of effects.

There remain, however, several areas in which additional research is needed. First, systematic dose-effect evaluations of phenylpropanolamine instead of the more common single-dose studies would be desirable. Such data would certainly aid our understanding of the clinical significance of the mood effects of phenylpropanolamine. Second, phenylpropanolamine should be assessed in a sleep-deprivation or fatigue situation since it is in such a fatigue setting that amphetamine-like, performance-enhancing effects are most readily detected. Third, since phenylpropanolamine has been widely marketed in combination with caffeine, it would be very useful to conduct studies comparing the behavioral, subjective, and physiological effects of phenylpropanolamine/caffeine combinations versus those of caffeine alone.

REFERENCES

Bigelow, G. E. et al. 1985. Progress report from the Division of Behavioral Biology, the Johns Hopkins University School of Medicine. In _Problems of drug dependence, 1984_, edited by L. S. Harris, National Institute on Drug Abuse research monograph series. Washington, D.C.: U.S. Government Printing Office.

Bigelow, G. E. et al. 1984. Assessment of phenylpropanolamine (PPA) abuse risk in weight control patients. _Fed Proc_ 43:571.

Bigelow, G. E. et al. 1982. Anorectic self-administration and preference during weight control treatment. Paper presented at the annual meeting of the American Psychological Association. Washington, D.C. August.

Bigelow, G. E. et al. 1980. Double-blind evaluation of reinforcing and anorectic actions of weight control medications. _Arch Gen Psychiatry_ 37:1118-23.

Chait, L. D., E. H. Uhlenhuth, and C. E. Johanson. 1984. Drug preference and mood in humans: mazindol and phenylpropanolamine. In Problems of drug dependence, edited by L. S. Harris, 327-28, National Institute on Drug Abuse research monograph series. Washington, D.C.: U.S. Government Printing Office.

Funderburk, F. 1984. Telephone conversation with author. June.

Griffith, J. D., J. G. Nutt, and D. R. Jasinski. 1975. A comparison of fenfluramine and amphetamine in man. Clin Pharmacol Ther 18:563-70.

Griffiths, R. R., G. E. Bigelow, and J. E. Henningfield. 1980. Similarities in animal and human drug-taking behavior. In Advances in substance abuse: behavioral and biological research, edited by N. K. Mello, 1-90. Greenwich, CT: JAI Press.

Griffiths, R. R., J. V. Brady, and J. D. Snell. 1978. Relationship between anorectic and reinforcing properties of appetite suppressant drugs: implications for assessment of abuse liability. Biol Psychiatry 13: 283-90.

Haertzen, C. A. 1974. An overview of Addiction Research Center Inventory (ARCI): an appendix and manual of scales. DHEW Publication No (ADM) 74-92. Washington, D.C.: U.S. Government Printing Office.

Jasinski, D. R. et al. 1975. Progress report on studies from the Clinical Pharmacology section of the Addiction Research Center. Committee on Problems of Drug Dependence. Washington, D.C.: National Academy of Sciences, National Research Council.

Jasinski, D. R., J. G. Nutt, and J. D. Griffith. 1974. Effects of diethylpropion and d-amphetamine after subcutaneous and oral administration. Clin Pharmacol Ther 16:645-52.

Johanson, C. E. 1984. Telephone coversation with author. June.

Johanson, C. E., K. Kilgore, and E. H. Uhlenhuth. 1983. Assessment of dependence potential of drugs in humans using multiple indices. Psychopharmacology 81:144-49.

Johanson, C. E. and E. H. Uhlenhuth. 1982. Drug preferences in humans. Fed Proc 41:228-33.

———. 1980. Drug preference and mood in humans: d-amphetamine. Psychopharamcology. 71:275-79.

Liebson, I. et al. 1982. An evaluation of the acute effects of phenylpropanolamine in normal volunteers: crossover design. Unpublished manuscript. Baltimore: Johns Hopkins University School of Medicine.

Martin, W. R. et al. 1971. Physiologic, subjective, and behavioral effects of amphetamine, methamphetamine, ephedrine, phenmetrazine, and methylphenidate in man. Clin Pharmacol Ther 12:245-58.

C. DOES PHENYLPROPANOLAMINE HAVE SIGNIFICANT ABUSE LIABILITY?

20

LOOK-ALIKE DRUGS AND DRUGS OF DECEPTION: EPIDEMIOLOGICAL, TOXICOLOGICAL, AND CLINICAL CONSIDERATIONS

David E. Smith

INTRODUCTION

Public concern about the toxic effects of over-the-counter (OTC) compounds containing phenylpropanolamine (PPA), particularly diet aid products, has paralleled broader concern over misuse, especially by adolescents and young adults, of "look-alike" drugs that sometimes contain phenylpropanolamine. Some consumer groups have attempted to equate the two phenomena. For example, the Center for Science in the Public Interest (CSPI) recently issued a press release stating, "Popular diet drugs containing phenylpropanolamine (PPA) have been linked with at least 17 cases of strokes and seizures among previously healthy dieters." According to CSPI's Dr. Bambi Batts Young, "These cases add to the already disturbing record of dangerous blood-pressure increases following PPA use." Citing as examples "half a dozen published medical reports describing phenylpropanolamine consumers who developed such high blood pressure as to risk life-threatening damage to the brain," she concluded, "The weight of the evidence has now grown so great that to dismiss it as coincidence would be reckless . . . ." Dr. Young also "warned that the drug could prove particularly hazardous for the estimated 30% of overweight Americans who already have serious high blood pressure." Thus, she recommended that, "Under the circumstances, nothing short of a ban on all OTC PPA-diet products will be sufficient to protect the consumer." The press release also contained a statement by Rep. Mary Rose Oakar (D-Ohio): "I see no reason why a teenager wanting to get high wouldn't simply turn to the large number of PPA diet products that are freely available in drug stores and supermarkets." (Center for Science in the Public Interest. 1984. Reprinted with permission.)

Banning a drug is more complex than it might appear, however, particularly when the targeted compound is as widely used as phenylpropanolamine, which is a major ingredient in OTC cough/cold and diet aid preparations. Before the desirability or even the practicality of banning phenylpropanolamine can be determined, several important issues should be considered. First, the therapeutic ratio of the drug must be examined, its therapeutic effectiveness weighed against its potential hazards. Millions of doses of phenylpropanolamine-containing compounds are taken on a regular basis by U.S. consumers, but only a tiny percentage of its users have experienced toxic side effects. A second consideration is that requiring a prescription to obtain a product currently available over-the-counter would contribute additional expense to the already high cost of health care. In addition, government regulatory agencies are often reluctant to ban therapeutically effective drugs, and the self-health care movement also frequently resists attempts to bring drugs under prescription control, since doing so would require a visit to the doctor to manage even the most minor of symptoms.

Yet even if all these obstacles were overcome, the goal of banning a medicinal might still not be achieved. A more effective tactic would instead be to alert those involved in drug abuse treatment that a large number of teenagers were diverting OTC compounds and abusing them. If such a belief could be established as true, then it would be simple to mobilize families, communities, and government regulatory agencies to deal with a "new drug abuse epidemic." In fact, the consumer groups seeking a ban on OTC phenylpropanolamine products who have raised such a specter of a teenage drug abuse epidemic have conducted no systematic studies of look-alike drug misuse and abuse, nor do they have an overview of the epidemiological, toxicological, and clinical issues regarding look-alikes in the United States.

The purpose of this paper is to help provide such an overview, to describe the look-alike drug phenomenon, including look-alike stimulants that contain phenylpropanolamine, and to examine whether the abuse of look-alikes justifies the banning of OTC products containing phenylpropanolamine.

A look-alike drug may be defined as a psychoactive preparation which is designed to resemble, in effects, appearance, or name, a powerful, often controlled psychoactive drug, but instead contains a completely different substance (or substances) which is usually neither a controlled nor a prescription drug. Some look-alikes may be accurately labeled, although not often at the point of final sale.

Others are clearly "drugs of deception," which are counterfeited to represent desired psychoactive drugs (e.g., Quaalude®), but actually contain another drug or combination of drugs (e.g., diazepam or doxylamine). They may even bear accurate manufacturers' names and logos, although on close inspection most will fail to replicate the product exactly. The substituted drugs usually have similar but less psychoactive effects and are available at a lower cost. As stressed by Morgan et al. (1984), "This is not just a cutting or dilution of a drug with an inactive substance which is so common as to be expected in an illicit marketplace."

Attempts to establish operative definitions for look-alikes and drugs of deception are of more than minor interest, because in recent years the look-alike drug phenomenon has become a major drug abuse issue in the United States. Yet it has been difficult to develop precise operational definitions and this has complicated the already arduous task of evaluating the epidemiological, toxicological, and clinical significance of look-alikes in the shifting drug culture. Moreover, the lack of consistent and accurate data resulting in part from imprecise analysis has introduced confusion into the legislative, law enforcement, medical, and drug treatment communities. In attempting to address some of these problems, the Haight-Ashbury Training and Education Project in association with the Haight-Ashbury Free Medical Clinic formed the Look-Alike Drug Research and Training Project.

The issue of fake or counterfeit medication is not new, but emerged simultaneously with the growth of the pharmaceutical industry in the 1940s. Black market medicine laboratories also were not new but they began to appear in greater numbers. They counterfeited legitimate pharmaceuticals and sold them profitably, even in the wholesale marketplace. Amphetamine products, for a variety of complicated reasons outlined by Morgan and Kagan (1979), became the most popular of the psychoactive counterfeits.

In the late 1960s, diversion of legitimately manufactured amphetamine escalated and contributed to the dimensions of the current problem (Ibid.). Increased use of pharmaceutical amphetamine and related stimulants helped to establish a social and cultural marketplace in which the appearance of a look-alike drug became one of its most important identifying characteristics. Both sellers and users came to rely on capsule shapes and colors, trademarks, and logos to assist them in buying, selling, and using such substances. For example, the legitimately manufactured Biphetamine®, when diverted to the drug culture, was identified by the markings and other characteristics of its capsule and was labeled "black beauty" by its users.

The look-alike explosion (Stock 1982a, 1982b; Morgan et al. 1984) did not really begin, however, until the passage of the Controlled Substances Act of 1970, when amphetamine production in the United States was slashed by almost 90%. In 1971, production of pharmaceutical amphetamines and related substances exceeded 30,000 kg. By 1980, less than 2 million prescriptions (supplied by 3,000 kg) for these drugs were processed in U.S. pharmacies.

It appears that illicit consumer demand for stimulants was easily diverted to the look-alikes when legitimate production and diversion were substantially reduced. A large consumer market for stimulants had been created with its own cultural definitions and identifying characteristics. Supply reduction alone could not resolve the problem. Clearly, the expansion of look-alikes occurred as a consequence of this vacuum. At the present time, the vast majority of products sold as amphetamine in the drug culture are not true amphetamine, but are really look-alikes (Morgan and Kagan 1979). The increased popularity of illicit cocaine and the development of legally produced cocaine look-alikes have also paralleled and aggravated the overall stimulant abuse problem.

The look-alike phenomenon represents, of course, more than consumer fraud and deception. It also introduces error and confusion into epidemiological, toxicological, and clinical analyses. For example, an individual who, after taking a look-alike drug mistakenly believed to be amphetamine, becomes ill or frightened and goes to an emergency room for treatment may atribute the problems to the drug, as may the emergency physician. A report of a case of amphetamine abuse will then be entered into one of the national data collection systems, such as the Drug Abuse Warning Network (DAWN), decreasing the reliability and accuracy of such systems (Ungerleider 1981).

The Look-Alike Drug Research and Training Project has found that, although look-alike drug experimentation is almost unheard of in some parts of the United States, concern over the look-alike drug problem has rapidly escalated in other areas. Much of the concern comes from school officials who are worried that the use of these substances may provide an introduction into the drug culture. Some adolescents, for example, learn to sell black beauties obtained by the thousands from "legitimate mail order houses" and derive profit from such sale. The economic and human costs associated with such early introduction to using and dealing in the drug culture are hard to quantify. It is also very difficult to assess the social and individual costs of the look-alike drug phenomenon since the ingredients contained in many of the compounds are of lower abuse potential than the alleged substances; relatively little clinical documentation of significant drug dependence, abuse, or toxicity exists at the present time. In order to more accurately determine the dangers associated with the look-alike phenomenon and to facilitate appropriate legislation, prevention training, and treatment activity, it is necessary to first assess the true toxicity of the look-alike drugs and drugs of deception by examining the clinical experience and research findings regarding them.

AN ANALYSIS OF LOOK-ALIKE TOXICITY IN A DRUG-AWARE COHORT

Much of the look-alike clinical analysis has been done by the Haight-Ashbury Free Medical Clinic Drug Detoxification and Aftercare Project, where approximately 125 drug-dependent individuals are treated on an outpatient basis each day. Approximately 50% of this population are involved with opiates, 30% with stimulants, and 20% with sedative/hypnotics, including alcohol. Approximately 10% have at some time used a look-alike drug, but only a very small percentage use them regularly, since they perceive look-alike stimulants as being weak and relatively ineffective. Adolescents are the primary users of look-alikes, especially of look-alike stimulants, which are usually taken when a more powerful stimulant such as amphetamine or cocaine cannot be located. Look-alikes may also be consumed by individuals who lack the experience to differentiate between a desired stimulant and a corresponding look-alike.

We have interviewed 100 individuals who use look-alike stimulants on a regular basis, and, although occasional anxiety reactions coupled with tachycardia and mild elevation of blood pressure have been reported, we have not seen a look-alike stimulant psychosis of the type associated with amphetamine or cocaine. We have identified 20 individuals who use look-alike stimulants in an upper/downer pattern to help counteract the effects of alcohol or other sedative/hypnotics such as barbiturates or street Quaalude® (usually counterfeit). In these situations, the individuals may take black beauties to facilitate performance during the day and then calm down with alcohol or other sedative/hypnotics at night. However, none of these dependence patterns involved OTC diet aid or cough/cold products containing phenylpropanolamine, which is viewed as a particularly weak stimulant and ranks very low on the drug preference scale of the drug culture. In fact, when one 18-year-old was asked whether he preferred black beauties obtained in the drug culture or OTC products containing phenylpropanolamine from the drugstore, he responded, "Maybe the black beauty will be the real thing. I know the stuff in the drugstore is not."

Dougherty (1982) has reported on drug use by adolescents and young adults, ages 13 to 25, in the central New York State area. He found that the three drugs most commonly abused were alcohol, marihuana, and "pseudospeed." Pseudospeed is his term for what is known in other regions of the United States as street speed or fake speed and refers to capsules and tablets containing various combinations of phenylpropanolamine, caffeine, and ephedrine. Dougherty estimated the street price of pseudospeed to be between one and three dollars per dose, somewhat higher than the price in the San Francisco Bay Area, which averages 50 cents to one dollar for a capsule of street speed. In comparison, a true amphetamine currently sells for approximately three dollars in the San Francisco Bay Area; this represents a significant decrease in amphetamine street pricing and reflects the availability of inexpensive counterfeit products.

Dougherty described teenagers swallowing five to six tablets of pseudospeed because they thought that the product, when combined with alcohol, would yield a stimulant rush which would be almost enough to produce an adequate high. In addition, some subjects in their early 20s used pseudospeed to facilitate performance in work settings in a way similar to the previous use of amphetamine. Dougherty attributed relatively little toxicity to this pattern of abuse, but speculated that a naive user might encounter greater toxicity if he happened to ingest true amphetamine.

It is interesting that the people using pseudospeed in the central New York area, relatively unsophisticated adolescents and young adults taking the drug to stimulate work performance, were similar to street speed consumers in the San Francisco Bay Area. In discussions with Dougherty (1984), another interesting similarity in the drug use patterns of the two populations was revealed. When the Food and Drug Administration (FDA) banned both the triple combination (phenylpropanolamine, caffeine, and ephedrine) and, more recently, the double combination (phenylpropanolamine and caffeine), some users tried phenylpropanolamine products alone. Users in both the San Francisco and New York groups found phenylpropanolamine alone to be ineffective and some would purchase OTC caffeine tablets to combine with phenylpropanolamine. This is especially noteworthy since a growing body of clinical evidence indicates that the effect of caffeine may be important to both the toxicity and dependence attributed to look-alike stimulants.

LOOK-ALIKE STIMULANTS

A majority of the recent look-alike stimulants contain phenylpropanolamine and caffeine, or phenylpropanolamine, caffeine, and ephedrine, although FDA restrictions have reduced the supply of double and triple combinations. These substances are manufactured to closely resemble amphetamine, but do not exactly duplicate the markings of controlled prescription psychoactive drugs. Allen (1982) has compiled a list of the street names of controlled stimulant drugs (table 20.1); the names of the corresponding look-alikes are similar to the street terms.

TABLE 20.1

Street names for controlled stimulant drugs

Controlled drug	Street names
Biphetamine® 20	Black Mollies, Dex, Dexies, Blacks, Speed, Black Beauties
Ianamin® 30	Yellows
Dexamyl® tablets	Greenhearts, 93s, Dex, Greens
Dexamyl® spansules	Green & Whites, Christmas Trees
Benzedrine® tablets	Orange Hearts, 92s, Oranges, Hearts, Peaches, Roses
Dexedrine® spansules	Uppers, Browns, Browns & Clears
Preludin®	Oranges, Sweeties
Adipex-P® tablets	Bird's Eggs, Robin's Eggs
Statobex® tablets	Bird's Eggs, Robin's Eggs

Source: Adapted from Allen, L. V., Jr. 1982. "Turkey drugs"--what you see is not what you get. U.S. Pharmacist 7:30. Reprinted with permission.

The more powerful the controlled substance, the more popular the look-alike designed to resemble it will be. Thus, even though the contents of two look-alikes may be identical, the value placed on each of them will depend on their names. For example, a look-alike black beauty, containing phenylpropanolamine, caffeine, and ephedrine, will sell at a high price in the drug culture because it is associated with Biphetamine®, which contains a high dose (20 mg) of amphetamine. If the same compound is given a different name associated with a less popular drug, it will sell for a lower price and will be perceived as less desirable by the user. This illustrates that an understanding of the look-alike drug phenomenon requires not only a knowledge of the pharmacology of the substance in question, but also a grasp of the psychological outlook, social climate, and cultural aura that surround its sale and use.

Caffeine

Increasing attention has been focused on the toxicity of the stimulant substances, including caffeine, contained in look-alikes. PharmChem Laboratories' analyses of stimulant look-alikes (Stock 1982a, 1982b) have indicated that they contain a wide range of caffeine varying between 37 and 323 mg. In comparison, the average brewed cup of coffee contains about 100 mg to 125 mg (see Greden, chapter 10, this volume). Varying amounts of caffeine are also found in certain OTC analgesics and allergy/cold preparations.

Caffeine is a member of the xanthine family, which also includes theobromine, the stimulant found in cocoa and chocolate (figure 20.1). Caffeine stimulates the central nervous system as well as the heart and the skeletal muscles, and dilates peripheral blood vessels while constricting cerebral blood flow. It requires about 100 to 125 mg of caffeine to produce stimulation in the average adult and, at this and even greater levels, the drug is considered safe. Excessive amounts may result in headaches, anxiety, sleep disturbances, cardiac arrhythmias, and, because of the stimulation of gastric acid, gastric irritation. Exceptionally high dosages can even cause stimulant-induced seizures and, like any stimulant, induce psychotic episodes. Caffeine consumption can also lead to dependence characterized by headaches and depression after its discontinuation. The lethal dose of caffeine is estimated to be about 10,000 mg. It would take approximately 30 look-alike stimulants ingested at one time to produce a potentially lethal overdose.

FIGURE 20.1

Chemical structure of caffeine

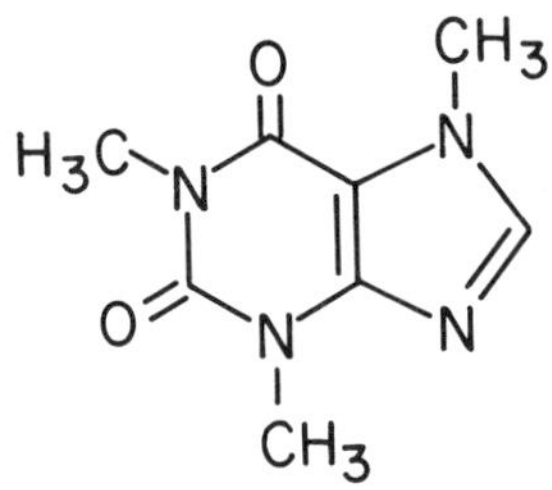

Source: Compiled by the author.

Caffeine poses an even greater risk for women who use birth control pills, as the pill appears to interfere with the elimination of caffeine (Patwardhan et al. 1980).

Clinical experience with look-alike drug abusers at the Haight-Ashbury Free Medical Clinic indicates that some individuals may become dependent on these products and ingest five to ten doses per day, putting them in the range of caffeine toxicity.

Ephedrine

Ephedrine is also present in many look-alikes, but is probably less common than caffeine. PharmChem Laboratories' analyses of stimulant look-alikes show that they often contain between 12.5 and 50 mg of ephedrine, the latter being the highest dosage permitted by law. Ephedrine is a sympathomimetic amine that releases endogenous stores of norepinephrine, provoking stimulation of alpha- and beta-adrenergic receptors (figure 20.2). Like caffeine, it is a CNS and peripheral stimulant which can produce an increase in blood pressure and heart rate and may induce cardiac arrhythmias. Prolonged high-dose abuse can produce a stimulant toxic psychosis, and massive overdose can be lethal as a result of stimulant-induced seizures and cardiac toxicity (Saxena and Kingston 1981; Lake et al., chapter 17, this volume).

FIGURE 20.2

Chemical structures of
phenylpropanolamine, ephedrine, and amphetamine

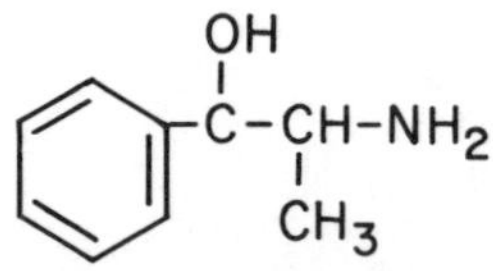

Phenylpropanolamine (PPA)

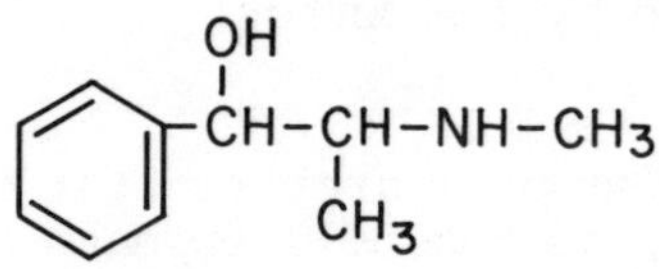

Ephedrine

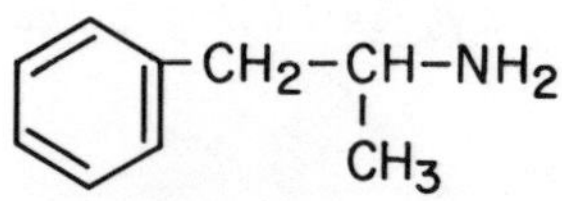

Amphetamine

Source: Compiled by the author.

Phenylpropanolamine

Phenylpropanolamine, which acts pharmacologically in a manner similar to ephedrine (figure 20.2), has recently been frequently found in look-alike stimulants, with the dosage varying between 25 and 50 mg, the latter being the highest legally permitted. Phenylpropanolamine is also contained in a wide variety of OTC decongestants and diet aids, but there is less street traffic in these products than in manufactured look-alikes. Phenylpropanolamine in high doses can cause anxiety, headaches, muscle tremors, heart palpitations, and elevation of blood pressure. Excessively high dosages pose a threat of drug-induced psychotic episodes, but relatively little evidence exists of stimulant-induced psychotic episodes and seizures associated with phenylpropanolamine alone. Hypertensive crises, seizures, and intracranial hemorrhages culminating in death have also been ascribed to phenylpropanolamine. However, the vast majority of clinical situations involving look-alike stimulants have been associated with the high-dose use of combinations of phenylpropanolamine with caffeine and/or ephedrine.

CLINICAL PROBLEMS IN LOOK-ALIKE ABUSE

The initial step in treating an overdose of a look-alike drug (as with any drug overdose) is to empty the stomach and administer activated charcoal to prevent drug absorption. If signs of clinical toxicity, such as elevated blood pressure, are present, propranolol or another antihypertensive drug may be administered. Symptoms of psychological toxicity, including acute anxiety reactions and transient stimulant psychosis, may be managed by reassuring the patient and, if indicated, by administering sedative/hypnotic medication. Rarely is an antipsychotic medication, such as haloperidol, needed in treating look-alike stimulant agitation.

LOOK-ALIKE COCAINE

Look-alike cocaine has also recently appeared. Look-alike cocaine may itself contain phenylpropanolamine, ephedrine, and caffeine as well as anesthetic agents such as lidocaine, tetracaine, or benzocaine. The white powder sold as cocaine will thus produce both an anesthetic effect and, because of the combination of caffeine with a sympathomimetic, a mild stimulant effect, which the user associates with pharmaceutical cocaine. It is interesting that Van Dyke and Byck (1982) found that, in a double-blind controlled study, experienced cocaine users could not tell the difference between low doses of cocaine and low doses of lidocaine, indicating that the placebo reaction and anticipation of drug effect are major factors in the acceptance of inexpensive look-alike cocaine sold as true cocaine. (It also may indicate that local anesthetics are psychoactive when inhaled.) The motivation for such transactions is obviously economic. Though widely cut, cocaine sells for 100 dollars per gram in the drug culture, whereas look-alike cocaine is much less expensive. Allen (1982) has compiled a clinically useful list of brand and street names used for legally manufactured look-alike cocaine (table 20.2).

TABLE 20.2

Names of commercially available turkey cocaine preparations and street names for cocaine

Commercial names of look-alike cocaine	Chattanooga Toot Toot Coco Sno Incense Incense King Toot Pseudocaine Incense Sno-Caine	Sno-Job Sno Seals Symma Caine Syn-Caine Toot
Street names of cocaine	Bernice Bernie's Flake Boy Burese C Charlie Coke Corine Corrine Dream Dust	Flake Girl Gold Dust Heaven Dust Her Him Joy Powder Lady Snow Star Dust White Stuff

Source: Adapted from Allen, L. V., Jr. 1982. "Turkey drugs"--what you see is not what you get. U.S. Pharmacist 7:36. Reprinted with permission.

As with other look-alikes, the epidemiological analysis of this situation is quite complicated. Legally manufactured look-alike cocaine contains noncontrolled substances and is therefore sold in establishments such as head shops, but it may also be diverted into the drug culture for recreational use and given a completely different name that associates and confuses look-alike cocaine with true cocaine in the user's mind. The addition of lidocaine does not alter, to any significant degree, the character and dose-effect responses of the ingredients in look-alike cocaine that are also found in the other look-alike stimulants. Its physiological and psychological toxicity seems primarily associated with the ephedrine/phenylpropanolamine/caffeine combination, with high dosages producing cardiac arrhythmias, elevated blood pressure, anxiety reactions, and transient stimulant agitation. Cocaine substitute products, however, do have a topical anesthetic, vasoconstricting, and drying effect on the nasal mucosa which might be quite irritating.

Cocaine look-alikes contain a variety of substances, some of which can produce adverse reactions as outlined in table 20.3. Some of these ingredients have a higher toxicity than others. For example, some cocaine smokers have reported that the smoking of pure lidocaine is similar to cocaine freebase. Lidocaine can produce cocaine-like seizure activity. In December 1982, one pure lidocaine overdose death and one pure lidocaine-induced stimulant psychosis were seen at the Haight-Ashbury Free Medical Clinic. Two additional cases of cocaine look-alike deaths were reported during 1983 in San Francisco. Cocaine and cocaine look-alike subarachnoid hemorrhages have also been reported (Lichtenfeld 1984).

LOOK-ALIKE DEPRESSANTS

Another component of the complicated look-alike drug scene involves look-alike depressants, particularly look-alike Quaalude®. Pharmaceutically produced Quaalude® (methaqualone*) is thought highly desirable in the drug culture and is sold for approximately five dollars a tablet. Methaqualone has a high abuse potential and can produce sedative/hypnotic overdose and cardiorespiratory depression. Chronic high dose abuse of methaqualone can lead to physical dependence, and abrupt cessation can cause withdrawal seizures. Look-alike Quaalude®, in contrast, usually contains the antihistamine doxylamine succinate, acetaminophen, and salicylamide. This combination of drugs has sedative effects that may weakly emulate the depressant effect desired by the user. However, as emphasized by Stock (1982a), abuse of these substances may produce excessive drowsiness and toxic physiological reactions ranging from skin rash to liver damage. Overdose symptoms include nausea, abdominal pain, coma, and convulsions. Mild overdoses are usually adequately managed by reassuring and observing the patient, but aggressive care is necessary in the case of massive overdoses in order to support the cardiorespiratory system and restore any electrolyte imbalance. Severe and life-threatening overdoses may require the administration of intravenous diazepam for seizures.

---

*The drug is no longer pharmaceutically produced in the United States, although it was at the time this article was prepared.

TABLE 20.3

Cocaine substitutes and reported adverse reactions

Product name	Principal ingredients	Reported adverse reactions
Cocafine® snuff	caffeine, citric acid	nasal irritation, tremors
Coca Leaf Incense®	procaine, tetracaine, caffeine, citric acid	nasal numbing and irritation
Cokesnuff®	ground tobacco (nicotine), menthol, fragrances	sneezing, insomnia, nausea
Iceberg® snuff	mannitol, benzocaine	nasal numbing
Ma-Huang® incense	ephedra (ephedrine)	nervousness, insomnia, palpitations
Mannite Conoscenti® and other mannite snuffs (e.g., Superior Cut®, Coke Cut®, Acut Above®, Perfect Cut®)	mannitol	diarrhea
Rock Crystal® snuff	mannitol, benzocaine, procaine	nasal numbing
Snort® snuff	dextrose, menthol, fragrances	nasal dryness
Yocaine® snuff	yohimbe hydrochloride, coryranthine	hypertension, nausea, vomiting
Zoom® tablets	guarana (caffeine)	stomach cramps, diarrhea

Source: Siegel, R. K. 1982. Cocaine free base use, part III. J Psychoactive Drugs. 14:312. Reprinted with permission.

The look-alike depressant situation, associated primarily with look-alike Quaalude®, is further complicated by drugs of deception. There is fake Quaalude® that does not contain the uncontrolled substances previously described, but instead contains other controlled substances, such as diazepam. There has been increasing use of look-alike street Quaalude® that contains amounts of diazepam as high as 200 mg. It appears that this diazepam is manufactured in bulk form in Europe, primarily Italy, and diverted to South America, particularly Colombia. There it is repackaged as street Quaalude®, then smuggled into the United States and sold at a very high price. Interviews with users of drug-of-deception Quaalude® indicate that they do not receive the same intense disinhibition euphoria associated with pharmaceutical Quaalude®; very often they complain of a prolonged drug effect, perhaps associated with the long-acting effects of diazepam.

Overdoses of street Quaalude®, even if it contains high doses of diazepam, are less life-threatening than overdoses of methaqualone and usually can be managed by observation or a life-support system. At the Haight-Ashbury Free Medical Clinic, however, cases of clinical confusion produced by street Quaalude® have been seen. If an individual abuses high doses of pharmaceutical Quaalude® containing methaqualone, physical dependence may result, with the peak liability for withdrawal seizures possibly occurring on the second day. With high-dose diazepam, however, the peak liability for withdrawal seizures following abrupt cessation is the fifth to seventh day, and the addition of alcohol may further delay withdrawal (Smith 1981a). A clinical situation has been reported (Ibid.) in which an individual ingested five to ten street Quaaludes® containing diazepam on a daily basis for 30 days. After stopping use, this individual used alcohol during the withdrawal period to calm anxiety and fight insomnia and had a withdrawal seizure ten days after the last dosage. The clinician dealing with depressant abuse must be aware of the complications added to the drug scene by the emergence of look-alike Quaalude® and drug-of-deception Quaalude®, both of which represent varying epidemiological, clinical, and toxicological patterns.

LOOK-ALIKE OPIOIDS

Drugs sold as heroin but containing other substances have long been available in the drug culture. The potentially greatest physiological danger associated with look-alike drugs and drugs of deception involves the look-alike opioids. For example, Smith (1981b) reported an increase in abuse of drugs called "set-ups" or "loads," which are sold as heroin but in fact contain codeine and glutethimide (Doriden®). This combination is quite powerful and has a high potential for overdose which, because of the mixed opioid/depressant effect, is only partially reversible by naloxone (Narcan®). In addition, abuse of set-ups or loads can result in a mixed opioid and sedative/hypnotic dependence which involves a more complicated withdrawal than pure opioid withdrawal. Glutethimide withdrawal can produce life-threatening seizures.

Ayres, Starsiak, and Sokolay (1981) have reported the appearance of "China white," which was sold as heroin, but actually contained 3-methyl fentanyl. Three-methyl fentanyl is a potent, illicit, synthetic narcotic, over 100 times more potent than heroin. Fentanyl is used medically as an obstetrical analgesic, but it appears that 3-methyl fentanyl is manufactured in clandestine laboratories and repackaged as high-quality heroin, which brings a high price in the drug culture. Three-methyl fentanyl has a great potential for overdose and can produce opioid dependence with severe withdrawal sequelae. The fentanyl overdose, like that of any opioid narcotic, can be reversed by naloxone, and withdrawal is mainly treated by either methadone substitution with graded reduction or symptomatic management detoxification not using opioids.

Of greater concern than any heroin deception discussed above has been the substitution of an illicitly synthesized meperidine analog, MPTP (1-methyl-4-phenyl-1,2,5,6-tetrahydropyridine), which is being sold as heroin in the drug culture. The abuser injects or snorts MPTP as if it were heroin and may develop an irreversible Parkinson-like syndrome within 48 hours to six weeks. The illness can progress to permanent disability and paralysis (Smith and Seymour 1984).

CONCLUSION

In summary, look-alikes and drugs of deception represent an extremely complicated and, in some instances, a hazardous phenomenon in the United States. This phenomenon has grown rapidly, influencing all aspects of the drug scene including stimulant, depressant, and opioid use. An understanding of look-alike drugs and drugs of deception is essential for accurate epidemiological and clinical analyses of drug abuse patterns and for effective diagnostic and treatment efforts.

A majority of the toxicity, abuse, and dependence is seen with the more powerful drugs of deception, which contain compounds that have substantial CNS effects and toxicity. Although misuse of the look-alike stimulants is widespread among adolescents and young adults in certain regions of the United States, significant toxicity and dependence are rare and confined to drug combinations. Phenylpropanolamine, although found in most look-alike stimulants, does not appear to be a major factor in their overall toxicity, abuse, or dependence.

This is not to say that the look-alike stimulant phenomenon is benign. Substantial concern must be voiced regarding the early induction of the adolescent into the drug culture that can result from his drug-seeking behavior. To address this problem, drug abuse prevention efforts aimed especially at adolescents need to be increased. Drug education at the family, school, and individual levels must be expanded, with particular emphasis on the individual susceptible to drug dependence. Diagnostic and treatment efforts should be improved in medical and drug treatment programs which deal with adolescents who are involved with the more powerful drugs. Regulatory efforts to reduce the production and publicizing of look-alike drugs should also be expanded, as well as law enforcement efforts to close down the clandestine labs which produce the more powerful drugs of deception--this is crucial.

In contrast, banning phenylpropanolamine, one of the least toxic of the drugs found in look-alikes and drugs of deception, will have no meaningful impact on the look-alike drug phenomenon and may have adverse effects in unrelated areas including therapeutics and the cost of medical care. Banning phenylpropanolamine in therapeutic preparations will not significantly reduce the use of look-alikes, but may create the illusion that something meaningful is being done by society to deal with the look-alike drug phenomenon, thereby diverting energy and resources away from more effective approaches. Furthermore, unsupported commentary on the dangerous abuse potential of phenylpropanolamine helps seduce drug experimenters more than it acts preventively.

REFERENCES

Allen, L. V., Jr. 1982. "Turkey drugs"--what you see is not what you get. U.S. Pharmacist 7:30-39.

Ayres, W. A., M. J. Starsiak, and P. Sokolay. 1981. The bogus drug: three methyl and alpha methyl fentanyl sold as "China white". J Psychoactive Drugs 13:91-93.

Center for Science in the Public Interest. 1984. Diet pills linked with 17 cases of strokes and seizures. News release. Washington, D.C. January 26.

Dougherty, R. J. 1984. Personal interview with author. April.

———. 1982. Pseudo-speed: look-alikes or pea-shooters. NY State J Med 82:74-75.

Lichtenfeld, P. 1984. Subarachnoid hemorrhage precipitated by cocaine snorting. Arch Neurol 41:223-24.

Morgan, J. P. et al. 1984. Duplicitous drugs: the history and current status of look-alikes. Unpublished manuscript.

Morgan, J. P. and D. V. Kagan. 1979. Street amphetamine quality and the Controlled Substances Act of 1970. In Amphetamine use, misuse and abuse, edited by D. E. Smith et al., 73-91. Boston: G. K. Hall.

Patwardhan, R. V. et al. 1980. Impaired elimination of caffeine by oral contraceptive steroids. J Lab Clin Med 95:603-8.

Saxena, K. and R. Kingston. 1981. Morbidity of street speed--an update. Vet Hum Toxicol 23:10-12.

Siegel, R. K. 1982. Cocaine free base use, part III. J Psychoactive Drugs 14:311-19.

Smith, D. E. 1981a. Prescription drugs and the alcoholic: the benzodiazepines--therapeutic and dependence considerations. In Alcoholism: a major challenge for the 1980's, proceedings of the Eisenhower Medical Center and the California Society for the Treatment of Alcoholism and Other Drug Dependencies conference, edited by J. J. Deller. Rancho Mirage, CA: Eisenhower Medical Center.

———. 1981b. Set-ups or loads. A new prescription drug abuse combination: glutethimide and codeine. Newsletter, California Society for the Treatment of Alcoholism and Other Drug Dependencies 8:3.

Smith, D. E. and R. B. Seymour. 1984. MTPT: abuse folio. High Times No. 103:30.

Stock, S. H. 1982a. The look-alike explosion, part I. PharmChem Newsletter 11:1-11.

———. 1982b. The look-alike explosion, part II. PharmChem Newsletter 11:3-4.

Ungerleider, J. T. 1981. DAWN, drugs and diplomacy. Street Pharmacologist 4:1-6.

Van Dyke, C. and R. Byck. 1982. Cocaine. Sci Am 246: 128-41.

21

PHENYLPROPANOLAMINE MENTIONS IN THE DRUG ABUSE WARNING NETWORK: NUMBERS PLUS INTERACTIONS

Donald R. Wesson and Susan Camber

DRUG ABUSE WARNING NETWORK

Statistics from the Drug Abuse Warning Network (DAWN), a database managed by the National Institute on Drug Abuse (NIDA), are often used to support drug regulatory decisions and legislation. DAWN data are generated from a nonrandom sample of hospital emergency rooms and medical examiner facilities in 26 metropolitan areas, covering about one-third of the U.S. population, throughout the continental United States (Anthony 1979).

The bulk of DAWN statistics is comprised of emergency room data. DAWN-reporting emergency rooms submit a report for each patient visit related to adverse effects of drugs. In 1982, over 120,000 emergency room visits were reported by 816 hospitals (National Institute on Drug Abuse 1982).

The raw datum for DAWN is the drug mention. A mention is an occurrence of drug use reported during an emergency room visit. The data report forms are completed from the patient's medical record, usually by a member of the emergency room or medical record staff. Generally the source of data is the patient's drug history, and usually no chemical or toxicological analysis of body fluid is carried out to confirm the claimed drug use (Ungerleider et al. 1980). A mention does not necessarily indicate abuse or drug dependency, as a mention may also result from an adverse medication reaction, the use of prescription drugs in a manner inconsistent with accepted medical practice, the use of over-the-counter (OTC) drugs contrary to approved labeling, or any use of an illicit drug. Since as many as six different drugs can be listed on each report form, one patient visit might create mentions of several different drugs, not all of which contributed to the emergency room visit. Since drug mentions in DAWN are based on emergency room visits rather than on particular patients, it is possible for one patient returning frequently to the emergency room to generate many mentions. In addition, a mention will be incorrect if the patient was mistaken or deceived regarding the actual identity of the drug taken or chose to mislead the emergency room staff for any reason.

Over the years, new emergency rooms have been recruited to report to the DAWN database while others have ceased reporting. Emergency rooms joining and leaving the reporting system introduce erratic fluctuations into the quantity and quality of reported data and, because different emergency rooms attract different types of patients, the character of the sample itself changes. For this reason, most time series analyses using DAWN data are based on the subset of data reported by the "consistent panel," a group of emergency rooms which have participated since the beginning of the DAWN network. Even when the consistent panel is used, however, some variation in quality, consistency, and thoroughness of data collection, recording, and reporting is to be expected as staff changes occur.

Some medical examiners submit information to DAWN about drug-related deaths, and there is a tendency to accept this as firm information. Even though NIDA encourages the use of specific, uniform reporting methods and provides training, some medical examiners include cases based on circumstantial evidence, whereas others may report only drug abuse deaths confirmed by toxicologic analyses (Gottschalk and Cravey 1980). For example, a case of suicide, in which the person took every drug available in the medicine cabinet, might involve six or more drugs. Some coroners would report all six drugs; others would report only the drug thought to be responsible for the death. Some regional variation in reporting is thus to be anticipated.

The data presented here are from the consistent panel emergency rooms. Although phenylpropanolamine (PPA) is contained in many cough/cold preparations, I have limited my consideration to mentions of diet medications and, for comparison, "speed" and aspirin. Speed was chosen both because it is a prototype of recreational stimulant use and because some mentions of it were probably of phenylpropanolamine-containing amphetamine "look-alikes." Aspirin was included as a common OTC medication, the use of which, because of its presence in almost every U.S. household, would be expected to occur at a relatively constant rate. Therefore, mentions of aspirin can be considered a measure of reporting volume.

OVER-THE-COUNTER DIET AIDS

The OTC diet aid category in DAWN captures mentions of OTC diet aids not specifically coded by trade name. Figure 21.1 shows the number of mentions by quarter between the last quarter of 1978 and the third quarter of 1983. The shaded area for the fourth quarter of 1982 and the first quarter of 1983 appearing in this and subsequent figures identifies an interval in which DAWN reporting from some sites was incomplete; these figures therefore reflect some underreporting.

FIGURE 21.1

Mentions of over-the-counter diet aids in the Drug Abuse Warning Network, 1978-83

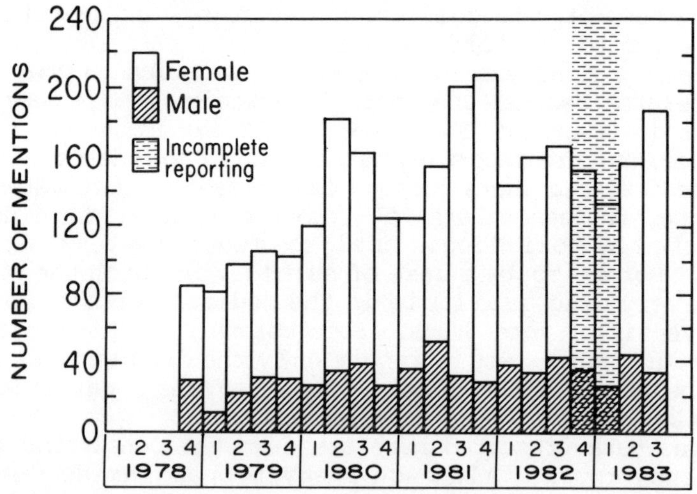

Source: Compiled by the authors. Data runs were provided by Edgar H. Adams, Assistant Director for Statistical and Epidemiological Analysis, National Institute on Drug Abuse, Rockville, MD.

Two conclusions can be drawn from the OTC diet aid reports in figure 21.1. First, the quarterly reporting volume for men is relatively constant, whereas for women increases with some fluctuations are apparent until late in 1981, after which the total number of mentions per quarter remains about constant. Second, the majority of users who generate DAWN mentions are women.

To analyze whether the growth in mentions might be an artifact due to variation in total reporting volume, I examined mentions of aspirin as a measure of reporting volume. Figure 21.2 shows the volume of aspirin mentions from the last quarter of 1978 through the third quarter of 1983. Like the OTC diet aid mentions, aspirin mentions were generated predominantly by women. The reporting rate was relatively constant for both males and females. Since the average rate of about 500 mentions per quarter for women and 400 per quarter for men was relatively constant throughout the five-year interval, I concluded that the increase in mentions of OTC diet aids observed from 1979 to 1980 was not due to changes in reporting volume.

FIGURE 21.2

Mentions of aspirin in the
Drug Abuse Warning Network, 1978-83

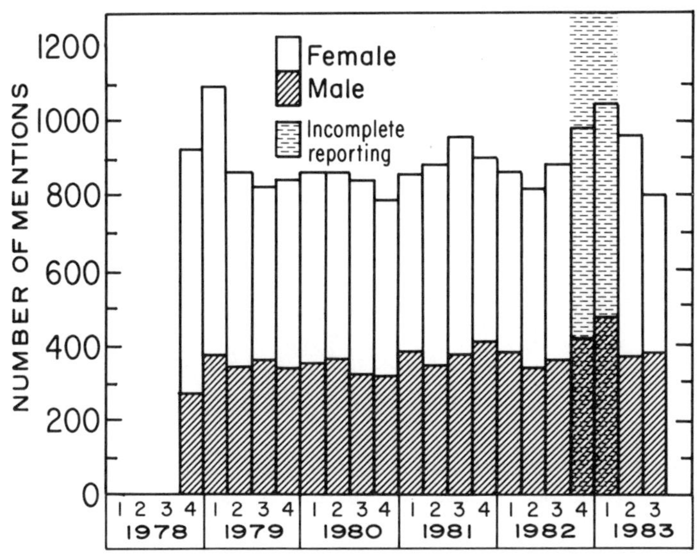

Source: Compiled by the authors. Data runs were provided by Edgar H. Adams, Assistant Director for Statistical and Epidemiological Analysis, National Institute on Drug Abuse, Rockville, MD.

SPEED

If OTC diet aids were being used in large amounts for recreational use as amphetamine substitutes, we might expect to see a sex distribution for speed mentions which would be similar to that for OTC diet aids. Speed mentions include amphetamine or products believed to be amphetamine (look-alikes). However, as illustrated in figure 21.3, the male/female ratio is actually the reverse of that in figure 21.1.

FIGURE 21.3

Mentions of speed in the Drug Abuse Warning Network, 1978-83

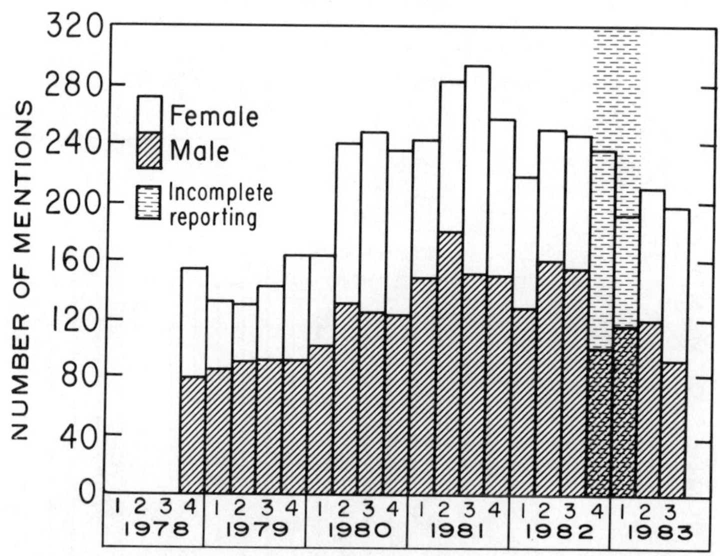

Source: Compiled by the authors. Data runs were provided by Edgar H. Adams, Assistant Director for Statistical and Epidemiological Analysis, National Institute on Drug Abuse, Rockville, MD.

The availability of actual amphetamine has declined due to regulatory changes placing production quotas and regulations on manufacturers of amphetamine. Production quotas allow U.S. pharmaceutical manufacturers to produce only a small fraction of the amount of amphetamine produced in the 1960s. Increased monitoring of shipping has reduced large-scale diversion of amphetamine into the drug black market. These and other factors have decreased the diversion of amphetamine from medical practice. We would therefore expect pharmaceutically manufactured amphetamine to be in short supply. Findings of street drug analysis programs support this (Morgan and Kagan 1978). One example of this shortage is that some people who claimed to have used street "black beauties" actually used amphetamine look-alikes containing OTC ingredients such as phenylpropanolamine, caffeine, or ephedrine. The number of speed mentions actually attributable to amphetamine look-alikes is unknown.

DEXATRIM™

Figure 21.4 shows the DAWN mentions of Dexatrim™, a widely used OTC diet aid containing phenylpropanolamine. The absolute magnitude of the Dexatrim™ mentions is about one-half that of OTC diet aids not specifically coded by trade name (figure 21.1). Importantly, the sex ratio of

FIGURE 21.4

Mentions of Dexatrim™ in the Drug Abuse Warning Network, 1978-83

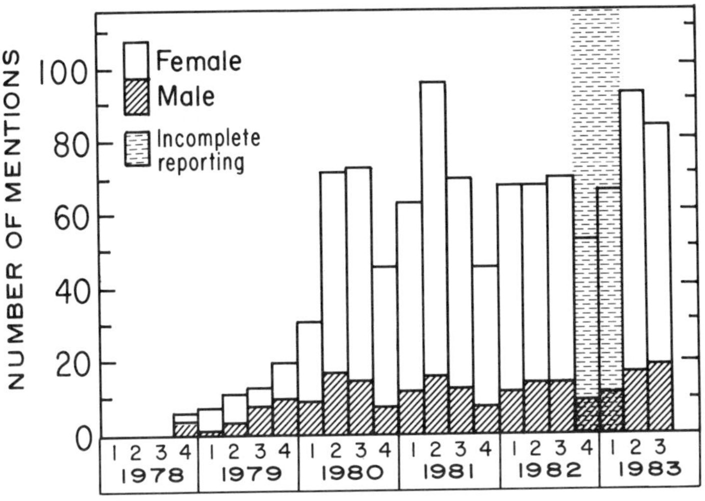

Source: Compiled by the authors. Data runs were provided by Edgar H. Adams, Assistant Director for Statistical and Epidemiological Analysis, National Institute on Drug Abuse, Rockville, MD.

Dexatrim™ mentions is similar to that observed with other OTC diet aids in having a predominance of female mentions. Again, if OTC diet aids were being used in great number as substitutes for speed, the sex distribution for Dexatrim™ might be similar to that for speed; it is, however, the reverse.

PSYCHIC EFFECTS

One of the data elements in DAWN coding is the stated reason for drug use. Possible responses include suicide, dependence, and psychic effects. The DAWN manual defines psychic effects as "euphoria, high, kicks, mood alteration, sexual enhancement, alleviation of unhappiness, trips, drug experiences for experimentation and fulfillment, use for social or recreational purposes or because of peer pressure" (National Institute on Drug Abuse 1982). Table 21.1 compares the psychic effects in mentions of OTC diet aids, Dexatrim™, speed, and aspirin.

TABLE 21.1

Drug Abuse Warning Network mentions of drugs taken for psychic effects: fourth quarter, 1978 through third quarter, 1982

Product	Males			Females		
	DAWN mentions (N)	Psychic effects (N)	%	DAWN mentions (N)	Psychic effects (N)	%
OTC diet aids	646	182	28	2,893	548	18
Dexatrim™	220	53	24	1,057	200	18
Speed	4,270	1,680	39	2,448	993	40
Aspirin	7,349	889	12	17,842	1,978	11

<u>Source</u>: Compiled by the authors. Data runs were provided by Edgar H. Adams, Assistant Director for Statistical and Epidemiological Analysis, National Institute on Drug Abuse, Rockville, MD.

Psychic effects were recorded as the reason for using speed by about 40% of both males and females. This figure seems surprisingly low since it would be reasonable to expect speed to be used principally for its psychic effects. For OTC diet aids, significantly more males (28%) are reported using them for psychic effects than are females (18%). In the case of aspirin, it is unexpected to find that about 10% of its use is reportedly to obtain psychic effects. There is, however, a probable explanation for this. Aspirin is commonly included in prescription pain relievers such as propoxyphene and codeine, and these medications are sometimes used for their psychic effects. Thus, aspirin may become a mention in abuse cases involving combination prescription drugs. This points out a potential pitfall if DAWN data are uncritically used as the basis for regulatory decisions. Aspirin exceeds speed in total volume of DAWN mentions. If regulatory decisions were based solely on volume, it would be more compelling to schedule aspirin than OTC diet aids.

CONCLUSION

Although DAWN statistics have some inherent limitations, they provide a useful window on the language and phenomena of drug misuse and abuse, particularly when correlated with other sources of data. DAWN data can be a useful resource in tracking trends in drug use patterns or a malleable set of numbers which can be marshalled to support drug regulatory decisions. Reasonable use of the database requires an understanding of what information is acquired and how the data are collected.

My analysis of DAWN data does not provide evidence that phenylpropanolamine-containing diet medications are widely used as amphetamine substitutes for recreational purposes. Further, the sex ratio of DAWN reports for legitimate phenylpropanolamine products varies significantly from the ratio for recreational speed. The frequency of phenylpropanolamine mentions in DAWN statistics does not necessarily indicate that it is being used as a recreational drug. Visibility of a medication in DAWN occurs in part because of its availability and widespread use, as illustrated by aspirin. Regulatory attention aimed at controlling OTC diet aids is misdirected if the intent is to curb recreational use of these medicinals.

REFERENCES

Anthony, J. L. 1979. The effect of federal drug law on the incidence of drug abuse. J Health Polit Policy Law 4:87-108.

Gottschalk, L. A. and R. H. Cravey. 1980. Toxicological and pathological studies on psychoactive drug-involved deaths, 35-59. Davis, CA: Biomedical Publications.

Morgan, J. P. and D. Kagan. 1978. Street amphetamine quality and the Controlled Substances Act of 1970. J Psychedelic Drugs 10:303-17.

National Institute on Drug Abuse. 1982. Annual data 1982: data from the Drug Abuse Warning Network, statistical series I, no. 1. Rockville, MD: National Institute on Drug Abuse.

Person, P. H., Jr. 1977. Indicators of drug abuse--DAWN. In The epidemiology of drug abuse: current issues, edited by L. R. Richards and L. B. Blevens, 135-37, National Institute on Drug Abuse research monograph no. 10. Rockville, MD: National Institute on Drug Abuse.

Ungerleider, J. T. et al. 1980. The Drug Abuse Warning Network (DAWN) program: toxicologic verification of 1,008 emergency room mentions. Arch Gen Psychiatry 37:106-9.

22

THE POISON CONTROL CENTER EXPERIENCE WITH PHENYLPROPANOLAMINE

Brent R. Ekins

POISON CONTROL CENTERS: THEIR PURPOSE AND OPERATION

Historical Perspective

The idea of a poison control center was first actualized in 1953 in Chicago as the need to obtain information about products involved in accidental poisonings was identified as an important public health concern. Through the cooperation of various health agencies, including the Illinois State Health Department, the Illinois Chapter of the American Academy of Pediatrics, and seven major hospitals, the first poison control center was established (Press and Mellins 1954).

The goal of this chemical and drug information center was to minimize the danger from poisonings through early and appropriate treatment and through poison prevention efforts. The idea caught on and other centers were established with similar purposes, with each center operating independently in compiling information, assessing toxicity, and recommending management techniques (Crotty and Verhulst 1970). It soon became apparent that a coordinating agency was needed to facilitate the collection and dissemination of information. The National Clearinghouse for Poison Control Centers (NCPCC) was organized in 1957. Its purpose was to coordinate efforts among the various poison control centers, to assemble, organize, and disseminate information about consumer products and other chemicals, and to gather data about the incidence of poisonings. When the NCPCC was created, there were 17 poison control centers already in existence in the United States. Within ten years, the number of poison control centers had increased to 460, and ultimately more than 600 recognized centers in the United States (Temple 1982) and approximately 200 in Canada and Europe were established (Govaerts 1970).

This rapid growth and the absence of a central directive organization contributed to a lack of uniformity in staffing, training, service, quality of information provided, and accessibility. As an alternative to this multiplicity of poison control centers, the concept of a larger, combined regional center was developed in the mid-1970s. This concept is now considered state-of-the-art for poison control centers. Consolidating resources, personnel, and expertise into one large regional poison control center is more efficient and cost-effective than the previous, haphazard delivery system. Regional centers have also been shown to be superior to nonregional centers in history-taking skills, treatment decisions, and overall case management (Thompson et al. 1983). The Food and Drug Administration's Poisoning Surveillance and Epidemiology Branch (PSEB) (formerly the NCPCC) continues to concentrate on data collection and analysis of poisoning occurrences.

The criteria for designation of a regional poison control center were first published by the American Association of Poison Control Centers (AAPCC) in 1978 and were most recently revised in April 1982 (American Association of Poison Control Centers 1978, 1982). By December 1982, 26 regional centers were listed by the PSEB as AAPCC-designated centers, far fewer than the over 600 poison control centers that once existed. As of February 1985, there were 31 certified regional centers.

The Operation of a Poison Control Center

Some centers are located in hospital emergency departments, where direct patient contact occurs; others are found in colleges of pharmacy, medical libraries, departments of hospital pharmacy, or in other settings where consultation is usually done only by telephone. The person receiving the call may be either a physician, pharmacist, nurse, or other trained individual. In regional poison control centers telephone coverage is provided 24 hours per day (American Association of Poison Control Centers 1982). Inquiries may originate with victims themselves, parents, friends, physicians or other health care professionals, school officials, or work supervisors. Ideally, in each case information about the victim is collected, resources are checked as needed, an assessment of the potential severity is quickly made, and management is suggested. Clinical consultation is available for all cases and specialists may be called for exposures involving uncommon poisons or toxins.

Operationally, a general exposure category is listed for each case: (1) nontoxic, (2) mildly toxic, or (3) severely toxic. For a nontoxic exposure, therapy is limited to reassurance or simple dilution and the patient remains at home. For a mildly toxic exposure in which no life-threatening effects are anticipated, management is also usually carried out at home with mild palliative therapy or emesis. Once treatment recommendations are given for home-managed cases, telephone contact is maintained until the case is completed and the written report finished. Telephone follow-up may detect unexpected or delayed side effects, symptoms of progressive toxicity, or treatment errors, or, importantly, may provide reassurance to a panic-stricken caller (Litovitz and Elshami 1982). With a severely toxic exposure, the patient is referred directly to the nearest emergency treatment facility. The poison control center notifies the facility and provides the history, assessment, and treatment information. A later call determines the outcome of each case.

Poison control centers generate information on the number of calls they receive, the chemicals involved in each case, the site of treatment, the medical outcome, and other data. A poison control center with additional expertise and staff is able to collect very detailed patient information for special projects. Such data may include, for example, more complete information about the dose ingested and the resultant symptoms experienced by the patient, the time course for blood concentrations of the drug, and other physical or biochemical findings. This information may be useful in estimating the toxicity and risks associated with new or existing drug products.

The current data collection system of the AAPCC was instituted as a pilot project in January and February of 1983 with the participation of nine regional poison control centers. During the remainder of 1983, a total of 16 centers were involved to some degree for a period of two to 12 months, with seven centers providing their total annual database to the system. The AAPCC database for calendar year 1983 included 251,012 total human exposures based on an annual service population of 25.8 million people. Extrapolating these figures to the current population of the United States indicates that the annual nationwide incidence of human exposures may be 2.3 million or more. Most of the cases in the database were acute poisonings, most were accidental in nature, and most involved children; only about 1% were adverse drug reactions (Veltri and Litovitz 1984). The data collection system of the AAPCC can track all cases involving specific brand name products, pharmacologically related compounds, or those used for the same purposes, such as all diet aids. Summary data of the cases can provide descriptors such as age, sex, type of exposure (accidental, intentional, adverse reaction, or other), and the medical outcome. The details of an individual case can be retrieved from the original contact form, if necessary.

THE POISON CONTROL CENTER EXPERIENCE WITH PHENYLPROPANOLAMINE

A Study of 70 Phenylpropanolamine Overdoses

Cases involving adverse reactions to diet aids have begun to appear in the data collected by the AAPCC as sales of over-the-counter (OTC) diet aid products have increased. An analysis was recently performed of 70 consecutive overdose cases involving diet aids containing phenylpropanolamine (PPA) reported to the Intermountain Regional Poison Control Center in Salt Lake City (Ekins and Spoerke 1983). The purposes of the study were threefold: (1) to estimate the minimum toxic dose of diet aids containing phenylpropanolamine or phenylpropanolamine/caffeine combinations ingested in an acute overdose; (2) to evaluate the signs and symptoms reported after such ingestions; and (3) to determine the medical outcome for each case.

The criteria for entrance into the study included a history of ingestion of a diet aid product and the ability to maintain contact with the victim or the physician managing the overdose. A patient was excluded if significant amounts of other drugs had been ingested, evidence indicated that his or her condition depended primarily on other diseases or events, or a complete history was not available.

Several factors limited the findings of the study. It was not a controlled study; most patients were not seen in a health care facility or by a physician (only 23% of cases were evaluated by a physician); some patients may have incorrectly estimated the number of tablets or capsules taken; and in most cases toxicologic analysis of the serum and urine was not done to confirm the presence and amount of the drug or to exclude other possible toxins.

In table 22.1, the 70 cases have been divided into four groups for analysis. Group I included 39 children ages five or less who had ingested a phenylpropanolamine-containing product, generally only one to two dosage units. Fourteen (36%) were treated with syrup of ipecac and cathartics, while 25 (64%) received no treatment. In the symptomatic cases, the average dose ingested was 10 mg/kg or 140 mg. Symptoms at this dosage included restlessness, shakiness, vomiting, and irritability as reported usually by the parent observer and usually lasted three to six hours. There were no serious toxicities in this group.

TABLE 22.1

Seventy cases of overdosage with diet aids containing phenylpropanolamine reported to a poison control center

Group	Number of cases	Percent	Age group/description
I	39	56	Children 5 years or younger.
II	2	3	Children ages 6-12.
III	7	10	Adults. Misuse of medicines to enhance therapeutic effect.
IV	22	31	Adults. Deliberate overdose.
Total	70		

Source: Adapted from Ekins, B. R. and D. G. Spoerke. 1983. An estimation of the toxicity of non-prescription diet aids from seventy exposure cases. Vet Hum Toxicol 25:81-85. Reprinted with permission.

Group II, which included two children ages eight and 11, was too small to analyze.

Group III consisted of adults and adolescents 13 and older who had taken the diet pills for the therapeutic benefit expected. The seven patients in this group reported having taken between one and three extra dosage units to increase the effect. Symptoms included central nervous system stimulation, peripheral numbness, headache, nausea, vomiting, weakness, tachycardia, dizziness, and restlessness and persisted eight to 12 hours. None of these patients required medical treatment, although two of the seven were seen in a hospital. In one of these two patients, blood pressure and heart rate were not documented. The other victim, who had ingested three dosage units, had a heart rate of 140 beats/min in a normal sinus rhythm.

TABLE 22.2

Three cases of significant phenylpropanolamine overdosage

Age (yr)	Product ingested	Amount taken (mg)	Comments
14	Control® (75 mg)	450	The patient vomited for 8 hours, was irritable and restless, but refused any medical care. Symptoms lasted 8 to 12 hours.
30	Hungrex® (25 mg)	1,550	Diaphoresis, respiratory difficulty, abdominal pain, nausea, and vomiting were noted. A heart rate of 100 and blood pressure of 110/80 mm Hg were the highest noted during hospitalization. Managed with induced vomiting, use of activated charcoal and cathartics, and supportive care in the hospital for 8 hours. Symptoms lasted 10 to 12 hours.
14	Dietac™ drops (25 mg)	1,875	Developed a tachycardia of 140 beats per minute, vomited for 6 hours, and complained of a headache and abdominal pain for 24 hours. Hospitalized for 2 days. Managed with IV fluids, phenobarbital, induced vomiting, and use of activated charcoal and cathartics. Symptoms persisted 30 to 36 hours.

Source: Adapted from Ekins, B. R. and D. G. Spoerke. 1983. An estimation of the toxicity of non-prescription diet aids from seventy exposure cases. Vet Hum Toxicol 25:81-85. Reprinted with permission.

Group IV included 22 adults or adolescents who had deliberately ingested an overdose of pills. Twelve patients had taken doses ranging from 165 to 450 mg, five from 500 to 750 mg, and the other five had allegedly ingested over 1,000 mg. All 22 were symptomatic, with the most common complaints being nausea or vomiting, nervousness, headache, dizziness, and a rapid heart rate. Approximately 50% of these patients were treated with ipecac, activated charcoal, and a saline cathartic. One patient received intravenous fluids and phenobarbital.

Only ten (14.3%) of the 70 cases involved products containing phenylpropanolamine alone. Six were children and five of the six were asymptomatic and received no treatment. All but one child had ingested only one dosage unit. This child had taken eight capsules and was given syrup of ipecac, which successfully induced vomiting. The child experienced no side effects except for brief vomiting episodes. Three of the four adults had taken intentional overdoses, allegedly 450, 1,550, and 1,875 mg of phenylpropanolamine. Data for these cases are summarized in table 22.2.

In summary, this study found that a child can take up to two dosages of products containing 75 mg of sustained-release phenylpropanolamine and not suffer any serious side effects. Often a small child takes only one dose set out for an adult to take but left unattended for a short time. In such a case, with or without treatment to remove the drug, it appears that a child can tolerate the dosage without serious harm. Adults who take one to three more pills than recommended to increase their therapeutic benefit will often suffer at least mild reactions, with the amount ingested determining the degree of toxicity. Adults who take large overdoses of phenylpropanolamine experience prominent toxicity. In only one of the 70 cases in this study did serious toxicity requiring aggressive treatment develop. No fatalities occurred among these 70 patients.

AAPCC Data on Phenylpropanolamine Exposures

Recent data from the AAPCC national data collection system regarding phenylpropanolamine exposures (table 22.3) provide an additional perspective (Veltri and Litovitz 1984). According to the preliminary data in this national reporting system, there were 965 exposures to phenylpropanolamine-containing diet aids per 251,012 total cases (0.384%) in 1983. Of these 965 cases, 80.0% were children under the age of six, 12.3% involved patients between six and 17 years of age, and the remaining 7.7% were adults or

TABLE 22.3

American Association of Poison Control Centers national data collection system cases involving phenylpropanolamine alone and in combination, 1983

	PPA only		Unknown OTC diet aid	
	No.	Percent	No.	Percent
Total reported	136	100	65	100
Age (years)				
< 6	104	76.5	48	73.8
6-17	22	16.2	13	20.0
> 17	3	2.2	1	1.5
Unknown	7	5.1	3	4.6
Exposure				
Accidental	111	81.6	48	73.8
Intentional	17	12.5	14	21.5
Adverse reaction	0	0	0	0
Unknown	8	5.9	3	4.6
Medical outcome*				
No effect	41	30.1	19	29.2
Minor effect	59	43.4	35	53.8
Major effect	8	5.9	4	6.2
Unknown	28	20.6	7	10.8
Death	0	0	0	0

*No effect: The patient developed no symptoms from the exposure.

Minor effect: Developed some symptoms, not serious, and had no residual disability or disfigurement.

Major effect: Developed life-threatening symptoms or had residual disability or disfigurement.

Look-alike diet aid		PPA plus caffeine		Total with PPA	
No.	Percent	No.	Percent	No.	Percent
49	100	715	100	965	100
25	51.0	595	83.2	772	80.0
9	18.4	75	10.5	119	12.3
2	4.1	18	2.5	24	2.5
13	26.5	27	3.8	50	5.2
26	53.1	568	79.4	753	78.0
11	22.4	115	16.1	157	16.3
1	2.0	3	0.4	4	0.4
11	22.4	29	4.1	51	5.3
7	14.3	191	26.7	258	26.7
19	38.8	360	50.3	473	49.0
7	14.3	73	10.2	92	9.5
16	32.7	91	12.7	142	14.7
0	0	1	0.1	1	0.1

Source: Adapted from Veltri, J. C. and T. L. Litovitz. 1984. 1983 annual report of the American Association of Poison Control Centers national data collection system. American Journal of Emergency Medicine 2:431, 442-43. Reprinted with permission.

patients whose ages could not be determined. Intentional overdoses comprised 16.3% of all reported cases, a figure consistent with the age breakdown. Two hundred fifty-eight patients (26.7%) developed no noticeable effects. Approximately half the patients developed minor effects either from the drug or the induction of emesis; no effort was made to distinguish between the two effects. Approximately 9.5% of the patients developed major effects, defined as cases in which prominent life-threatening symptoms were present, hospitalization was necessary, or residual disability or disfigurement occurred.

There was one death reported involving a phenylpropanolamine/caffeine combination. This case involved a woman in her early 20s who had taken an undetermined number of pink, triangular-shaped tablets marked with the letters "PDK." The patient suffered a cardiopulmonary arrest and died a short time after she had arrived at the hospital. Phenylpropanolamine and caffeine were both found in the urine toxicology drug screen performed. A high level of caffeine was found in the blood, but a quantitative blood level of phenylpropanolamine was unfortunately not available. In this case as in others involving drug combinations, it is not possible to implicate either drug as the sole causative agent; at this time both drugs would have to be considered responsible. As more information becomes available about the role of each agent, a more definitive statement can be made about the toxicity or safety of phenylpropanolamine, caffeine, and their combinations.

With 60 poison control centers providing data during 1984, it is anticipated that reports of 1.25 million cases of human exposure to drugs, chemicals, and other toxins will be collected in the United States. If the proportion of cases remains the same in 1984 as in 1983, there will be at least 4,800 cases of phenylpropanolamine-containing drug overdoses reported to the nation's poison control centers, compared to 965 in 1983. This increase is an artifact of a larger database and does not necessarily indicate a higher incidence of poisoning exposures to these agents. This expanded database can be expected to provide additional critical information about phenylpropanolamine overdoses and toxic reactions.

CONCLUSION

The data of the national data collection system of the AAPCC are in agreement with other published reports of overdoses involving phenylpropanolamine. Phenylpropanolamine when taken alone or in combination with caffeine in an accidental or intentional overdose does not result in death or permanent disability in most cases.

This conclusion is not intended to minimize the potential risks from overdosage with any substance and especially not with phenylpropanolamine alone or in combination with other drugs. Case reports of serious toxicity associated with phenylpropanolamine, such as persistent neurologic deficits, cardiovascular toxicity, and death, cannot be discounted. Until all the responsible factors can be fully elucidated, these effects must remain a concern for the health care community.

In summary, the poison control center experience with products containing phenylpropanolamine is not consistent with the isolated case reports of severe toxicity. With the removal of caffeine from these products at the manufacturing level in December 1983 and with more uniform and sophisticated analytical support in managing overdoses, a clearer picture of phenylpropanolamine's toxicity will continue to evolve.

REFERENCES

American Association of Poison Control Centers. 1982. Criteria for designation as a regional poison center. April.

------. 1978. Regionalization criteria. Vet Hum Toxicol 20:117-18.

Crotty, J. J. and H. L. Verhulst. 1970. Organization and delivery of poison information in the United States. Pediatr Clin North Am 17:741-46.

Ekins, B. R. and D. G. Spoerke. 1983. An estimation of the toxicity of non-prescription diet aids from seventy exposure cases. Vet Hum Toxicol 25:81-85.

Govaerts, M. 1970. Poison control in Europe. Pediatr Clin North Am 17:729-39.

Litovitz, T. L. and J. E. Elshami. 1982. Poison center operations: the necessity of follow-up. Ann Emerg Med 11:348-52.

Press, E. and R. B. Mellins. 1954. A poisoning control program. Am J Public Health 44:1515-25.

Temple, A. R. 1982. History and present status of American poison control centers. <u>Vet Hum Toxicol</u> 24 (Supplement):2-4.

Thompson, D. F. et al. 1983. Evaluation of regional and nonregional poison centers. <u>N Engl J Med</u> 308:191-94.

Veltri, J. C. and T. L. Litovitz. 1984. 1983 annual report of the American Association of Poison Control Centers national data collection system. <u>American Journal of Emergency Medicine</u> 2:420-43.

23

AN OVERVIEW OF PHENYLPROPANOLAMINE MISUSE LIABILITY

Charles Winick

INTRODUCTION

Any chemical substance that can be abused or misused or on which dependence can develop is subject to a wide range of use, from experimental to occasional to regular to heavy to dysfunctional. There are also varying degrees of maladaptation or dysfunction, interpretable in medical, social, or psychological terms. For example, most psychological and psychiatric approaches view drug dependence as a function of individual pathology; in contrast, sociologically oriented approaches, such as that of the World Health Organization, are more concerned with the effects of drug dependence on the person's ability to function (Kramer and Cameron 1975).

The question of whether phenylpropanolamine (PPA) is abused or misused can be discussed at various levels of generalization, depending on the concepts that are used. If only the traditional criteria of abuse and addiction potential, i.e., habituation, dependence, tolerance, and a withdrawal reaction, are considered, phenylpropanolamine would not appear to qualify as a substance of abuse. However, it is a truism that there are no really hard drugs, but that any drug can be used in a hard, as opposed to a soft, way. Only by examining actual user experiences with phenylpropanolamine will it be possible to draw valid conclusions about the degree of its potential for misuse or abuse.

Other criteria traditionally used to define a substance of abuse, misuse, or dependence include generation of a "high," significant dysfunctional effects, function as a "gateway" drug, and social and occupational impairment. Data on whether and to what extent a substance is being misused or abused are provided by drug abuse treatment agencies, sample surveys and epidemiological conferences, street surveys, the Drug Abuse Warning Network (DAWN), poison control centers, and other sources of information on the incidence of morbid events associated with the drug. Data from each of these sources will be discussed below in order to examine the extent to which phenylpropanolamine is being used in a hard, or personally and socially destructive, way. By the very nature of the methodologies employed, observational, survey, and interview data represent a different, though not a lesser, level of validity than do experimental and clinical studies.

REPORTS FROM DRUG ABUSE TREATMENT CENTERS

A substantial proportion of drug abusers seek treatment at a variety of outpatient and inpatient facilities--therapeutic communities, maintenance day centers, counseling centers, hospitals, and the like. Patients of such facilities are asked about their drug use in a situation in which they are likely to answer candidly. What have people in treatment reported about their use of phenylpropanolamine products? If there is significant abuse of phenylpropanolamine, it should emerge among those persons whose drug use is so dysfunctional that it leads them to seek treatment. If phenylpropanolamine is a drug of abuse, then there should be evidence of its being taken by drug abusers.

The most comprehensive national source of information on drugs taken by persons in treatment is the Drug Abuse Epidemiology Data Center (DAEDEC) (1983), which operated at Texas Christian University from 1973 through 1981 and is now at Texas A & M University. The more than half million drug abusers whose treatment during the period from 1973 through 1981 was supported by the National Institute on Drug Abuse provided background information on the substances that they used. According to DAEDEC records, the number of persons who reported using phenylpropanolamine was not significant.

Inquiries regarding phenylpropanolamine abuse were made in 1984 at several well-established and representative treatment centers in New York City, including Phoenix House, the country's largest therapeutic community for drug abusers; Beth Israel Hospital, which provides the country's largest methadone maintenance program; the Lower East Side Service Center, which runs the country's largest free-standing, multimodality treatment program for polydrug-dependent persons; and the Central Labor Rehabilitation Council of New York, which administers the country's leading labor-oriented, employee-assistance program (Winick 1985). These agencies have each been continuously providing services for drug abusers for over 20 years and are very sensitive to changes in the substances taken by their clients.

None of them reported even one patient who was or had been taking phenylpropanolamine. Key personnel at some of these agencies have seen many thousands of drug abusers. The intake psychiatrist at Beth Israel Hospital, for example, had interviewed an average of 40 drug abusers a day for 17 years; when interviewed at intake, not one of these had mentioned a phenylpropanolamine problem.

Inquiries were also made at treatment centers and data collection programs, such as the Client Oriented Data Acquisition Program (CODAP), in other parts of the country (National Institute on Drug Abuse 1982). None of the major drug abuse treatment centers questioned reported a significant number of phenylpropanolamine users receiving care.

There have been, however, two reports of persons from the upstate New York area seeking treatment for problems related to phenylpropanolamine use. Dougherty (1982) has cited a number of cases of young people who sought help for problems relating to pseudospeed, a "look-alike" product that resembles legitimately produced pharmaceutical amphetamine but actually contains phenylpropanolamine, caffeine, and ephedrine. This is the sole published report describing dependence on look-alike drugs containing phenylpropanolamine. The young people indicated that pseudospeed produced a high when combined with alcohol. In the fall of 1982, the Food and Drug Administration (FDA) essentially outlawed these three-ingredient preparations and 43 states have since followed suit. In the fall of 1983, the FDA similarly moved against two-ingredient products containing any two of the above three ingredients.

Dougherty (1984) has also reported that some middle-aged women in "empty nest" situations in the Syracuse area have sought treatment after taking diet pills containing phenylpropanolamine to help them deal with their emotional problems. The typical woman in this study had children away at school, was depressed, and originally overused diet aid products to increase their appetite suppressant effects but then began to more seriously abuse them. This kind of abuse has not been reported in other parts of the country.

SURVEY FINDINGS

The sample survey is probably the subfield of substance abuse research that has expanded the most vigorously and achieved the greatest methodological sophistication in recent years. When earlier approaches are compared with more recent ones, it is clear that substantive data have increasingly replaced conjecture and subjective impressions (Winick 1981, 1965).

The survey is the primary tool used to determine who is using what substances, for what purposes, with what effects, and for what length of time. Surveys may be conducted nationally, regionally, or among subgroups of the population, and may elicit information on the use of any substance, whether it be prescription or over-the-counter (OTC), licit or illicit, taken with or without medical supervision (Parry 1979). Program officials find that surveys are useful not only in documenting trends but also in providing legislators with convincing justifications for budget requests.

Contemporary reliance on surveys for guidance in planning and policy matters originated with the work of the National Commission on Marihuana and Drug Abuse (1973), which conducted the first of a major series of national household surveys in which a large sample of U.S. residents were asked about their use of various substances, including illicit drugs and prescription and other psychotherapeutic products taken for nonmedical purposes. From the first survey in 1973 through the eighth in 1982, phenylpropanolamine was never reported as a drug of abuse. It was not cited in the most recent (1982) survey, although the survey had a special focus on discovering forms of drug use that had not previously come to the attention of medical or legal authorities (Miller 1983).

Another major national survey was conducted among young men ages 20 to 30, who represent a high-risk group for drug experimentation and use (O'Donnell et al. 1976). This survey included measures of lifetime prevalence and current use of selected drugs, including alcohol, cigarettes, stimulants, sedatives, and illegal substances. Phenylpropanolamine was not reported as a drug of abuse in this population.

Beginning in the spring of 1975, the University of Michigan has annually surveyed the substance use patterns of a national sample of successive cohorts of high school seniors, as part of its Monitoring the Future study. The most recent 1982 survey for the first time included questions on nonprescription diet aid pills, such as Dietac™, Dexatrim™, and Prolamine™. Diet aids had been used by 21% of the students in the previous year and by 10% in the month preceding the interview. Apparently they had been taken for appetite suppression purposes since the diet aid pills were not cited as sources of highs, although many other substances were (Johnston, Bachman, and O'Malley 1982). Lending further support to the probability that diet aids had been used for weight reduction rather than stimulation purposes is the finding that nearly 2.5 times more women then men (42% versus 17%) had taken these products sometime during their lives. Many other studies have documented that women are several times more likely than men to wish to lose weight.

The relatively high level of use of phenylpropanolamine for weight loss purposes seems to continue into the college years. In one study, over three-tenths (30.1%) of a sample of women undergraduates and 3.7% of a sample of men undergraduates at Michigan State University had used an OTC phenylpropanolamine appetite suppressant in the previous year (Krupka and Vener 1983).

In addition to such national and school-specific studies, various states and regions systematically conduct surveys on drug use and abuse among their residents. The most thorough statewide survey of the prevalence of substance abuse is conducted by the New York State Division of Substance Abuse Services (1981), which since 1967 has periodically interviewed a large sample of the state's residents in order to establish their patterns of drug abuse. In the most recent study in 1981, none of the 3,487 state residents who were asked about their use of a large number of licit and illicit substances cited phenylpropanolamine as a substance of abuse. Every previous New York survey also failed to identify phenylpropanolamine as a drug of abuse.

Additional data from New York are provided by the laboratories of the Division of Substance Abuse Services, which analyze 40,000 to 45,000 urine samples every month, as part of the largest urine testing program in the United States. Most of these urine tests are performed for drug abuse treatment programs but some are done as part of preemployment screening examinations. The number of tests with phenylpropanolamine-positive results was so insignificant—a small fraction of 1%—that testing for phenylpropanolamine was abandoned (Mulé 1984). In those few cases in which phenylpropanolamine was detected, it was being used for legitimate medical purposes, usually as a decongestant.

The concept of a gateway drug, a substance whose use may lead to attempts to gain a more gratifying level of satisfaction from a stronger drug, has been developed by Kandel (1984). Over a period of many years, she has conducted the most intensive and extensive studies of substance abuse by young people and has not found phenylpropanolamine to be significant either as a gateway substance or as a drug of abuse. Nor has any other survey of drug use by the young ever identified phenylpropanolamine as a drug of abuse (O'Donnell and Clayton 1982; Donovan and Jessor 1982).

Indeed, no survey, on any level, has found phenylpropanolamine to be an important substance of abuse. Since so many surveys, conducted using sophisticated sampling techniques under different auspices and for varied purposes, all concur, it can certainly be concluded that survey results suggest that phenylpropanolamine is not being abused or misused either by the general population or by any subgroups, including high-risk groups.

REPORTS FROM CONFERENCES OF EPIDEMIOLOGISTS

Even a sophisticated and carefully conducted survey may overlook some instances of drug abuse, if, for example, the interval between surveys is too long, if an isolated pocket of drug abuse activity is too small to be detected, or if sampling or callback procedures are inadequate. Therefore, in order to identify newly emerging trends, specific regional situations, minor drugs of abuse, and other problems in the epidemiology of substance abuse, the National Institute on Drug Abuse (NIDA) semiannually convenes a meeting of public and private sector specialists from throughout the United States to discuss patterns in drug abuse, based on all available indicators. These indicators include ethnographic studies, special population surveys, treatment admissions, patient information, street data, drug arrests, and overdoses. At these meetings, regional officials who have primary responsibility for tracking epidemiological trends in their areas submit whatever quantitative and qualitative data are available and make oral presentations on special highlights of the situation during the previous six months. During the eight years these meetings have occurred, phenylpropanolamine has never been cited as a significant substance of abuse.

At four of the most recent meetings, in December 1982, June 1983, December 1983, and December 1984, presentations were given by representatives from 19 different cities. These epidemiology experts, constituting the Community Epidemiology Work Group, met at NIDA headquarters to discuss drugs of abuse in their communities. Phenylpropanolamine was not mentioned in the reports of any of the meetings as a significant drug of abuse, nor in the summary reports from each of the communities (Division of Epidemiology and Statistical Analysis 1984, 1983a, 1983b, 1982).

Phenylpropanolamine was referred to only twice during the meetings, in any context. In 1982 and 1983, the representative from Illinois briefly discussed look-alike pills containing phenylpropanolamine, which had accounted for about 1% of the 20 substances found in toxicology laboratory reports in the state. With the recent FDA designation of the combination of phenylpropanolamine, caffeine, and ephedrine as a new drug, it may be anticipated that this look-alike combination will be cited even less frequently in future reports.

The other citation of phenylpropanolamine was from King County, Washington, at the 1982 meeting. Of 714 men and 264 women who were asked about their use of 21 other substances in addition to alcohol within the three hours preceding their arrests for driving while intoxicated (DWI), 0.7% of the men and 1.5% of the women said they had taken a diet pill during this period. Since they had been arrested for being under the influence of alcohol, their use of diet pills was probably fortuitous and as unrelated to their arrests as the fact that 37.4% of the men and 55.3% of the women had used tobacco during the same period. The irrelevance of phenylpropanolamine to abuse can be inferred from the fact that it was not mentioned at all by Washington epidemiologists as a drug of abuse in the state.

These two citations--of look-alikes from Illinois and diet pills from Washington--were the only references made to phenylpropanolamine in this thorough analysis of the epidemiology of the drug abuse problem in the United States. It would be reasonable to conclude that state epidemiological officials, whose work involves monitoring drug abuse trends, do not regard phenylpropanolamine as a significant drug of abuse. Other epidemiological surveys also do not cite phenylpropanolamine (Winick 1981).

EVIDENCE FROM STREET SURVEYS

Another source of information on drugs which are being misused or abused is the street survey, in which drug users who are not in treatment are observed in a context of ordinary social living by participant observers and other investigators. Street surveys have been conducted in various cities to monitor trends in the use of illicit substances or the use of licit substances for psychoactive or mood modification purposes (Crawford 1977).

Different communities favor different mood modifiers at different times. During the last decade, no street survey or investigator in any community has reported significant phenylpropanolamine use.

It is reasonable to expect that if there were to be any substantial use of phenylpropanolamine by street users, it would occur in communities with a major street amphetamine problem. At times when amphetamine products became temporarily unavailable, a natural experiment would be created.

Would phenylpropanolamine use increase in such communities at such times?

Since 1976, reported illicit use of methamphetamine sulphate ("crank"), methamphetamine hydrochloride ("crystal"), and various "Mexican" amphetamine products has been widespread in many cities. Substantial illegal amphetamine use has been reported in Chicago, Dallas, Denver, Detroit, Miami, Minneapolis, New Orleans, San Francisco, and Washington. Street surveys and less formal studies in these cities have failed to find any significant phenylpropanolamine use among amphetamine users who had been temporarily deprived of their drug of choice. Interviews I have conducted over a period of 14 years in several cities with amphetamine users who, seeking a replacement high, have tried phenylpropanolamine have consistently found that the users are disappointed by the effects of phenylpropanolamine.

Occasionally legislation or other social change also creates a natural experiment in which the replacement of amphetamine by phenylpropanolamine can be examined. In 1981, amphetamine use in New York state was made illegal except in treatment of a limited number of medical conditions such as narcolepsy. The most common indication for prescribing, to cause anorexia, was disallowed. If phenylpropanolamine provided cognate gratifications to amphetamine users, street observation units would be expected to detect a sharp increase in street activity involving phenylpropanolamine, as former amphetamine users lost access to their drug of choice. No such shift to phenylpropanolamine-containing products or even to look-alikes occurred. Informal questioning of amphetamine users in the state indicated that many tried phenylpropanolamine but found that it did not provide a stimulant effect of any kind. "That stuff is no good at all," said one regular amphetamine user of the phenylpropanolamine he had tried.

In a major review of the abuse of amphetamines and anorexiants, Ellinwood (1979) discussed various amphetamine-like products but did not cite phenylpropanolamine as being one of them. More recently, he has indicated that phenylpropanolamine is not significantly abused either as a drug of choice or as an amphetamine substitute (Ellinwood 1985). The leading ethnographer of street drug abuse in the United States, Edward Preble (1981), has never found phenylpropanolamine to be a drug of abuse in his many investigations.

After amphetamine was reclassified by the Drug Enforcement Administration as a Schedule II controlled substance in 1971, the street supply of the drug decreased because of the dramatic decline in the amount of licit amphetamine available for diversion. This decline was not followed by a corresponding rise in the popularity of phenylpropanolamine, which would have been expected had the effects of the two drugs been similar. Since many laboratory studies have found that phenylpropanolamine does not produce euphoria, there is no reason to believe that the effects of amphetamine and phenylpropanolamine are similar.

Street studies can also provide information on substances that users believe have a booster effect that increases the intoxicating effects of another drug. For example, users may consume alcohol because they think it has such an effect on methadone. No studies or formal or informal reports have ever cited phenylpropanolamine as producing a booster effect.

Since 1957, I have been interviewing drug abusers who are not in treatment, have not been arrested, and are not otherwise known to law enforcement, treatment, or other authorities (Winick 1974). These persons constitute a panel of drug abusers who are reinterviewed on a regular basis in order to plot their changing drug habits and social and personal adaptations. A total of 6,230 persons have been on the panel. Not one of them has reported using phenylpropanolamine.

In summary, street studies, which provide a unique and important dimension of information on drugs of abuse, have uniformly failed to find evidence that phenylpropanolamine is a drug of abuse.

DRUG ABUSE WARNING NETWORK DATA

Another important source of data on drug misuse and abuse is the Drug Abuse Warning Network (DAWN), which collects information on persons with drug problems from 816 hospital emergency rooms and 84 medical examiners in 24 major metropolitan areas.

People seeking help for acute drug-related problems often have ingested a number of different substances, so that it is difficult to ascribe symptoms to any one drug. However, the contribution of phenylpropanolamine to such emergency situations can be inferred from the national figures on the incidence of phenylpropanolamine mentions (see Wesson and Camber, chapter 21, this volume, for a discussion of drug mentions in DAWN statistics). During the July-September 1982 quarter, for example, phenylpropanolamine ranked 102nd in frequency of mentions of substances reported to DAWN, accounting for less than 0.2% of the mentions (National Institute on Drug Abuse 1983a). In comparison, aspirin, the fifth most frequently cited substance, was reported in 5.17% of the mentions.

In 1981 and 1982, aspirin, acetaminophen, and sleep aids were consistently cited more often than phenylpropanolamine in DAWN reports of adverse effects associated with ingestion of OTC products. For the full year 1982, the use of OTC diet aids was reported in 0.88% of the total episodes and phenylpropanolamine in 0.14% (National Institute on Drug Abuse 1983b).

In over three-fourths (75.4%) of the diet aid cases, patients contacted emergency rooms because of overdoses. Perhaps the overdoses contributed to the fact that a suicide attempt was the most frequent occasion (54% in 1982) for phenylpropanolamine being reported to DAWN; however, aspirin, acetaminophen, and OTC sleep aids were more frequently cited than phenylpropanolamine in the total number of suicide attempts. Phenylpropanolamine was not one of the 50 drugs that medical examiners most frequently cited in reports of suicides in 1982. Acetaminophen was involved in 130 suicide deaths in 1982, aspirin in 102, OTC sleep aids in four, and phenylpropanolamine in one. It is probable that persons who attempt suicide are more likely to ingest large quantities of whatever substances are available than to seek out specific substances believed to be lethal.

These data do not indicate that the ingestion of any of these four categories of products is an especially effective way to commit suicide, but that a large percentage of those who attempt suicide do so by taking a mixture of readily available drugs. In fact, the survival rate of persons who attempt suicide by taking diet aids, including phenylpropanolamine products, is very high; phenylpropanolamine does not appear to lend itself to committing suicide.

The number of phenylpropanolamine mentions in DAWN statistics can be expected to decline as the product is more widely used and people become more familiar with it. From the October 1980-September 1981 period to the October 1981-September 1982 period, there was a 5.6% decrease in the number of OTC diet aid mentions reported by DAWN emergency rooms (from 1,048, or 0.566%, of the 185,230 total drug mentions in 1980-81 to 989, or 0.518%, of the 190,819 total drug mentions in 1981-82). This is a small drop but, although the total number of drug mentions increased slightly, the number of OTC diet aids mentions decreased both absolutely and as a proportion of the whole. A continuing small decline in each of the next several years can be anticipated.

REPORTS FROM POISON CONTROL CENTERS

In 1981, the Bulletin of the National Clearinghouse for Poison Control Centers (NCPCC) called attention to an increase in poison control center cases of adverse reactions following ingestion of phenylpropanolamine. Soon after this, two physicians reported that three patients had experienced severe cardiovascular and central nervous system problems after taking relatively small doses of phenylpropanolamine (Bernstein and Diskant 1982). More recently, the Poison Control Center in Utah reported that symptoms tended to be mild and short-lived in the 70 phenylpropanolamine-related cases seen there and raised questions about the serious reactions cited in earlier reports (Ekins and Spoerke 1983). Other centers that do not participate in the NCPCC have also reported their experiences with phenylpropanolamine-related cases (New York City Department of Health 1984).

The cases reported to poison control centers vary widely in severity and type. A telephone information request and a serious, incapacitating reaction are each counted as one mention. What is recorded as a hospitalization outcome may be a brief visit to an emergency room. The most frequent kind of case involves young children who accidentally ingest something harmful. Most ingestions are of multiple products. Whatever substances are reported are recorded, with little opportunity to confirm the identity and quantity of the substances actually ingested. A number of substances cited in the first major NCPCC report (1981) as containing phenylpropanolamine do not actually contain it. Poison control center data clearly must be interpreted with caution, especially since so many cases involve multi-ingredient products or ingestion of multiple products.

Look-alikes figure prominently in the phenylpropanolamine-related cases reported to the centers. There are also frequent reports of persons who use phenylpropanolamine products to lose weight but take several times the recommended dosages in order to accelerate the weight loss process, reasoning that if one pill is good, three or four at a time will be even better. Such overdoses can obviously result in symptoms that may lead people to call poison control centers.

Reports from poison control centers also have to be viewed from the perspective of what is known about the public's changing perceptions of a drug as it becomes better known. When a drug is introduced, first becomes widely used, or is used for new purposes, unexpected reactions to it are often interpreted as pathological and may lead to panic and the seeking of hospital or other emergency institutional help. For example, in the first few years after marihuana became popular in the United States, a large number of its users appeared at hospital emergency rooms for the treatment of psychotic reactions. However, once marihuana use had become routinized and users were familiar with the range of its effects, reports of psychotic reactions vanished completely (Becker 1967).

The enormous surge in the use of phenylpropanolamine in OTC appetite suppressants over the last decade, from practically nothing to a billion doses annually, has included millions of people taking the product for the first time. Unexpected reactions could, and did, lead some users to call poison control centers for information or assistance. As the product becomes better known and achieves an experienced user base, it is likely that the number of such calls will sharply decline and that wider understanding of its effects will minimize the naive overdose accidents often reported to poison control centers.

INFORMATION FROM OTHER SOURCES

Other sources of information on possible misuse or abuse of phenylpropanolamine are counterculture publications, "head" folklore, the popular media, surveys dealing with mood modification, and studies of the use of look-alikes and act-alikes.

During the 1960s and 1970s, more than 1,000 newspapers and magazines were published by and for the many members of the counterculture. Publications such as the *Berkeley Barb*, *Los Angeles Free Press*, *Boston Phoenix*, and New York's *East Village Other* regularly carried stories and features that encouraged the use of drugs for recreational purposes. With the end of the war in Vietnam and the increasing acceptance by the dominant culture of the use of mood-modifying substances, most of the underground newspapers and magazines ceased publication as their two most prominent themes became less significant.

The leading counterculture publication today is the monthly magazine *High Times*, which first appeared in 1974. It regularly monitors and reports drug use developments and has a loyal readership that regards it as a kind of countercultural *Consumer Reports*. The magazine's articles are widely discussed, carefully researched, and authoritative. In 1983, *High Times* carried a three-part report on phenylpropanolamine, which concluded that phenylpropanolamine is worthless as a psychoactive substance and has no stimulant or other mood-modifying effects (Latimer 1983a, 1983b, 1983c). Such a conclusion is important because of the publication's reputation for integrity and its commitment to countercultural values.

Some persons seeking a new stimulant drug may try phenylpropanolamine because of media publicity about its presumed psychoactive qualities. Most will try it once or twice and and stop when they realize that it does not produce the desired effects. A few, however, may have unexpected reactions and come to the attention of DAWN or other institutions that record negative experiences with drugs.

It has been reported that some young people have taken as many as 20 look-alike capsules daily, along with considerable quantities of alcohol (Dougherty 1982). Like other experimenters with multiple drugs, persons ingesting such combinations could experience adverse reactions, which might reflect drug interactions or extreme caffeinism, as well as phenylpropanolamine overdose. Yet in toxicity reports, such cases are often listed as reactions to phenylpropanolamine.

Although look-alikes containing phenylpropanolamine, caffeine, and ephedrine have been barred in most states and by the FDA, they remain available in many areas. As recently as December 1983, look-alikes containing this combination were plentiful in cities like Chicago, with young people paying 50 cents to one dollar per pill (Division of Epidemiology and Statistical Analysis 1983b). At the time this article was prepared, a number of small firms were still manufacturing these products and distributing them via direct mail, at truck stops, and through retail stores, in defiance of the law (National Institute on Drug Abuse 1983c).

Act-alike drugs, which contain ingredients similar to look-alikes but do not simulate controlled substances, have recently been manufactured in an attempt to avoid the prohibition against look-alikes. Act-alikes may be sold as speed with the implied assurance that they are licit and safe. No data indicate that young people who use either look-alikes or act-alikes employ them as steppingstones to other substances. It is possible, however, that a user might inadvertently take genuine amphetamine instead of a look-alike or act-alike and encounter an unexpected reaction (Saxena and Kingston 1981), although amphetamine itself is not particularly dangerous in acute overdose.

It is most unlikely that the phenylpropanolamine component in look-alikes or act-alikes contributes significantly to a high for the user. If phenylpropanolamine did actually provide a rush or high, there would have been a sharp upward trend in its use which the many indicators of drug abuse would have detected.

A logical question is why look-alikes and act-alikes contain phenylpropanolamine, if it has only a minimal stimulant effect. Interviews with some manufacturers and purveyors of look-alikes suggest that a number of them erroneously believed phenylpropanolamine to be a potent stimulant which would make a good combination with the known stimulants ephedrine and caffeine. One reason for their belief is that, since phenylpropanolamine is classified as a sympathomimetic drug, it was assumed to have an excitatory effect on the central nervous system. However, although most sympathomimetics do stimulate the central nervous system, phenylpropanolamine essentially does not. Phenylpropanolamine was also mistakenly thought to have euphorigenic qualities because of its association with the sympathomimetics.

Another reason that phenylpropanolamine was included in look-alikes is that, until a few years ago, it was sometimes incorrectly identified and referred to as cathine (e.g., Zelger and Carlini 1980). Cathine is, in fact, a stimulant but phenylpropanolamine and cathine are distinct stereoisomers and are chemically different. This confusion between phenylpropanolamine and cathine apparently led some manufacturers to assume that phenylpropanolamine has the stimulant effects of cathine.

Since phenylpropanolamine is a component of many look-alikes, there is a sense in which it may be considered to be unwittingly abused, even though it has no apparent stimulant or euphorigenic effects. Persons seeking a stimulant high who take these look-alikes are also taking phenylpropanolamine, even if they do not know that the drug is included in the products. There are other situations in which an ingredient contained in a street drug may be unknowingly abused. Sellers may, for example, dilute an expensive drug with a less costly substance. Thus, many regular heroin users doubtless become unwitting quinine abusers because quinine is so often employed to "cut" street heroin. Relatively few street drug users are aware of the actual composition of the substances they buy or of the degree to which ingredient substitution routinely occurs.

Another indirect indicator of a drug of abuse is the extent to which a body of folklore has emerged in connection with the substance and its properties. Any drug that is popular as a mood modifier generates a mystique and a set of beliefs, with references to it found in anecdotes, popular music, verse, fiction, movies, and television programs. Changing beliefs about substances like alcohol, marihuana, cocaine, and heroin and trends in their use can be tracked via such folklore (Winick 1985, 1976; Schwartz, Feinglass, and Drucker 1973).

No substance of abuse has ever become popular without such folklore developing. Phenylpropanolamine is not the subject of any special folklore, suggesting that its use has never become an integral part of any group's life style or subculture. No "hustle" is associated with it and, because it is so easily available and provokes little opposition, it does not share the appeal of forbidden substances such as cocaine and marihuana, whose attraction for many people, especially young people, lies in society's attempts to proscribe them.

DISCUSSION

What does it mean to say that a substance is a drug of misuse or abuse? It suggests that use of the drug may lead to psychological dependence, physical addiction, or the use of other drugs or may result in organ damage or morbidity. It may additionally indicate that the drug is a mood modifier or is euphorigenic or that it produces stimulation, depression, pharmacogenic orgasm, or some other consistent sensation. A drug of abuse may also be associated with a special life style or subculture or provide an escape from reality and an entry to a fantasy world. Phenylpropanolamine has none of these characteristics.

The major effort to develop theory-free and operational definitions of drug misuse was made by the American Psychiatric Association (1980) in the 3rd edition of its _Diagnostic and Statistical Manual of Mental Disorders_ (DSM-III). Diagnostic criteria for substance abuse include pathological use, impairment of social or occupational functioning, and minimum duration of disturbance of one month. Substance dependence, a more serious condition, is further characterized by withdrawal or tolerance. Phenylpropanolamine does not meet these criteria for either abuse or dependence.

If we examine all the criteria for a substance of abuse and misuse and the several different methods for identifying such substances--formal or informal criteria, institutional or more individual definitions, operational or more casual approaches, or medical or social life style indicators--the data clearly show that phenylpropanolamine is not a reinforcing substance and does not induce drug-seeking behavior. It has not been found to be addicting, habituating, or a source of highs, nor does it contribute to an altered or deviant life style or involvement in the subculture of drug abuse. Results from sample surveys, epidemiological studies, street surveys, DAWN reports, poison control center data, and all other sources agree with and provide additional confirmation of the consistent animal, clinical, and laboratory findings that phenylpropanolamine has no potential for abuse and misuse or for serious psychological and physiological effects.

REFERENCES

American Psychiatric Association. 1980. Diagnostic and statistical manual of mental disorders, 3rd ed. Washington, D.C.: American Psychiatric Association.

Becker, H. S. 1967. History, culture, and subjective experience: an explanation of the social bases of drug-induced experiences. J Health Soc Behav 8:163-76.

Bernstein, E. and B. M. Diskant. 1982. Phenylpropanolamine: a potentially hazardous drug. Ann Emerg Med 11:311-15.

Crawford, G. A. 1977. Non-survey observational techniques. In The epidemiology of drug abuse: current issues, edited by L. G. Richards and L. B. Blevens, 73-77. Washington, D.C.: U.S. Government Printing Office.

Division of Epidemiology and Statistical Analysis. 1984. Community epidemiology work group conference proceedings. Rockville, MD: National Institute on Drug Abuse. December 4-7.

———. 1983a. Community epidemiology work group conference proceedings. Rockville, MD: National Institute on Drug Abuse. June 21-24.

———. 1983b. Community epidemiology work group conference proceedings, Rockville, MD: National Institute on Drug Abuse. December.

———. 1982. Community epidemiology work group conference proceedings. Rockville, MD: National Institute on Drug Abuse. December 8-9.

Donovan, J. E. and R. Jessor. 1983. Problem drinking and the dimension of involvement with drugs: a Guttman Scabgram analysis of adolescent drug use. Am J Public Health 73:543-52.

Dougherty, R. J. 1984. Statement at public hearings on phenylpropanolamine, New York State Committee on Drug Abuse. New York City. January 30.

———. 1982. Pseudo-speed: look-alikes or pea-shooters. NY State J Med 82:74-75.

Drug Abuse Epidemiology Data Center. 1983. Original data file directory and user's guide. College Station, TX: Behavioral Research Program.

Ekins, B. R. and D. G. Spoerke. 1983. An estimation of the toxicity of nonprescription diet aids from seventy cases. Vet Hum Toxicol 25:81-85.

Ellinwood, E. H. 1979. Amphetamines/anorectics. In Handbook on drug abuse, edited by R. I. DuPont, A. Goldstein, and J. O'Donnell, 221-32. Washington, D.C.: U.S. Government Printing Office.

———. 1985. Telephone conversation with author. May 3.

Johnston, L. D., J. G. Bachman, and P. M. O'Malley. 1982. Student drug use, attitudes, and beliefs: national trends, 1975-1982, National Institute on Drug Abuse research report. Washington, D.C.: U.S. Government Printing Office.

Kandel, D. B. 1984. Problems of drug use from adolescence to young adulthood: II. Sequences of progression. Am J Public Health 74:668-72.

Kramer, J. S. and D. C. Cameron. 1975. A manual on drug dependence compiled on the basis of WHO expert reports, WHO expert groups and other WHO public sources. Geneva: World Health Organization.

Krupka, L. R. and A. M. Vener. 1983. Over-the-counter appetite suppressants containing phenylpropanolamine hydrochloride (PPA) and the young adult: usage and perceived effectiveness. Journal of Drug Education 13:141-52.

Latimer, D. 1983a. The peashooter perplex, part I. High Times August: 60-65.

———. 1983b. The peashooter perplex, part II. High Times September: 40-45.

———. 1983c. The peashooter perplex, part III. High Times October: 45-48, 65-68, 97.

Miller, J. D. 1983. National survey on drug abuse: main findings, 1982. Washington, D.C.: U.S. Government Printing Office.

Mulé, S. J. 1984. Telephone coversation with author. September 17.

National Clearinghouse for Poison Control Centers. 1981. Bulletin 25:16-18.

National Commission on Marihuana and Drug Abuse. 1973. Drug use in America: problem in perspective. Washington, D.C.: U.S. Government Printing Office.

National Institute on Drug Abuse. 1983a. Data from the Drug Abuse Warning Network, statistical series G, no. 12. Rockville, MD: National Institute on Drug Abuse.

———. 1983b. Data from the Drug Abuse Warning Network, statistical series I, no. 2. Rockville, MD: National Institute on Drug Abuse.

———. 1983c. Look-alike and act-alike drug products. NIDA Capsules. September.

———. 1982. Data from the Client Oriented Data Acquisition Process, 1978-81, series E, no. 24, Rockville, MD: National Institute on Drug Abuse.

New York City Department of Health. 1984. Over-the-counter diet pills. City Health Information 3(5):1-3.

New York State Division of Substance Abuse Services. 1981. Drug use among New York State's household population. Albany: New York State Division of Substance Abuse Services.

O'Donnell, J. A. and R. R. Clayton. 1982. The stepping-stone hypothesis: a reappraisal. Clinical Dependencies 4:229-41.

O'Donnell, J. A. et al. 1976. Young men and drugs: a nationwide survey. National Institute on Drug Abuse research monograph no. 5. Washington, D.C.: U.S. Government Printing Office.

Parry, H. J. 1979. Sample surveys of drug abuse. In Handbook on drug abuse, edited by R. I. DuPont, A. Goldstein, and J. O'Donnell, 381-94. Washington, D.C.: U.S. Government Printing Office.

Preble, E. 1981. Personal interview with author. March 23.

Saxena, K. and R. Kingston. 1981. Morbidity of street speed--an update. Vet Hum Toxicol 23:10-12.

Schwartz, E. S., S. J. Feinglass, and C. Drucker. 1973. Popular music and drug lyrics: analysis of a scapegoat. In Social responses to drug use, second report of the National Commission on Marihuana and Drug Abuse, 718-48. Washington, D.C.: U.S. Government Printing Office.

Winick, C. 1985. A labor approach to alcohol and other substance abuse. In Yearbook of substance use and abuse, vol. 3, 115-39, edited by L. Brill and C. Winick. New York: Human Sciences Press.

———. 1983. Drinking and disinhibition in popular culture. In Alcohol and disinhibition: nature and meaning of the link, edited by R. Room and G. Collins, 347-401. Washington, D.C.: U.S. Government Printing Office.

———. 1981. Epidemiology of substance abuse. In Substance abuse: clinical problems and perspectives, edited by J. H. Lowinson and P. Ruiz, 24-34. Baltimore: Williams & Wilkins.

———. 1976. Drug education and the content of mass media dealing with "dangerous drugs" and alcohol. In Communication research and drug education, edited by R. E. Ostman, 437-52. Beverly Hills, CA: Sage.

———. 1974. Some aspects of careers of chronic heroin users. In Drug use: epidemiological and sociological approaches, edited by E. Josephson and E. E. Carroll, 105-28. New York: John Wiley.

———. 1965. Epidemiology of narcotics use. In Narcotics, edited by D. M. Wilner and G. G. Kassebam. New York: McGraw-Hill.

Zelger, J. L. and E. A. Carlini. 1980. Anorexigenic effects of two amines obtained from Catha edulis Forsk. (khat) in rats. Pharmacol Biochem Behav 12:701-5.

DISCUSSION

John P. Morgan

INTRODUCTION

In addition to the formal talks at the phenylpropanolamine conference, there was time allotted for queries, comments, and argument from those attending it. All of the remarks, formal and informal, were taped and later transcribed. Participants often aligned themselves clearly with pro or con positions regarding phenylpropanolamine usage and control. Most of the viewpoints expressed during the discussions have already been fully covered in the preceding chapters, but some of them have not. In the discussion comments that follow, I have included a number of these, selected, edited, and organized to reflect points of view that have not been adequately discussed or emphasized in the chapters themselves. In addition, a few of the following remarks (indicated by asterisks) did not originate in floor debate, but have been taken from discussions I had with some of the conference participants. Although statements are followed by references to the chapters to which they apply, they are presented without attribution to the speakers. Since they have been extensively edited and grouped in somewhat arbitrary categories, I assume full responsibility for their accuracy and placement.

CLINICAL TRIALS OF ANOREXIANTS

Many participants wished to comment on the testing of anorexiants in reference to the presentations by both Dr. Weintraub and Dr. Bray:

Dr. Weintraub seems to have had two goals. He commented on the very poor execution of clinical trials of phenylpropanolamine, yet congratulated those who carried them out for working in good faith. This is damning with faint praise. (chapter 5)

Clinical trials of the sort Dr. Weintraub describes do not mimic or even describe clinical practice. One does not learn about patient-clinician communication or the characteristics of patients who are likely to be highly successful when they feel very supported. These factors are not reflected in clinical trial statistics. (chapter 5)

(Response) Indeed the clinical trial cannot mimic clinical practice. It assesses whether under controlled conditions in a matched group of subjects the treatment statistically varies from the control. Most trials are also by necessity short-term and cannot yield useful information on long-term efficacy. (chapter 5)

Other further important points can be made about clinical trials with anorexiant agents. It is relatively easy to recruit subjects even into trials with rigid entry criteria and it is easy to make up comparable groups using a few or many stratification characteristics. (chapter 5)

Dropouts are always a problem but they do not necessarily occur because of active treatment toxicity. Subjects move and change jobs or schedules. Placebo subjects drop out because they do not have anorexia and are not losing weight after a short time. (chapter 5)

*Dr. Weintraub was critical of flaws in the clinical designs of many of the phenylpropanolamine studies he reviewed. Most of the trials he assessed were parallel group studies. The Review Panel of the U.S. Food and Drug Administration in fact had earlier recommended conducting some crossover studies of phenylpropanolamine. (chapter 5)

CLINICAL APPLICATIONS OF WEIGHT LOSS AND DIETS

The character of weight loss and the performance and efficacy of anorexiants and dieting also provoked comment:

Most anorexiant drugs seem to provoke similar amounts of weight loss, and dose-ranging studies do not indicate much increased effect from increased dose. The adrenergic (or stimulant-responsive system) may have a very limited range over which it can modulate body weight. Few people ever lose more than 10 kg on these drugs. Whether there is a preexistent "set point" for individuals is uncertain but it is a useful concept. Further, if people are maintained on medication, such treatment often works to hold the set point and tachyphylaxis does not regularly occur. (chapter 7)

People may hold at certain points after weight loss because a previous diet providing a certain number of calories per kilogram now provides more calories per kilogram at the new, lower weight, and weight loss will continue only if a more restrictive diet is imposed. In patients at plateau, significant weight gain follows stopping of the drug. Tachyphylaxis is not the real problem. (chapter 7)

Weight loss is a first-order process; that is, it proceeds as a fraction of beginning weight over time. The rate of weight loss therefore diminishes over time and invariably reaches a plateau or very small decrements hidden in a plateau. (chapters 5, 7)

In altering meal patterns, particularly in encouraging a larger breakfast and a smaller evening meal, we may introduce significant family turmoil because of the importance of the evening meal to the family. (chapter 7)

Humans may have a rhythmic network of neuroendocrine processes. Many symptoms--irritability, sleep disturbances, depression, anxiety, and others--may respond to synchronization of eating patterns, exercise, sleep, etc. Chronobiology is an infant science but it may provide solutions to many problems that result from pattern-programmed disruptions. (chapters 7, 10)

CAFFEINE AND ITS EFFECTS

The impact of caffeine was taken seriously:

In the studies described by Dr. Weintraub, prestudy queries were directed at any use of other anorexiants. However, there was no attempt to identify or exclude users of other stimulants, including caffeine. Although unproved, it is possible or even likely that subjects who begin diets consume more caffeine. (chapter 10)

The caffeine present in the earlier versions of anorexiant products may have combatted the lethargy caused by dieting as well as the lethargy sometimes associated with phenylpropanolamine. (chapters 7, 10)

Phenylpropanolamine, in a recent study in stimulant users, did not provoke euphoria but, if anything, a slight physically referred dysphoria. Phenylpropanolamine may make people a little tired or dragged out and the caffeine then yields a lift. (chapter 10)

Many of the symptoms attributed to medication (phenylpropanolamine or caffeine) may truly be related to feelings or symptoms caused by fasting or stringent dieting. (chapters 7, 10)

Certainly fasting people manifest one stimulant symptom, anorexia. However, the most prominent psychological symptom in fasting is depression. (chapter 7)

Dr. Mueller's dosage pattern would translate to a dosage of 1,800 mg of caffeine in humans. The findings of cerebral hemorrhage in the rats could be due only to that. The study might be expanded to additional groups using phenylpropanolamine and caffeine alone. The rats were also somewhat elderly and the fasting procedure may have been debilitating. (chapter 14)

PHENYLPROPANOLAMINE, ASPIRIN, AND THE DRUG ABUSE WARNING NETWORK

Another commonplace drug was discussed:

Dr. Wesson noted a high incidence of aspirin in Drug Abuse Warning Network (DAWN) reports. This does not necessarily indicate that aspirin was used for psychic effect but that it may have been in combination with agents which were (e.g., propoxyphene, pentazocine, etc.). Also, even though phenylpropanolamine may be taken in greater than one billion doses, aspirin ingestion probably exceeds 17 billion. (chapter 21)

Aspirin was not really singled out as a misused drug but as a drug present in every home and taken in suicide attempts. The aspirin mentions were examined as an index because any great variation in mentions would indicate problems with the reporting system. (chapter 21)

*Although popular over-the-counter (OTC) drugs like phenylpropanolamine and aspirin are used in suicide attempts, the Poison Control Center Bulletin (August 1981) indicated that the risk of a fatal ingestion of phenylpropanolamine is minimal. The report stated that there were 739 telephone inquiries concerning overuse of phenylpropanolamine diet aids in 1980; of those, 42% involved children under the age of five, only 21 individuals required a hospital visit, and there were no fatalities. In 1978 there were 204 suicide attempts with phenylpropanolamine reported, but no deaths. (chapters 10, 21, 22)

BLOOD PRESSURE EFFECTS OF PPA

The most intense commentary examined the relationship between phenylpropanolamine and increased blood pressure:

If phenylpropanolamine causes an increase in blood pressure, the therapeutic dilemma is that even if it diminishes one risk factor (obesity), it may magnify another. (chapters 13, 16)

Studies have been done looking at phenylpropanolamine's effect on blood pressure after steady state using sustained-release preparations. These studies demonstrated no hypertensive effect with phenylpropanolamine after four days. This may reinforce Dr. Reidenberg's suggestion that continued dosage causes tachyphylaxis at least to hypertensive effects. (chapters 12, 13, 16)

One of the studies reviewed by Dr. Krakoff (the effect of phenylpropanolamine in controlled hypertension) has been extended. Fifty-two such patients were treated with 75 mg sustained-release preparations and no effect was noted on the mean pretreatment diastolic blood pressure of 94 mm Hg. (chapter 13)

In a study of medications that cause small changes in blood pressure, the usual blood pressure cuff may be inadequate. Modern, wearable, automated equipment may ultimately yield more information. (chapters 12, 13, 16)

In any study of hypertensive patients on treatment, the diuretic used may blunt the effect of a sympathomimetic drug. (chapters 12, 13, 16)

Humans who exercise strenuously in hot climates may elevate their diastolic pressures by 20-30 mm Hg. It is very hard to believe that the small increases noted in these phenylpropanolamine studies can matter. This appears true even if we grant that OTC availability means that some individuals will consume too much. We now know by telemetric-monitoring studies that the diastolic pressure of normal human beings may vary nearly as much as in those who exercise as above. There is much more daily variation in blood pressure in a single individual than in any of the cited phenylpropanolamine studies. (chapters 12, 13, 16)

Perhaps the increased blood pressure secondary to sympathomimetic vasoconstriction is more damaging than any increased blood pressure secondary to increased cardiac output, such as that seen after exercise. (chapters 12, 13, 16)

The risk of blood pressure elevation is continuous. There is a greater risk from higher blood pressure even if the increase is small and the measurement is casual. (chapter 13)

The blood pressure elevation caused by sympathomimetics is dose-related and the safety margin of most of them has not been particularly well-studied. This includes phenylpropanolamine and norpseudoephedrine. Since many people take these agents (along with caffeine), sometimes to excess, the risk of deleterious consequences due to OTC availability may be great or much greater than supposed. (chapters 12, 13)

The use of phenylpropanolamine may provoke a very slight--even statistically significant--increase in blood pressure but there is little reason to believe that such change is biologically significant. (chapters 12, 13, 16)

The possibility that phenylpropanolamine interacts with prostaglandin synthetase inhibitors has been raised by Dr. Krakoff. In a clinical study sponsored by Johnson & Johnson, Pugliese carried out a 30-day double-blind study of 68 patients (published in the Federal Register, September 9, 1976). Subjects were given daily either 2,600 mg of a nonsteroidal anti-inflammatory agent (aspirin) in combination with 200 mg of phenylpropanolamine, 200 mg of phenylpropanolamine alone, 2,600 mg of aspirin alone, or placebo. No adverse effects relative to blood pressure or other vital signs were reported. (chapters 2, 13)

PSYCHIATRIC DISORDERS REPORTED WITH PHENYLPROPANOLAMINE USE

The subjects reported in Dr. Dietz' paper were not examined by him, there were no toxicological confirmations that phenylpropanolamine had been ingested, and the retrospective chart review may not be probative enough to rule out the consumption of other medicines or drugs. (chapter 18)

PPA PREPARATIONS AND PRODUCTS

The issue of the constituents of Trimolets is unresolved:

Phenylpropanolamine is made in large quantities by a relatively few chemical suppliers who then sell it to the drug industry or other chemical firms for use in further syntheses. Essentially all the phenylpropanolamine made in the United States is racemic ($\pm$)-phenylpropanolamine. There are practical processes by which the isomers may be separated but there is little use for the isomeric products. (chapters 2, 11)

Despite some confusion, the Trimolets products contained immediate-release preparations although some were labeled "take one daily." There has been significant argument about the probable isomeric format of Trimolets. Some formats of the Trimolets products almost certainly contained an ingredient that is not present in the phenylpropanolamine used in the United States. Dosage, chemical composition, and the release characteristics are dissimilar. The Australian Trimolets product may not be comparable with the phenylpropanolamine manufactured in the United States over the last 40 years. (chapters 2, 11, 12)

The studies reviewed by Dr. Krakoff all used a Thompson Medical Company product, which, in the 75 mg preparation, is made sustained-release by the bead formulation methodology. This product has been studied and demonstrates appropriate bioavailability. (chapters 2, 13)

*Dr. Wertheimer commented that destructive behavior by consumers can be prevented with improved package labeling. But the current labels for phenylpropanolamine appetite suppressants do list cautions, directions, and warnings, including drug interaction precautions. They state, for example: do not take if you are presently taking another medication containing phenylpropanolamine; read before using; for adult use only; do not give this product to children under 12 years of age; persons between ages 12-18 or over age 60 should consult their physicians or pharmacists before using; and taking greater than recommended amounts of this or any other drug can cause untoward health complications. Although these products may at times be used carelessly, at least the labeling is responsible and informative. (chapter 4)

PHENYLPROPANOLAMINE AVAILABILITY: RX, OTC, OR . . . ?

Should other possibilities of phenylpropanolamine control and distribution be considered?

Phenylpropanolamine is probably not an appropriate choice for markedly obese patients and those with cardiovascular and metabolic complications of obesity, particularly if phenylpropanolamine is self-selected and the diet is self-designed and self-imposed. Such patients probably need prescription anorexiants as part of a comprehensive, designed approach to weight loss. The most important issue is not that prescription products are more effective than phenylpropanolamine, but that the program of treatment should be closely supervised. (chapters 5, 7)

The case reports of phenylpropanolamine toxicity should be balanced against a large number of clinical safety studies and efficacy studies that have been submitted to the Food and Drug Administration. The drug may well be used intermittently by consumers who in that pattern may maintain weight loss more easily than if they had to return to physicians to obtain prescription medications. (chapter 7)

INDEX

ABOUT THE AUTHORS

Sheryle W. Alagna, Ph.D. Assistant Professor, Department of Medical Psychology. F. Edward Hébert School of Medicine of the Uniformed Services University of the Health Sciences. Bethesda, MD.

George E. Bigelow, Ph.D. Associate Professor of Behavioral Biology, Departments of Psychiatry and Behavioral Sciences. The Johns Hopkins University School of Medicine. Baltimore, MD.

Harvey Blumberg, Ph.D. Professor of Quantitative Methods; Chairman, Departments of Finance and Quantitative Methods. Montclair State College. Montclair, NJ.

George A. Bray, M.D. Professor, Department of Medicine; Chief, Division of Diabetes and Clinical Nutrition. University of Southern California School of Medicine. Los Angeles, CA.

Susan Camber, M.A. Research Coordinator. Merritt Peralta Institute, Chemical Dependency Recovery Hospital. Oakland, CA.

Albert J. Dietz, Jr., M.D., Ph.D. Associate Professor, Department of Medicine; Chief, Division of Clinical Pharmacology. University of North Dakota School of Medicine. Fargo, ND.

Brent R. Ekins, Pharm.D. Director, Fresno Regional Poison Control Center. Fresno, CA.

David S. Freeman, Ph.D. Assistant Professor, Department of Pharmaceutical Sciences. North Dakota State University College of Pharmacy. Fargo, ND.

John F. Greden, M.D. Professor and Chairman, Department of Psychiatry; Director, Clinical Studies Unit. University of Michigan Medical School. Ann Arbor, MI.

Jack P. Green, M.D., Ph.D. Professor and Chairman, Department of Pharmacology. Mount Sinai School of Medicine of the City University of New York. New York, NY.

John D. Horowitz, M.D., Ph.D. Senior Research Fellow, Department of Cardiology. Faculty of Medicine, Austin Hospital of the University of Melbourne. Parkville, Victoria, Australia.

Lawrence R. Krakoff, M.D. Professor, Department of Medicine; Chief, Hypertension Division. Mount Sinai School of Medicine of the City University of New York. New York, NY.

Lawrence R. Krupka, Ph.D. Professor, Department of Natural Science. Michigan State University, East Lansing, MI.

C. Raymond Lake, M.D., Ph.D. Professor, Departments of Psychiatry and Pharmacology. F. Edward Hébert School of Medicine of the Uniformed Services University of the Health Sciences. Bethesda, MD.

William J. Louis, M.B.B.S., M.D. Professor, Department of Clinical Pharmacology and Therapeutics. Faculty of Medicine, Austin Hospital of the University of Melbourne. Parkville, Victoria, Australia.

Edward O. Magarian, Ph.D. Associate Professor and Chairman, Department of Pharmaceutical Sciences. North Dakota State University College of Pharmacy. Fargo, ND.

Kathleen M. Moriarty, B.A. Assistant Editor, Journal of Hospital and Community Psychiatry. American Psychiatric Association. Washington, D.C.

Shirley M. Mueller, M.D. Associate Professor, Departments of Neurology and Physiology; Chief, Adult Neurology Service. Wishard Memorial Hospital. Indiana University School of Medicine. Indianapolis, IN.

Karoline S. Puder. Medical Student. City University of New York Medical School. New York, NY.

Rosemarie S. Quirk, B.S. Research Chemist, Department of Psychiatry. F. Edward Hébert School of Medicine of the Uniformed Services University of the Health Services. Bethesda, MD.

Audrey A. Reid, M.S. Research Chemist, Department of Psychiatry. F. Edward Hébert School of Medicine of the Uniformed Services University of the Health Services. Bethesda, MD.

Marcus M. Reidenberg, M.D. Professor, Departments of Medicine and Pharmacology; Head, Division of Clinical Pharmacology. Cornell University Medical College. New York, NY.

Harold I. Silverman, D.Sc. (At the time of the conference) Professor and Associate Dean, Massachusetts College of Pharmacy and Allied Health Sciences; Executive Director, Pfeiffer Pharmaceutical Sciences Laboratories. Boston, MA. (Currently) Vice President and Scientific Director. Thompson Medical Company. New York, NY.

David E. Smith, M.D. Medical Director and Founder, Haight-Ashbury Free Medical Clinic; Research Director, Merritt Peralta Chemical Dependency Institute; Associate Clinical Professor of Toxicology, University of California School of Medicine. San Francisco, CA.

Arthur M. Vener, Ph.D. Professor, Department of Social Science. Michigan State University. East Lansing, MI.

Murray Weiner, M.D. Clinical Professor, Departments of Medicine and Pharmacology; Acting Director, Division of Clinical Pharmacology and Toxicology. University of Cincinnati College of Medicine. Cincinnati, OH.

Michael Weintraub, M.D. Associate Professor, Department of Preventive Family and Rehabilitation Medicine. University of Rochester School of Medicine and Dentistry. Rochester, NY.

Albert I. Wertheimer, Ph.D. Professor and Chairman, Department of Social and Administrative Pharmacy. University of Minnesota. Minneapolis, MN.

Donald R. Wesson, M.D. Research Director, Look-Alike Research and Physician Training Project; Assistant Clinical Professor, Departments of Psychiatry. University of California and Veterans Administration Medical Center. San Francisco, CA.

Charles Winick, Ph.D. Professor, Department of Sociology. City College and Graduate School, City University of New York. New York, NY.

ABOUT THE EDITORS

Jane S. Brody, M.A. Research Associate, Pharmacology Program. City University of New York Medical School. New York, NY; Ph.D. candidate, Yale University. New Haven, CT.

Doreen V. Kagan, M.S. Research Associate, Pharmacology Program. City University of New York Medical School. New York, NY.

John P. Morgan, M.D. Medical Professor and Director, Pharmacology Program. City University of New York Medical School; Associate Professor, Departments of Medicine and Pharmacology. Mount Sinai School of Medicine of the City University of New York. New York, NY.